Gene Therapy

Editors

DANIEL E. BAUER
DONALD B. KOHN

HEMATOLOGY/ONCOLOGY CLINICS OF NORTH AMERICA

www.hemonc.theclinics.com

Consulting Editors
GEORGE P. CANELLOS
H. FRANKLIN BUNN

October 2017 • Volume 31 • Number 5

ELSEVIER

1600 John F. Kennedy Boulevard • Suite 1800 • Philadelphia, Pennsylvania, 19103-2899

http://www.theclinics.com

HEMATOLOGY/ONCOLOGY CLINICS OF NORTH AMERICA Volume 31, Number 5
October 2017 ISSN 0889-8588, ISBN 13: 978-0-323-54668-3

Editor: Stacy Eastman
Developmental Editor: Kristen Helm

Hematology/Oncology Clinics (ISSN 0889-8588) is published bimonthly by Elsevier Inc., 360 Park Avenue South, New York, NY 10010-1710. Months of issue are February, April, June, August, October, and December. Business and Editorial Offices: 1600 John F. Kennedy Blvd., Ste. 1800, Philadelphia, PA 19103–2899. Customer Service Office: 3251 Riverport Lane, Maryland Heights, MO 63043. Periodicals postage paid at New York, NY and at additional mailing offices. Subscription prices are $397.00 per year (domestic individuals), $742.00 per year (domestic institutions), $100.00 per year (domestic students/residents), $453.00 per year (Canadian individuals), $919.00 per year (Canadian institutions) $536.00 per year (international individuals), $919.00 per year (international institutions), and $255.00 per year (international and Canadian students/residents). International air speed delivery is included in all *Clinics* subscription prices. All prices are subject to change without notice. **POSTMASTER:** Send address changes to *Hematology/Oncology Clinics of North America*, Elsevier Health Sciences Division, Subscription Customer Service, 3251 Riverport Lane, Maryland Heights, MO 63043. Customer Service (orders, claims, online, change of address): Elsevier Health Sciences Division, Subscription **Customer Service, 3251 Riverport Lane, Maryland Heights, MO 63043. Tel: 1-800-654-2452 (U.S. and Canada); 314-447-8871 (outside U.S. and Canada). Fax: 314-447-8029. E-mail: journalscustomerservice-usa@elsevier.com (for print support); journalsonlinesupport-usa@elsevier.com (for online support)**.

Reprints. For copies of 100 or more, of articles in this publication, please contact the Commercial Reprints Department, Elsevier Inc., 360 Park Avenue South, New York, New York 10010-1710; Tel.: 212-633-3874, Fax: 212-633-3820, E-mail: reprints@elsevier.com.

Hematology/Oncology Clinics of North America is covered in *MEDLINE/PubMed (Index Medicus), EMBASE/ Excerpta Medica, and BIOSIS.*

Contributors

CONSULTING EDITORS

GEORGE P. CANELLOS, MD
William Rosenberg Professor of Medicine, Department of Medical Oncology, Dana-Farber Cancer Institute, Boston, Massachusetts, USA

H. FRANKLIN BUNN, MD
Professor of Medicine, Division of Hematology, Brigham and Women's Hospital, Harvard Medical School, Boston, Massachusetts, USA

EDITORS

DANIEL E. BAUER, MD, PhD
Staff Physician, Division of Pediatric Hematology/Oncology, Dana-Farber/Boston Children's Cancer and Blood Disorders Center, Assistant Professor of Pediatrics, Harvard Medical School, Principal Faculty, Harvard Stem Cell Institute, Associate Member, Broad Institute of MIT and Harvard, Boston, Massachusetts, USA

DONALD B. KOHN, MD
Professor, Department of Microbiology, Immunology and Molecular Genetics, Division of Hematology/Oncology, Departments of Pediatrics and Molecular and Medical Pharmacology, UCLA Eli & Edythe Broad Center of Regenerative Medicine & Stem Cell Research, UCLA Jonsson Comprehensive Cancer Center, David Geffen School of Medicine at UCLA, University of California, Los Angeles, Los Angeles, California, USA

AUTHORS

ULRIKE ABRAMOWSKI-MOCK, PhD
Molecular and Cellular Immunology Unit, University College London, UCL Great Ormond Street Institute of Child Health, London, United Kingdom

JENNIFER E. ADAIR, PhD
Fred Hutchinson Cancer Research Center, University of Washington School of Medicine, Seattle, Washington, USA

DALE ANDO, MD
President, Gene Editing and Gene Therapy Consulting

TAKIS ATHANASOPOULOS, PhD
Head of Transgene Delivery, Cell and Gene Therapy Discovery Research, Platform Technology and Sciences, GSK Medicines Research Centre, Stevenage, Hertfordshire, United Kingdom

LUCA BIASCO, PhD
Gene Therapy Program, Dana-Farber/Boston Children's Cancer and Blood Disorders Center, Harvard Medical School, Boston, Massachusetts, USA; University College London, UCL Great Ormond Street Institute of Child Health, UCL Faculty of Population Health Sciences, London, United Kingdom

ALESSANDRA BIFFI, MD
Director, Gene Therapy Program, Dana-Farber/Boston Children's Cancer and Blood Disorders Center, Associate Professor of Pediatrics, Harvard Medical School, Boston, Massachusetts, USA

PAULA M. CANNON, PhD
Department of Molecular Microbiology and Immunology, Keck School of Medicine of University of Southern California, Los Angeles, California, USA

MARINA CAVAZZANA, MD
Biotherapy Department, Necker Children's Hospital, Imagine Institute, Paris Descartes University, Paris, France

MORTON J. COWAN, MD
Professor Emeritus, Pediatric Allergy Immunology and Blood and Marrow Transplant Division, UCSF Benioff Children's Hospital, San Francisco, San Francisco, California, USA

ANDREW M. DAVIDOFF, MD
Department of Surgery, St. Jude Children's Research Hospital, Memphis, Tennessee, USA

JULIETTE M. DELHOVE, PhD
Molecular and Cellular Immunology Unit, University College London, UCL Great Ormond Street Institute of Child Health, London, United Kingdom

CHRISTOPHER C. DVORAK, MD
Associate Professor, Pediatric Allergy Immunology and Blood and Marrow Transplant Division, UCSF Benioff Children's Hospital, San Francisco, San Francisco, California, USA

GIULIANA FERRARI, PhD
San Raffaele-Telethon Institute for Gene Therapy (SR-TIGET), Istituto Scientifico Ospedale San Raffaele, Vita-Salute San Raffaele University, Milan, Italy

H. BOBBY GASPAR, MBBS, PhD
GOSHCC Professor of Paediatrics and Immunology, Consultant in Paediatric Immunology, Infection, Immunity, Inflammation, Molecular and Cellular Immunology Section, University College London, UCL Great Ormond Street Institute of Child Health, London, United Kingdom

SUJAL GHOSH, MD
Infection, Immunity, Inflammation, Molecular and Cellular Immunology Section, University College London, UCL Great Ormond Street Institute of Child Health, London, United Kingdom; Department of Pediatric Oncology, Hematology and Clinical Immunology, Medical Faculty, Center of Child and Adolescent Health, Heinrich-Heine-University, Düsseldorf, Germany

OLIVIER HUMBERT, PhD
Senior Fellow, Clinical Research Division, Fred Hutchinson Cancer Research Center, Seattle, Washington, USA

HANS-PETER KIEM, MD, PhD
Professor, Clinical Research Division, Fred Hutchinson Cancer Research Center, Department of Medicine, University of Washington School of Medicine, Seattle, Washington, USA

DONALD B. KOHN, MD
Professor, Department of Microbiology, Immunology and Molecular Genetics, Division of Hematology/Oncology, Departments of Pediatrics and Molecular and Medical Pharmacology, UCLA Eli and Edythe Broad Center of Regenerative Medicine and Stem Cell Research, UCLA Jonsson Comprehensive Cancer Center, David Geffen School of Medicine at UCLA, University of California, Los Angeles, Los Angeles, California, USA

SARA P. KUBEK, PhD
Fred Hutchinson Cancer Research Center, University of Washington School of Medicine, Seattle, Washington, USA

ANDRÉ LIEBER, MD, PhD
Professor, Division of Medical Genetics, Department of Pathology, University of Washington, Seattle, Washington, USA

JANEL LONG-BOYLE, PharmD, PhD
Associate Professor, Department of Clinical Pharmacy, University of California San Francisco, San Francisco, California, USA

CHRISTOPHER T. LUX, MD, PhD
Acting Instructor, Department of Pediatrics, Cancer and Blood Disorders Center, Seattle Children's Hospital, Seattle, Washington, USA

FULVIO MAVILIO, PhD
Department of Life Sciences, University of Modena and Reggio Emilia, Modena, Italy

KATHLEEN MEYER, MPH, PhD
Vice President, Nonclinical Development, Sangamo Therapeutics, Richmond, California, USA

CAROL MIAO, PhD
Professor, Department of Pediatrics, University of Washington, Research Institute, Seattle Children's Hospital, Seattle, Washington, USA

MUSTAFA M. MUNYE, PhD
Scientific Investigator, Transgene Delivery, Cell and Gene Therapy Discovery Research, Platform Technology and Sciences, GSK Medicines Research Centre, Stevenage, Hertfordshire, United Kingdom

AMIT C. NATHWANI, MBChB, FRCP, FRCPath, PhD
Department of Academic Haematology, UCL Cancer Institute, Katharine Dormandy Haemophilia and Thrombosis Centre, London, United Kingdom; National Health Service Blood and Transplant, Watford, Hertfordshire, United Kingdom

THALIA PAPAYANNOPOULOU, MD
Professor, Division of Hematology, University of Washington, Seattle, Washington, USA

WASEEM QASIM, MBBS, PhD
Professor, Molecular and Cellular Immunology Unit, University College London, UCL Great Ormond Street Institute of Child Health, London, United Kingdom

MAXIMILIAN RICHTER, PhD
Senior Fellow, Division of Medical Genetics, University of Washington, Seattle, Washington, USA

GEOFFREY L. ROGERS, PhD
Department of Molecular Microbiology and Immunology, Keck School of Medicine of University of Southern California, Los Angeles, California, USA

MICHAEL ROTHE, PhD
Institute of Experimental Hematology, REBIRTH Cluster of Excellence, Hannover Medical School, Hannover, Germany

AXEL SCHAMBACH, MD, PhD
Institute of Experimental Hematology, REBIRTH Cluster of Excellence, Hannover Medical School, Hannover, Germany; Division of Hematology/Oncology, Boston Children's Hospital, Harvard Medical School, Boston, Massachusetts, USA

ANDREW M. SCHARENBERG, MD
Professor, Department of Pediatrics, Adjunct Professor, Department of Immunology, Seattle Children's Hospital, Seattle, Washington, USA

JULIANE W. SCHOTT, PhD
Institute of Experimental Hematology, REBIRTH Cluster of Excellence, Hannover Medical School, Hannover, Germany

DANIEL STONE, PhD
Senior Fellow, Vaccine and Infectious Disease Division, Fred Hutchinson Cancer Research Center, Seattle, Washington, USA

EDWARD G.D. TUDDENHAM, MD
Department of Academic Haematology, UCL Cancer Institute, Katharine Dormandy Haemophilia and Thrombosis Centre, London, United Kingdom

RAFAEL J. YÁÑEZ-MUÑOZ, PhD
Professor of Advanced Therapy, Advanced Gene and Cell Therapy Laboratory (AGCTlab.org), Centre for Biomedical Sciences, School of Biological Sciences, Royal Holloway, University of London, Egham, Surrey, United Kingdom

Contents

Preface: Gene Therapy xiii

Daniel E. Bauer and Donald B. Kohn

Historical Perspective on the Current Renaissance for Hematopoietic Stem Cell
Gene Therapy 721

Donald B. Kohn

Gene therapy using hematopoietic stem cells (HSCs) has developed over
the past 3 decades, with progressive improvements in efficacy and safety.
Autologous transplantation of HSCs modified with murine gammaretroviral
vectors first showed clinical benefits for patients with several primary immune deficiencies, but some of these patients suffered complications from
vector-related genotoxicity. Lentiviral vectors have been used recently for
gene additions to HSCs and have yielded clinical benefits for primary immune deficiencies, metabolic diseases, and hemoglobinopathies, without
vector-related complications. Gene editing using site-specific endonucleases is emerging as a promising technology for gene therapy and is moving into clinical trials.

Integrating Vectors for Gene Therapy and Clonal Tracking of Engineered
Hematopoiesis 737

Luca Biasco, Michael Rothe, Juliane W. Schott, and Axel Schambach

Gene therapy using autologous or allogeneic cells offers promising possibilities to treat inherited and acquired diseases, ideally leading to a long-
lasting therapeutic correction. This article summarizes efforts that use
integrating vectors derived from retroviruses and transposons, and briefly
explains integrating vector biology and integration site analysis and recent
successful application of this technology in clinical trials. Moreover, the
article outlines how these vectors can be used for cancer gene discovery
and clonal tracking of benign and malignant hematopoiesis to gain insights
into the dynamics of hematopoiesis.

Nonintegrating Gene Therapy Vectors 753

Takis Athanasopoulos, Mustafa M. Munye, and Rafael J. Yáñez-Muñoz

Gene delivery vectors that do not rely on host cell genome integration offer
several advantages for gene transfer, chiefly the avoidance of insertional
mutagenesis and position effect variegation. However, unless engineered
for replication and segregation, nonintegrating vectors will dilute progressively in proliferating cells, and are not exempt of epigenetic effects. This
article provides an overview of the main nonintegrating viral (adenoviral,
adeno-associated viral, integration-deficient retro-lentiviral, poxviral),
and nonviral (plasmid vectors, artificial chromosomes) vectors used for
preclinical and clinical cell and gene therapy applications. Particular
emphasis is placed on their use in hematologic disease.

In Vivo Hematopoietic Stem Cell Transduction   771

Maximilian Richter, Daniel Stone, Carol Miao, Olivier Humbert,
Hans-Peter Kiem, Thalia Papayannopoulou, and André Lieber

> Current protocols for hematopoietic stem cell (HSC) gene therapy, involving the transplantation of ex vivo lentivirus vector-transduced HSCs into myeloablated recipients, are complex and not without risk for the patient. In vivo HSC gene therapy can be achieved by the direct modification of HSCs in the bone marrow after intraosseous injection of gene delivery vectors. A recently developed approach involves the mobilization of HSCs from the bone marrow into the peripheral blood circulation, intravenous vector injection, and re-engraftment of genetically modified HSCs in the bone marrow. We provide examples for in vivo HSC gene therapy and discuss advantages and disadvantages.

Therapeutic Gene Editing Safety and Specificity   787

Christopher T. Lux and Andrew M. Scharenberg

> Therapeutic gene editing is significant for medical advancement. Safety is intricately linked to the specificity of the editing tools used to cut at precise genomic targets. Improvements can be achieved by thoughtful design of nucleases and repair templates, analysis of off-target editing, and careful utilization of viral vectors. Advancements in DNA repair mechanisms and development of new generations of tools improve targeting of specific sequences while minimizing risks. It is important to plot a safe course for future clinical trials. This article reviews safety and specificity for therapeutic gene editing to spur dialogue and advancement.

Gene Editing: Regulatory and Translation to Clinic   797

Dale Ando and Kathleen Meyer

> The clinical application and regulatory strategy of genome editing for ex vivo cell therapy is derived from the intersection of 2 fields of study: viral vector gene therapy trials and clinical trials with ex vivo purification and engraftment of CD34$^+$ hematopoietic stem cells, T cells, and tumor cell vaccines. This article covers the regulatory and translational preclinical activities needed for a genome editing clinical trial modifying hematopoietic stem cells and the genesis of this current strategy based on previous clinical trials using genome-edited T cells. The SB-728 zinc finger nuclease platform is discussed because this is the most clinically advanced genome editing technology.

Opening Marrow Niches in Patients Undergoing Autologous Hematopoietic Stem Cell Gene Therapy   809

Morton J. Cowan, Christopher C. Dvorak, and Janel Long-Boyle

> Successful gene therapy for genetic disorders requires marrow niches to be opened to varying degrees to engraft gene-corrected hematopoietic stem cells. For example, in severe combined immunodeficiency, relatively limited chimerism is necessary for both T-cell and B-cell immune reconstitution, whereas for inborn errors of metabolism, maximal donor chimerism is the goal. Currently, alkylating chemotherapy is used for this purpose. Significant pharmacokinetic variability exists in drug clearance in children

younger than 12 years. Thus, pharmacokinetic monitoring is needed to achieve the targeted exposure goal for busulfan.

Gene Therapy Approaches to Immunodeficiency   823

Sujal Ghosh and H. Bobby Gaspar

Transfer of gene-corrected autologous hematopoietic stem cells in patients with primary immunodeficiencies has emerged as a new therapeutic approach. Patients with various conditions lacking a suitable donor have been treated with retroviral vectors and a gene-addition strategy. Initial promising results were shadowed by the occurrence of malignancies in some of these patients. Current trials, developed in the past decade, use safer viral vectors to overcome the risk of genotoxicity and have led to improved clinical outcomes. This article reflects the progress made in specific disorders, including adenosine deaminase deficiency, X-linked severe combined immunodeficiency, chronic granulomatous disease, and Wiskott-Aldrich syndrome.

Gene Therapy Approaches to Hemoglobinopathies   835

Giuliana Ferrari, Marina Cavazzana, and Fulvio Mavilio

Gene therapy for hemoglobinopathies is currently based on transplantation of autologous hematopoietic stem cells genetically modified with a lentiviral vector expressing a globin gene under the control of globin transcriptional regulatory elements. Preclinical and early clinical studies showed the safety and potential efficacy of this therapeutic approach, as well as the hurdles still limiting its general application. In addition, for both beta-thalassemia and sickle cell disease, an altered bone marrow microenvironment reduces the efficiency of stem cell harvesting and engraftment. These hurdles need to be addressed for gene therapy for hemoglobinopathies to become a clinical reality.

Gene Therapy for Hemophilia   853

Amit C. Nathwani, Andrew M. Davidoff, and Edward G.D. Tuddenham

The best currently available treatments for hemophilia A and B (factor VIII or factor IX deficiency, respectively) require frequent intravenous infusions of highly expensive proteins that have short half-lives. Factor levels follow a sawtooth pattern that is seldom in the normal range and falls so low that breakthrough bleeding occurs. Most individuals with hemophilia worldwide do not have access to even this level of care. In stark contrast, gene therapy holds the hope of a cure by inducing continuous endogenous expression of factor VIII or IX after transfer of a functional gene to replace the hemophilic patient's own defective gene.

Hematopoietic Gene Therapies for Metabolic and Neurologic Diseases   869

Alessandra Biffi

Increasingly, patients affected by metabolic diseases affecting the central nervous system and neuroinflammatory disorders receive hematopoietic cell transplantation in an attempt to slow the course of their disease, delay or attenuate symptoms, and improve pathologic findings. The possible replacement of brain-resident myeloid cells by the transplanted cell progeny contributes to clinical benefit. Genetic engineering of the cells to be transplanted (hematopoietic stem cells) may endow the brain myeloid progeny of these cells with enhanced or novel functions, contributing to therapeutic effects.

Gene Therapy Approaches to Human Immunodeficiency Virus and Other Infectious Diseases   883

Geoffrey L. Rogers and Paula M. Cannon

Advances in gene therapy technologies, particularly in gene editing, are suggesting new avenues for the treatment of human immunodeficiency virus and other infectious diseases. This article outlines recent developments in antiviral gene therapies, including those based on the disruption of entry receptors or that target viral genomes using targeted nucleases, such as the CRISPR/Cas9 system. In addition, new ways to express circulating antiviral factors, such as antibodies, and approaches to harness and engineer the immune system to provide an antiviral effect that is not naturally achieved are described.

Hematopoietic Stem Cell Approaches to Cancer   897

Jennifer E. Adair, Sara P. Kubek, and Hans-Peter Kiem

Hematopoietic stem cells (HSCs) are unique in their ability to self-renew and generate all blood lineages for the entire life. HSC modification affects red blood cells, platelets, lymphocytes, and myeloid cells. Chemotherapy can result in myelosuppression, limiting effective chemotherapy administration. For diseases like glioblastoma, high expression of methylguanine methyltransferase can inactivate alkylating agent chemotherapy. Here we discuss how HSCs can be modified to overcome this resistance, permitting sensitization of tumors to chemotherapy while simultaneously protecting the hematopoietic system. We also discuss how HSCs can be harnessed to produce powerful tumor-killing T cells, potentially benefiting and complementing T-cell–based immunotherapies.

Gene Modified T Cell Therapies for Hematological Malignancies   913

Ulrike Abramowski-Mock, Juliette M. Delhove, and Waseem Qasim

This article focuses on clinical applications of T cells transduced to express recombinant T-cell receptor and chimeric antigen receptor constructs directed toward hematological malignancies, and considers newer strategies incorporating gene-editing technologies to address graft-versus-host disease and host-mediated rejection. Recent data from clinical trials are reviewed, and an overview is provided of current and emerging manufacturing processes; consideration is also given to new developments in the pipeline.

HEMATOLOGY/ONCOLOGY CLINICS OF NORTH AMERICA

FORTHCOMING ISSUES

December 2017
Hematology/Oncology Emergencies
John C. Perkins and Jonathan E. Davis,
Editors

February 2018
Castleman Disease
Frits van Rhee and Nikhil C. Munshi,
Editors

April 2018
Thalassemia
Ali Taher, *Editor*

RECENT ISSUES

August 2017
The Treatment of Myeloid Malignancies
with Kinase Inhibitors
Ann Mullally, *Editor*

June 2017
Upper Gastrointestinal Malignancies
Manish A. Shah, *Editor*

April 2017
T-Cell Lymphoma
Eric D. Jacobsen, *Editor*

Preface

Gene Therapy

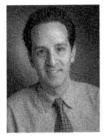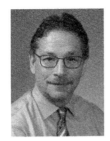

Daniel E. Bauer, MD, PhD   Donald B. Kohn, MD
Editors

This issue of *Hematology/Oncology Clinics of North America* addresses the current status of gene therapy as it applies to hematologic diseases and hematopoietic stem cell–based treatments. It documents the exciting advances that have been accomplished in recent years to provide clinical benefits for patients suffering from a wide range of disorders. Improvements in methods for hematopoietic stem cell processing, ex vivo and in vivo gene transfer with viral vectors, and gene editing are described. Opportunities for further improvements in gene addition and editing, stem cell engraftment, and in vivo genetic manipulation are explored. The scope includes the scientific, regulatory, and ethical issues that must be addressed to develop innovative therapies. The authors are all experts in the areas they cover and provide clear and knowledgeable summaries. We greatly appreciate the work done by each of them to provide their articles. We hope you will enjoy reading these articles as much as we did.

Daniel E. Bauer, MD, PhD
Division of Pediatric Hematology/Oncology
Dana-Farber/Boston Children's Cancer and Blood Disorders Center
Harvard Medical School
Harvard Stem Cell Institute
Broad Institute of MIT and Harvard
Karp 8211, 1 Blackfan Circle
Boston, MA 02115, USA

Hematol Oncol Clin N Am 31 (2017) xiii–xiv
http://dx.doi.org/10.1016/j.hoc.2017.07.001
0889-8588/17/© 2017 Published by Elsevier Inc.

hemonc.theclinics.com

Donald B. Kohn, MD
Department of Microbiology
Department of Immunology & Molecular Genetics
Department of Pediatrics
Department of Molecular & Medical Pharmacology
UCLA Eli & Edythe Broad Center
of Regenerative Medicine &
Stem Cell Research
David Geffen School of Medicine
University of California, Los Angeles
3163 Terasaki Life Science Building
610 Charles E. Young Drive East
Los Angeles, CA 90095, USA

E-mail addresses:
daniel.bauer@childrens.harvard.edu (D.E. Bauer)
dkohn1@mednet.ucla.edu (D.B. Kohn)

Historical Perspective on the Current Renaissance for Hematopoietic Stem Cell Gene Therapy

CrossMark

Donald B. Kohn, MD[a,b,c,d,e,*]

KEYWORDS

- Gene therapy • Hematopoietic stem cells • Gammaretroviral vector
- Lentiviral vector • Gene editing • Site-specific endonucleases
- Homologous recombination

KEY POINTS

- Gene therapy using gammaretroviral vectors into hematopoietic stem cells led to immune reconstitution for several primary immunodeficiency disorders, but produced leukoproliferative complications in some cases.
- Lentiviral vectors have become the predominant gene addition tool for hematopoietic stem cells and are showing efficacy and safety for numerous genetic blood cell diseases.
- Gene editing through the use of site-specific endonucleases is an emerging technology that may be applied for gene therapy using hematopoietic stem cells.

Disclosures: D.B. Kohn is a member of the Scientific Advisory Board of Orchard Therapeutics and an inventor on intellectual property licensed to them from University of California, Los Angeles.

Disclaimer: Due to word limits, only essential references are included.

[a] Department of Microbiology, Immunology and Molecular Genetics, David Geffen School of Medicine, University of California, Los Angeles, Los Angeles, CA, USA; [b] Division of Hematology/Oncology, Department of Pediatrics, David Geffen School of Medicine, University of California, Los Angeles, Los Angeles, CA, USA; [c] Department of Molecular and Medical Pharmacology, David Geffen School of Medicine, University of California, Los Angeles, Los Angeles, CA, USA; [d] UCLA Eli and Edythe Broad Center of Regenerative Medicine and Stem Cell Research, David Geffen School of Medicine at UCLA, University of California, Los Angeles, Los Angeles, CA, USA; [e] UCLA Jonsson Comprehensive Cancer Center, David Geffen School of Medicine, University of California, Los Angeles, Los Angeles, CA, USA

* Corresponding author. 3163 Terasaki Life Science Building, 610 Charles E. Young Drive East, Los Angeles, CA 90095.

E-mail address: dkohn1@mednet.ucla.edu

IN THE BEGINNING

It took more than 3 decades, but now gene therapy for blood cell diseases has become a clinical reality, as documented in the articles of this issue. From a bold vision proclaimed in editorials in the 1970s to 1980s,[1,2] steady incremental improvements in the underlying technology and successive series of clinical trials have advanced the state of the field so that a first hematopoietic stem cell (HSC)-based gene therapy product has been licensed for marketing in the European Union, with several more likely to follow there and in the United States.

The origins of gene therapy lie within the origins of modern molecular biology. The capacity to clone human genes as complementary DNA (cDNA) led to isolation of clinically relevant genes such as *beta-globin*, *HPRT*, *ADA*, and *DHFR*. Gene transfer to mammalian cells began with the development of calcium phosphate transfection methods, using selectable marker genes such as HSV *TK* and *DHFR*.[3] Early viral vectors derived from SV40 and Polyoma were also examined. Plasmids carrying the HSV *TK* gene or a human *beta-globin* cDNA were transfected into murine bone marrow (BM) cells and detected in vivo after cells were reinjected into mice.[4]

The field of gene therapy for blood cell disorders suffered an early setback when an initial attempt was made to translate the results from murine studies to clinical gene therapy for beta-thalassemia. The method used was ex vivo transfection of BM cells using a plasmid containing a human beta-globin cDNA. Two patients with beta-thalassemia major with severely advanced clinical complications were treated.[5] No clinically beneficial effects were detected, but no adverse effects resulted either (these results were never published). The study was performed in Italy and Israel at a time when there was no institutional review board approval to perform the studies at the primary US institution, due to concerns about insufficient preclinical efficacy data. The subsequent investigations led to censure of the lead scientist.[6]

The history of gene therapy cannot be fully told without a tribute to the role that the National Institutes of Health (NIH) Recombinant DNA Advisory Committee (RAC) played for the clinical translation of gene therapy, at least in the United States.[7] The RAC was formulated at NIH in the mid-1970s to provide guidance on policies to protect public safety as recombinant DNA technology was emerging, especially as potential biohazards were addressed by the scientific community at the landmark Asilomar meetings.[8] Following the violation of rules in the initial beta-globin gene transfer study, the Human Gene Therapy Subcommittee (HGTS) of the RAC was tasked by NIH Director Donald Fredrickson with formulating rules for review and conduct of federally funded clinical trials of gene therapy. Over the next decade, the HGTS developed a process for applying for permission from the NIH to perform clinical investigations of gene therapy. The existence of this highly rational and well-considered body obviated passage of legislation to govern this activity. The RAC played a very active role in shaping the conduct of gene therapy trials in the early days under public purview. Its role has been successively rolled back over time as greater experience was gained with clinical gene therapy, and the RAC has increasingly focused on novel issues of biosafety, and less on details of clinical trial design and performance.

GAMMARETROVIRAL VECTORS EMERGE

In the 1980s, recombinant versions of murine gammaretroviral vectors (gRV), primarily derived from the Moloney murine leukemia virus, were developed to carry genes into mammalian cells.[9,10] Several studies followed demonstrating that these vectors were capable of introducing foreign genetic material, often in the form of the neomycin phosphotransferase marker gene into HSC in murine BM cells.[11–13] Transplantation of gRV-treated murine BM led to the production of mature blood cells containing the integrated vector sequences. The unique integration site of the vector in each individual transduced HSC provided a clonal marker that could be detected using Southern blot analysis of a unique restriction fragment length polymorphism; these types of analyses showed that the same integrant was present in both myeloid and lymphoid cells, demonstrating gene transduction of pluripotent HSC capable of producing both dichotomous lineages of blood cells. gRV were developed to carry genes of direct relevance to human diseases, such as adenosine deaminase (ADA) to treat severe combined immune deficiency (SCID), glucocerebrosidase, the gene responsible for Gaucher disease, genes encoding cytokines for cancer immunotherapy, and others.[14,15] The use of the envelope glycoprotein from the murine amphotropic retrovirus broadened the host range of the vectors and allowed them to transduce human and other mammalian cells. Adding to the excitement were in vitro studies with human BM, demonstrating relatively efficient gene transfer to colony-forming progenitor cells, taken as a surrogate marker for the ability to transduce pluripotent long-term stem cells.[16] These positive results raised expectations for rapid translation to human applications for gene therapy for blood cell diseases.

However, subsequent studies performed in large animal models (canine and nonhuman primate) did not reproduce the high-level gene transduction of long-term HSC that had been seen in the murine models.[17] The frequencies of gene-marked blood cells that were achieved were in the range of 0.01% to 0.1%, much too low to be expected to have efficacy in a clinical application. This low level of in vivo gene marking led to the realizations that (1) murine HSC were more susceptible to transduction by gRV vectors than were HSC from larger primates, and presumably humans; and (2) progenitor cells that could be measured by in vitro colony-formation assays were poor predictors of long-term engrafting stem cells, which were more difficult to transduce.

During this time, the gRVs and stable packaging cell lines to produce them were developed that could make relatively high titer vectors in the absence of replication-competent retrovirus (RCR).[18,19] The absence of RCR was thought to be an essential safety factor to prevent spread of vector sequences within a subject and from treated subjects to others (health care workers, family members, other contacts). In fact, the importance of ensuring absence of RCR was shown in some studies in which nonhuman primates received autologous BM transplants of cells treated with vector preparations that were later found to be contaminated with high levels of RCR.[20] Several of the animals developed leukoproliferative complications (lymphoma) that were determined to be due to insertional oncogenesis by the RCR spreading and multiply-infecting proliferating stem and progenitor cells, leading to malignant transformation.

Initial clinical trials using gRV-mediated gene transfer to human BM were performed in the early 1990s for ADA-deficient SCID, Gaucher disease, chronic granulomatous disease, and leukocyte adhesion deficiency.[21–25] The stem cell processing methods used in these clinical all produced very low levels of gene-corrected cells that were mostly short lived. Inklings of efficacy were seen with preferential accumulation of gene-corrected T lymphocytes in ADA SCID patients, but this was highly pauciclonal with only small numbers of engrafted HSC.[26] These unsuccessful trials fed the general skepticism about gene therapy that was emerging in the mid 1990s, leading then NIH Director, Harold Varmus, to appoint a committee to review the status of the field and make recommendations (http://osp.od.nih.gov/office-biotechnology-activities/orkin-motulsky-report).

Nevertheless, at the same time, ongoing research led to several incremental technical improvements in the methods for HSC gene therapy that would lead to a second era in which clinical efficacy was achieved for several disorders. Additional vector pseudotypes, such as the Gibbon ape leukemia virus envelope, further improved gene transfer efficacy to human HSC.[27] Multiple aspects of the culture conditions used for ex vivo transduction of HSC were improved. Newly identified hematopoietic growth factors that stimulated proliferation of early human HSC, essential for gRV transduction, became available as recombinant proteins. Although still not unanimously agreed upon even today, combinations such as ckit ligand, flt-3 ligand, and thrombopoietin (S/F/T) were shown to favor transduction of early HSC with minimal push to differentiation and loss of long-term pluripotency. David Williams and colleagues[28] showed that the extracellular matrix protein fibronectin could be used to coat the tissue culture dishes and similarly augment transduction. Working with Takara Shuzo in Japan that had produced several recombinant fibronectin fragment molecules, they identified one in particular, called CH296 and marketed as Retronectin, which facilitated transduction, presumably by binding and colocalizing both the HSC and the retroviral vector particles.[29] Retronectin also was shown to play a role preserving HSC capacity during ex vivo transduction, possibly by engaging cellular integrins and providing antiapoptotic signals.[30] At this time, serum-free media were developed that would provide more uniform culture conditions, compared with the variability imposed by animal sera, such as fetal calf serum, that could contain variable levels of cytokines, for example, transforming growth factor-β and tumor necrosis factor, that affected HSC survival and differentiation. The development of methods to mobilize HSC into peripheral blood using granulocyte colony-stimulating factor (G-CSF) (peripheral blood stem cells, or PBSC) provided a more abundant source of HSC that could be used instead of BM harvested cells. One additional concept that was incorporated from the field of clinical HSCT was that of "reduced intensity conditioning": the use of subablative levels of chemotherapy or total body irradiation to make some space for engraftment of donor stem cells but with reduced toxicity risks. Subsequent studies of gene transfer/HSCT combining these individual improvements for the transduction of HSC from large animals led to significantly improved levels of engraftment of gene-transduced HSC, into the 1% to 10% range, when given to animals subjected to fully ablative conditioning.[31,32] The improved levels of engraftment of gene-modified HSC achieved in these large animal studies presaged the successes that would follow in clinical trials.

Following the period of technological development, clinical trials began to show efficacy. The first was a report from France where 2 young boys with X-linked SCID were treated using a gRV to introduce a normal IL2RG cDNA into BM CD34$^+$ cells.[33] The cells were reinfused without preparative conditioning. The patients developed T cells expressing the introduced IL2RG gene and displayed appropriate immunologic function. This trial represented the first achievement of a clinical benefit for any patients using gene therapy, and the results brought great excitement to the field. They extended their series to 10 subjects, with the majority realizing good T-cell immunity.[34] B-cell functional recovery (antibody production) was more variable, likely because the absence of pretransplant conditioning minimized engraftment of gene-corrected HSC, which may be necessary for B-cell correction. Investigators in London, United Kingdom reported similar results using a similar approach with a gRV.[35]

Shortly thereafter, successful results were reported for ADA-deficient SCID by investigators in Italy.[36] They also used a gRV for ADA gene transfer to BM CD34$^+$ cells, but added the use of reduced intensity conditioning (busulfan 4 mg/kg) to "make space" in the marrow and enhance engraftment. They have gone on to treat least 18 ADA SCID patients by this approach, with the majority achieving good to excellent immunity.[37] They licensed their vector/cell product to GlaxoSmithKline, and it has been approved by the European Medicines Agency in

2016 as Strimvelis, only the second licensed gene therapy product in the West. Groups in the United Kingdom and the United States also successfully treated ADA SCID patients using similar approaches with gRVs and low-dose busulfan conditioning.[38-40]

However, in the XSCID studies from France and England, 5 of 20 who had been treated developed a T-lymphoproliferative complication 2 to 3 years after the treatment.[41] Investigations revealed that the process of insertional oncogenesis has occurred, in which the integrated vector *trans*-activated a nearby protooncogene, causing clonal expansion. Four of the 5 who developed clonal expansions were successfully treated with anti–leukemia chemotherapy and remain in remission to the present time, but one patient died of the complication. Other clinical trials performed for X-linked chronic granulomatous disease (XCGD) and Wiskott-Aldrich Syndrome (WAS) similarly led to initial successful immune reconstitution, followed by later development of leukemia-like complications in most of the patients (see Luca Biasco and colleagues' article, "Integrating Vectors for Gene Therapy and Clonal Tracking of Engineered Hematopoiesis"; and Sujal Ghosh and H. Bobby Gaspar's article, "Gene Therapy Approaches to Immunodeficiency," in this issue, for more in-depth discussion of these events).[42,43] Thus, although the proof of efficacy had been obtained, the genotoxicity that occurred (except in the setting of ADA deficiency for unknown but fortuitous reasons) led to a general turning away from gRVs with intact long-terminal repeat (LTR) enhancers to the use of self-inactivated (SIN) vectors, lacking LTR enhancers, from either gRVs or lentiviral vectors (LV).

RISE OF THE LENTIVIRAL VECTORS

Early in the development of LVs, the SIN configuration in which the LTR enhancers are eliminated was adopted.[44] The SIN configuration allows transcription of the transgene to be driven by an internal promoter that may be selected for safety and/or lineage specificity of expression. Core promoters such as *PGK* and *EF1-alpha* have relatively strong, constitutive, ubiquitous promoter activity, but have minimal enhancer activity, which greatly reduces risks of *trans*-activation of adjacent cellular genes at the sites of integration. Promoters from cellular genes may be used to impose specificity of expression, such as the *beta-globin* gene promoter for erythroid-specific expression for hemoglobinopathies, the Wiskott-Aldrich Syndrome Protein (*WASP*) gene promoter for pan-hematopoietic expression in the treatment of WAS, or a chimeric cathepsin G enhancer/*cfes* promoter for myeloid-restricted expression for the treatment of XCGD.[45-47]

LVs were shown to have greatly increased capacity to transduce nondividing cells, including primitive human CD34$^+$/CD38-stem/progenitor cells, making them more effective than gRVs for HSC-directed gene therapies.[48] Lentiviral transduction can be performed optimally in 36 to 48 hours of ex vivo culture, whereas gRVs require 72 to 96 hours for maximal transduction, and the longer culture time leads to higher loss of stem cell activity.[49] LVs have now been used for human subjects in at least a dozen clinical trials (**Table 1**).

Significant clinical efficacy has been demonstrated in many of these studies. There has been effective gene transfer to engrafting stem cells, long-term persistence of the gene-corrected stem cells, and production of gene-containing cells of multiple lineages. The absence of vector-related open-reading frames obviates risks of immunologic responses to vector-related proteins in the transplanted cells. In the first of these trials, for X-linked adrenoleukodystrophy, there was neurologic stabilization and outcomes at least equivalent to those with an unrelated marrow donor, without the risks

Table 1
Clinical trials using lentiviral vectors with hematopoietic stem cells

Disease	Transcriptional Control/Gene	Responsible Party	Clinical Trials.gov #
X-adrenoleukodystrophy	MND retroviral LTR U3, *ALDP* NM_000033.3	Aubourg P Bluebird bio	NCT01801709 NCT01896102
Metachromatic leukodystrophy	Human phosphoglycerate kinase gene, *ASA* NC_000023.11/NC_000022.11	Biffi A	NCT01560182
Beta-Thalassemia	*Beta-Globin* enhancer/promoter/locus control region, *HBB* NC_000011.10	Cavazzana M/Leboulche P Memorial Sloan Kettering Cancer Center Bluebird bio Bluebird bio Ferrari G Bluebird bio	Preceded CT.gov NCT01639690 NCT01745120 NCT02140554 NCT02453477 NCT02906202
Sickle cell disease	*Beta-Globin* Enh/Prom/LCR-*HBB* or *HBG* NC_000011.10	Bluebird bio Bluebird bio Malik P Kohn D	NCT02140554 NCT02151526 NCT02186418 NCT02247843
ADA-deficient SCID	*EF1alpha* short (EFS), *ADA* NC_000006.12/NC_000020.11	Gaspar HB Kohn D Garabedian E/Candotti F/Kohn D Kohn D	NCT01380990 NCT01852071 NCT02022696 NCT02999984
X-linked SCID	*EF1alpha* short (EFS), *IL2RG* NC_000006.12/NC_000023.11	De Ravin S Sorrentino B/Mamcarz E	NCT01306019 NCT01512888
WAS	Human *WASP* gene promoter, *WASP* NC_000023.11	Thrasher A Fischer A/Cavazzana M Williams D/Pai S Aiuti A	NCT01347242 NCT01347346 NCT01410825 NCT01515462
XCGD	Cathepsin G enhancer/*cFES* promoter, *CYBB* NC_000014.9/NC_000015.10 NC_000023.11	Thrasher A/Reichenbach J/Serve P Kohn D Blanche S	NCT01855685 NCT02234834 NCT02757911
HIV-associated lymphoma NC_000011.10 NC_000003.12 NC_000012.12 NC_000011.10	H1 RNA pol III promoter-TAR Decoy/CCR5RZ H1 RNA pol III promoter-shRNA to CCR5 and Ubiquitin promoter-C46 fusion inhibitor CCR5 shRNA/TRIM5alpha/TAR Decoy	Krishnan A Kiem HP Kiem HP AIDS Malignancy Consortium	NCT00569985 NCT02343666 NCT02378922 NCT02797470

of graft-versus-host disease.[50] For metachromatic leukodystrophy, the neurologic outcomes were vastly superior to those seen from earlier allogeneic transplantations, presumably because the capacity to overexpress the gene product from the LV led to cross-correction of neuronal cells that exceeded what may occur with normal donor cells expressing only the normal amount of the transgene product.[51] Robust and sustained immune reconstitution has been accomplished for WAS, ADA SCID, and XSCID at multiple centers.[52–55]

Results of the hemoglobinopathies have been somewhat less salutary. The standard design of the vectors constructed to express *beta-globin* (either wild-type for replacement in beta-thalassemia or anti-sickling variants [T87Q, Beta-AS3, gamma-globin-exon substituted] for sickle cell disease) have included mini-gene cassettes with the *beta-globin* gene exons, introns, 5′ and 3′ flanking sequences, and combinations of several upstream erythroid-specific DNase I hypersensitive sites that compose a master chromatin regulatory element referred to as the locus control region (LCR). These elements were all found to be necessary for copy-dependent, position-independent expression of beta-globin transgenes in mice.[56] Early efforts to carry them in gRVs were unsuccessful, because of relatively weak expression and frequent rearrangements with loss of sequences during retroviral vector genome RNA production and reverse transcription.

Sadelain and colleagues[45] first demonstrated that these same components could be transmitted with high integrity using LV backbones. This basic vector design has been used in all of the subsequent trials for beta-thalassemia and sickle cell disease.[57–59] With the beta-globin LVs, the maximum titers achieved during large-scale production have been suboptimal as has been the resulting efficacy of gene transfer to CD34+ cells. These low titers necessitate large amounts of vector material per patient dose that may be limiting in large-scale applications. Efforts to improve vector design and titer or enrich the target HSCs may facilitate more widespread application.[60]

There has been an excellent safety profile with the use of SIN LVs in these clinical studies. One transient clonal expansion was seen in a beta-thalassemia trial subject, but this did not progress to myelodysplastic syndrome, and subsequently receded.[57] The relatively consistent pattern of LV integration in the drug product (LV-transduced CD34+ cells from BM or mobilized peripheral blood) and in blood cell and BM cell samples from subjects across all the trials has not shown any predisposition to integration near protooncogenes nor expansion of clones with specific integration sites.[50,51,61]

THIS IS THE DAWNING OF THE AGE OF GENE EDITING

The major alternative approach to gene addition for gene therapy is gene editing. Initial attempts to perform gene editing through homologous recombination (HR) by addition of complementary nucleic acids sequences (oligonucleotides, short hairpins, RNA/DNA hybrids, or plasmids) established proof of principle but achieved only very low frequencies of gene correction with primary HSCs.[62] A major advance came with the discovery that a large increase in HR can be induced at a locus by introduction of a nearby double-stranded DNA break (DSB).[63] A succession of site-specific endonucleases have been developed for targeted genome editing, including zinc finger nucleases, homing endonucleases, TALENs, and more recently the highly malleable CRISPR/Cas endonuclease system. Technical developments over the past decade have defined methods to transiently introduce the necessary gene editing reagents (nuclease, homologous donor) into primary HSCs, often by a combination of electroporation and viral vector transduction.

The methods allow several types of gene edits to be introduced. Gene inactivation can be achieved by applying the nuclease only and allowing the error-prone nonhomologous end-joining pathway to introduce nested insertions and deletions at the cleavage site, disrupting the gene sequence. Gene inactivation has been applied to efforts to eliminate CCR5, an HIV-1 coreceptor from HSC to produce an antiviral effect (see Geoffrey L. Rogers and Paula M. Cannon's article, "Gene Therapy Approaches to HIV and Other Infectious Diseases," in this issue).[64] Trials using gene disruption of a repressor of gamma-globin expression, BCL11A, to induce fetal hemoglobin production for the treatment of beta-thalassemia and sickle cell disease are planned.[65] Gene correction by replacing single base-pairs and short sequences has been accomplished in preclinical studies for several disease-related loci, and the efficiency continues to increase.[66–70] Targeted gene insertion using a transgene cassette flanked by homology arms complementary to the sequences at the nuclease target site can add a normal cDNA into its endogenous locus to be expressed from the endogenous promoter and thereby override any downstream mutations.

Not all gene editing relies on introducing a DSB. Nucleases can be modified to only cleave one strand, producing DNA nicks, which can also promote HR and may have lower genotoxicity risks than DSB. Liu and colleagues[71] tethered cytosine deaminase to a catalytically inactive Cas9 protein to convert individual cytosine residues to uracil and hence thymidine (or change a G to an A by targeting the cytosine on the other strand). The repertoire of molecular editing tools is likely to expand.

The critical issues for assessing different nucleases are their endonuclease activity, their specificity for the target sequence versus off-target endonuclease activity, and the types of cut ends they leave (blunt vs overhanging), which may affect editing outcomes. Further information is needed about the potential genotoxicity from either disrupting the target locus and/or acting at off-target sites. In addition, the process of adding the gene-editing reagents may impose some degree of cytotoxicity by induction of apoptosis and loss of stem cells, which could even limit engraftment capacity. All of these issues are being studied as gene editing in HSC moves forward to clinical applications (see Christopher Lux and Andrew M. Scharenberg's article, "Therapeutic Gene Editing Safety and Specificity"; and Dale Ando and Kathleen Meyer's article, "Gene Editing—Regulatory and Translation to Clinic," in this issue).

ONGOING CHALLENGES

There is a critical need to develop methods to expand HSC to a clinically meaningful extent (eg, 3- to 10-fold) to improve the outcomes from gene therapy. HSC are rare and fragile. Their isolation from clinical cell sources leads to some degree of cell loss. Ex vivo manipulations, for example, electroporation for gene editing, may lead to further decreases in viable numbers of engraftable HSC. The lower limits for an effective cell dose for gene-modified autologous CD34+ cells has not been formally studied, but there is a dose effect, with CD34+ cell dosages under 1 to 2 million per kilogram leading to poorer engraftment and disease modification. Although the available HSC from adult patients (usually G-CSF mobilized PBSC) have been sufficient in many trials, the quality and frequency of HSC are definitely higher with younger age donors. Some conditions where the numbers of available HSC are reduced, for example, Fanconi anemia and osteopetrosis, may have limited potential for treatment through gene therapy, unless the HSC can be expanded. Several small molecules have been identified that may support modest degrees of HSC expansion,[72,73] but the ideal drug or combination has not yet been reported that is capable of expanding the numbers of HSC to improve effectiveness of gene therapy. HSC expansion remains a Holy Grail.

The limited numbers of HSC available from patients may be completely overcome if methods can be developed to produce high numbers of transplantable HSC from pluripotent cell sources, such as induced pluripotent stem cells (iPSC). As with HSC expansion, successful derivation of clinically relevant numbers of HSC from iPSC has been elusive.[74,75] Once solved, sourcing large numbers of HSC from iPSC would provide greatly improved capacities for gene therapy. Besides the increased supply of cells, gene-modified iPSC can be cloned and characterized to obtain the desired genetic modification without measurable off-target changes and then be used to produce corrected HSC.

CD34$^+$ cell selection has been the standard approach to enriching HSC to reduce the numbers of cells from BM or PBSC that need to be treated with vector, representing ~50-fold enrichment of cells to be transduced and concordant reductions in needed vector amounts. Further purification of HSC to produce a more stem cell–enriched population than bulk CD34$^+$ cells (eg, CD34$^+$/CD38$^-$, CD34$^+$/CD133$^+$, CD34$^+$/CD90$^+$) would reduce further the amounts of vector needed to make each patient's cell dose. It is likely that additional purification steps would come at the cost of additional cell losses of HSC.[60] An optimal compromise between enrichment and recovery will need to be struck.

Transduction of CD34$^+$, and hence HSC, is achieved to the necessary level that provides clinical benefit with most LVs. However, human HSC are relatively restrictive to LV transduction, compared with many cell lines and primary nonhematopoietic cell types, resulting in the seemingly high multiplicity of infection of LV needed for CD34$^+$ cells (eg, 20–100), based on titers determined on permissive cell lines. Several small molecules have been reported to increase transduction, either by affecting the effectiveness of binding of vector to the CD34$^+$ cells or by overcoming putative intracellular inhibitory factors (eg, cyclosporine A, rapamycin, proteasome inhibitors).[76–78] Combinations of these reagents may support a clinically useful increase in CD34$^+$ transduction, also lowering the needed amounts of vector.

Expression from LVs has not been a significantly observed problem. Vectors with constitutive promoters, such as PGK and EF1alpha, have not suffered noticeable silencing of expression. Lineage-specific promoters, such as those from the human genes for *beta-globin* and *WASP*, have expressed their transgenes sufficiently to provide clinical benefits, but they do not drive fully normal levels of gene expression, compared with their endogenous counterparts.[79] Further development of transcriptional control elements guided by genomic, epigenetic, and chromatin information may produce vectors with more physiologic levels and patterns of expression. Of course, gene editing would leave the relevant gene in its normal chromosomal context, and expression should precisely follow the normal pattern.

Pretransplant conditioning remains another area where progress is vitally needed (see Morton J. Cowan and colleagues' article, "Opening Marrow Niches in Patients Undergoing Autologous Hematopoietic Stem Cell Gene Therapy," in this issue). Although reduced intensity conditioning with busulfan has been well tolerated in the short term, there remain potential late effects from this alkylating agent. More intense regimens used for some disorders where highest levels of engraftment are needed would be expected to have further increased risks. Thus, development of conditioning methods not based on chemotherapy is another crucial challenge. The recent advancements using monoclonal antibodies in combinations and as immunotoxin conjugates are promising and exciting.[80–82]

Ideally, methods will be developed that allow direct in vivo transduction of HSC, without the necessity to harvest and process them ex vivo (see Maximilian Richter and colleagues' article, "In Vivo Hematopoietic Stem Cell Transduction," in this issue). Current LVs have not led to high-level transduction when administered directly in vivo. New vector pseudotypes with high tropism and specificity for HSC and capacity to effective transduce them, even if primarily quiescent, may allow this to be accomplished.

Gene therapy carries risks of immune responses to new transgene products, even if from the normal gene, when expressed in a genetically null recipient. Hypothetically, transplantation of gene-modified HSC may lead to development of immunologic tolerance, from expression of the transgene product in thymic dendritic cells or another cell that induces tolerance such as regulatory T cells or myeloid dendritic cells. Conditioning with busulfan as a single agent would not be expected to be potently immune suppressive, so that preexisting immunity would likely persist and could lead to rejection of transduced cells expressing the transgene product. To date, this has not been observed to any appreciable extent, although it is not routinely monitored. Gene therapy in patients with compromised cellular immunity (eg, SCID) may have reduced risks of immune rejection, but this complication has not been seen even in disorders with relatively intact cellular immunity, such as the leukodystrophies or XCGD. Some trials have added immune suppressive agents, such as fludarabine, to conditioning regimens for gene therapy, especially for conditions such as WAS where preexisting autoimmunity may persist through transplantation and remain problematic.

Commercialization of the production of gene-modified HSC will hold many challenges. As a patient-specific cell product, each patient requires a unique lot of the cell product, with costly release testing. The fragility of primary HSC imposes strict boundaries around the logistics of cell transport, processing, and formulation. Alternative models are emerging for clinical cell processing. Several companies are establishing centralized high-level good manufacturing practice facilities to receive cell products collected at various remote clinical sites, process the cells under pharmaceutical standards, and then return the cryopreserved final cell product to the clinical site for transplantation. Centralized cell processing will require shipping of the fresh cell product, which has risks for delays in cell product delivery with late processing causing a decrease in HSC content. A different approach is based on devices being developed to perform all of the stages of cell processing within a closed system at local treatment sites and not require specialized laboratory facilities. It remains to be seen which of these business models will prevail. It is a sign of the maturity of this area of medicine and the effectiveness of gene therapy for so many disorders that such issues of scale-up and product distribution are coming to the fore.

REFERENCES

1. Friedmann T, Roblin R. Gene therapy for human genetic disease? Science 1972; 175(4025):949–55.
2. Anderson WF, Fletcher JC. Sounding boards. Gene therapy in human beings: when is it ethical to begin? N Engl J Med 1980;303(22):1293–7.
3. Williamson B. Reintroduction of genetically transformed bone marrow cells into mice. Nature 1980;284(5755):397–8.
4. Mercola KE, Stang HD, Browne J, et al. Insertion of a new gene of viral origin into bone marrow cells of mice. Science 1980;208(4447):1033–5.
5. Jacobs P, the Los Angeles Times. Doctor tried gene therapy on 2 humans. The Washington Post 1980.

6. Schmeck HM Jr. U.S. agency disciplines gene-splicing researcher. New York Times 1981.

7. Wivel NA. Historical perspectives pertaining to the NIH Recombinant DNA Advisory Committee. Hum Gene Ther 2014;25(1):19–24.

8. Fredrickson DS. Asilomar and recombinant DNA: the end of the beginning. In: Institute of Medicine (US) Committee to Study Decision Making, Hanna KE, editors. Biomedical Politics. Washington (DC): National Academies Press (US); 1991. p. 258–308. Available at: https://www.ncbi.nlm.nih.gov/books/NBK234217/?report=classic.

9. Cone RD, Mulligan RC. High-efficiency gene transfer into mammalian cells: generation of helper-free recombinant retrovirus with broad mammalian host range. Proc Natl Acad Sci U S A 1984;81:6349–53.

10. Armentano D, Yu SF, Kantoff PW, et al. Gene expression in mice after high efficiency retroviral-mediated gene transfer. Science 1985;230:1395–8.

11. Williams DA, Lemischka IR, Nathan DG, et al. Introduction of new genetic material into pluripotent haematopoietic stem cells of the mouse. Nature 1984;310: 476–80.

12. Eglitis MA, Kantoff P, Gilboa E, et al. Gene expression in mice after high efficiency retroviral-mediated gene transfer. Science 1985;230:1395–8.

13. Dick JE, Magli MC, Huszar D, et al. Introduction of a selectable gene into primitive stem cells capable of long-term reconstitution of the hemopoietic system of W/Wv mice. Cell 1985;42(1):71–9.

14. Belmont JW, Henkel-Tigges J, Chang SM, et al. Expression of human adenosine deaminase in murine haematopoietic progenitor cells following retroviral transfer. Nature 1986;322:385–7.

15. Karlsson S, Bodine DM, Perry L, et al. Expression of the human beta-globin gene following retroviral-mediated transfer into multipotential hematopoietic progenitors of mice. Proc Natl Acad Sci U S A 1988;85(16):6062–6.

16. Gruber HE, Finley KD, Hershberg RM, et al. Retroviral vector-mediated gene transfer into human hematopoietic progenitor cells. Science 1985;230:1057–61.

17. Schuening FG, Kawahara K, Miller AD, et al. Retrovirus-mediated gene transduction into long-term repopulating marrow cells of dogs. Blood 1991;78:2568–76.

18. Miller AD, Buttimore C. Redesign of retrovirus packaging cell lines to avoid recombination leading to helper virus production. Mol Cell Biol 1986;6:2895–902.

19. Markowitz D, Goff S, Bank A. A safe packaging line for gene transfer: separating viral genes on two different plasmids. J Virol 1988;62:1120–4.

20. Donahue RE, Kessler SW, Bodine D, et al. Helper virus induced T cell lymphoma in nonhuman primates after retroviral mediated gene transfer. J Exp Med 1992; 176:1125–35.

21. Bordignon C, Notarangelo LD, Nobili N, et al. Gene therapy in peripheral blood lymphocytes and bone marrow for ADA- immunodeficient patients. Science 1995;270(5235):470–5.

22. Kohn DB, Weinberg KI, Nolta JA, et al. Engraftment of gene-modified umbilical cord blood cells in neonates with adenosine deaminase deficiency. Nat Med 1995;1(10):1017–23.

23. Dunbar CE, Kohn DB, Schiffmann R, et al. Retroviral transfer of the glucocerebrosidase gene into CD34+ cells from patients with Gaucher disease: in vivo detection of transduced cells without myeloablation. Hum Gene Ther 1998;9(17): 2629–40.

24. Malech HL, Maples PB, Whiting-Theobald N, et al. Prolonged production of NADPH oxidase-corrected granulocytes after gene therapy of chronic granulomatous disease. Proc Natl Acad Sci U S A 1997;94(22):12133–8.

25. Bauer TR, Schwartz BR, Liles WC, et al. Retroviral-mediated gene transfer of the leukocyte integrin CD18 into peripheral blood CD34+ cells derived from a patient with leukocyte adhesion deficiency type 1. Blood 1998;91(5):1520–6.

26. Schmidt M, Carbonaro DA, Speckmann C, et al. Clonality analysis after retroviral-mediated gene transfer to CD34+ cells from the cord blood of ADA-deficient SCID neonates. Nat Med 2003;9(4):463–8.

27. Miller AD, Garcia JV, von Suhr N, et al. Construction and properties of retrovirus packaging cells based on gibbon ape leukemia virus. J Virol 1991;65(5):2220–4.

28. Moritz T, Patel VP, Williams DA. Bone marrow extracellular matrix molecules improve gene transfer into human hematopoietic cells via retroviral vectors. J Clin Invest 1994;93(4):1451–7.

29. Pollok KE, Hanenberg H, Noblitt TW, et al. High-efficiency gene transfer into normal and adenosine deaminase-deficient T lymphocytes is mediated by transduction on recombinant fibronectin fragments. J Virol 1998;72(6):4882–92.

30. Dao MA, Hashino K, Kato I, et al. Adhesion to fibronectin maintains regenerative capacity during ex vivo culture and transduction of human hematopoietic stem and progenitor cells. Blood 1998;92(12):4612–21.

31. Kurre P, Morris J, Horn PA, et al. Gene transfer into baboon repopulating cells: a comparison of Flt-3 ligand and megakaryocyte growth and development factor versus IL-3 during ex vivo transduction. Mol Ther 2001;3(6):920–7.

32. Wu T, Kim HJ, Sellers SE, et al. Prolonged high-level detection of retrovirally marked hematopoietic cells in nonhuman primates after transduction of CD34+ progenitors using clinically feasible methods. Mol Ther 2000;1(3):285–93.

33. Cavazzana-Calvo M, Hacein-Bey S, de Saint Basile G, et al. Gene therapy of human severe combined immunodeficiency (SCID)-X1 disease. Science 2000; 288(5466):669–72.

34. Hacein-Bey-Abina S, Hauer J, Lim A, et al. Efficacy of gene therapy for X-linked severe combined immunodeficiency. N Engl J Med 2010;363(4):355–64.

35. Gaspar HB, Parsley KL, Howe S, et al. Gene therapy of X-linked severe combined immunodeficiency by use of a pseudotyped gammaretroviral vector. Lancet 2004;364(9452):2181–7.

36. Aiuti A, Slavin S, Aker M, et al. Correction of ADA-SCID by stem cell gene therapy combined with nonmyeloablative conditioning. Science 2002;296(5577):2410–3.

37. Cicalese MP, Ferrua F, Castagnaro L, et al. Update on the safety and efficacy of retroviral gene therapy for immunodeficiency due to adenosine deaminase deficiency. Blood 2016;128(1):45–54.

38. Gaspar HB, Cooray S, Gilmour KC, et al. Hematopoietic stem cell gene therapy for adenosine deaminase-deficient severe combined immunodeficiency leads to long-term immunological recovery and metabolic correction. Sci Transl Med 2011;3(97):97ra80.

39. Candotti F, Shaw KL, Muul L, et al. Gene therapy for adenosine deaminase-deficient severe combined immune deficiency: clinical comparison of retroviral vectors and treatment plans. Blood 2012;120(18):3635–46.

40. Shaw KL, Garabedian E, Mishra S, et al. A phase II clinical trial of gene therapy for adenosine deaminase-deficient severe combined immune deficiency using a gamma-retroviral vector and reduced intensity conditioning. J Clin Invest 2017; 120:3635–46.

41. Hacein-Bey-Abina S, Von Kalle C, Schmidt M, et al. LMO2-associated clonal T cell proliferation in two patients after gene therapy for SCID-X1. Science 2003;302(5644):415–9.

42. Stein S, Ott MG, Schultze-Strasser S, et al. Genomic instability and myelodysplasia with monosomy 7 consequent to EVI1 activation after gene therapy for chronic granulomatous disease. Nat Med 2010;16(2):198–204.
43. Braun CJ, Boztug K, Paruzynski A, et al. Gene therapy for Wiskott-Aldrich syndrome–long-term efficacy and genotoxicity. Sci Transl Med 2014;6(227):227ra33.
44. Zufferey R, Dull T, Mandel RJ, et al. Self-inactivating lentivirus vector for safe and efficient in vivo gene delivery. J Virol 1998;72(12):9873–80.
45. May C, Rivella S, Callegari J, et al. Therapeutic haemoglobin synthesis in beta-thalassaemic mice expressing lentivirus-encoded human beta-globin. Nature 2000;406(6791):82–6.
46. Charrier S, Stockholm D, Seye K, et al. A lentiviral vector encoding the human Wiskott-Aldrich syndrome protein corrects immune and cytoskeletal defects in WASP knockout mice. Gene Ther 2005;12(7):597–606.
47. Santilli G, Almarza E, Brendel C, et al. Biochemical correction of X-CGD by a novel chimeric promoter regulating high levels of transgene expression in myeloid cells. Mol Ther 2011;19(1):122–32.
48. Case SS, Price MA, Jordan CT, et al. Stable transduction of quiescent CD34(+) CD38(-) human hematopoietic cells by HIV-1-based lentiviral vectors. Proc Natl Acad Sci U S A 1999;96(6):2988–93.
49. Mazurier F, Gan OI, McKenzie JL, et al. Lentivector-mediated clonal tracking reveals intrinsic heterogeneity in the human hematopoietic stem cell compartment and culture-induced stem cell impairment. Blood 2004;103(2):545–52.
50. Cartier N, Hacein-Bey-Abina S, Bartholomae CC, et al. Hematopoietic stem cell gene therapy with a lentiviral vector in X-linked adrenoleukodystrophy. Science 2009;326(5954):818–23.
51. Biffi A, Montini E, Lorioli L, et al. Lentiviral hematopoietic stem cell gene therapy benefits metachromatic leukodystrophy. Science 2013;341(6148):1233158.
52. Aiuti A, Biasco L, Scaramuzza S, et al. Lentiviral hematopoietic stem cell gene therapy in patients with Wiskott-Aldrich syndrome. Science 2013;341(6148): 1233151.
53. Hacein-Bey Abina S, Gaspar HB, Blondeau J, et al. Outcomes following gene therapy in patients with severe Wiskott-Aldrich syndrome. JAMA 2015;313(15): 50–63.
54. Gaspar HB, Buckland K, Carbonaro DA, et al. Immunological and metabolic correction after lentiviral vector gene therapy for ADA deficiency. Mol Ther 2015;23(Suppl 1):S102.
55. De Ravin SS, Wu X, Moir S, et al. Lentiviral hematopoietic stem cell gene therapy for X-linked severe combined immunodeficiency. Sci Transl Med 2016;8(335): 335ra57.
56. Grosveld F, van Assendelft GB, Greaves DR, et al. Position-independent, high-level expression of the human beta-globin gene in transgenic mice. Cell 1987; 51(6):975–85.
57. Cavazzana-Calvo M, Payen E, Negre O, et al. Transfusion independence and HMGA2 activation after gene therapy of human β-thalassaemia. Nature 2010; 467(7313):318–22.
58. Roselli EA, Mezzadra R, Frittoli MC, et al. Correction of beta-thalassemia major by gene transfer in haematopoietic progenitors of pediatric patients. EMBO Mol Med 2010;2(8):315–28.
59. Urbinati F, Hargrove PW, Geiger S, et al. Potentially therapeutic levels of anti-sickling globin gene expression following lentivirus-mediated gene transfer in sickle cell disease bone marrow CD34+ cells. Exp Hematol 2015;43(5):346–51.

60. Baldwin K, Urbinati F, Romero Z, et al. Enrichment of human hematopoietic stem/progenitor cells facilitates transduction for stem cell gene therapy. Stem Cells 2015;33(5):1532–42.

61. Biasco L, Pellin D, Scala S, et al. In vivo tracking of human hematopoiesis reveals patterns of clonal dynamics during early and steady-state reconstitution phases. Cell Stem Cell 2016;19(1):107–19.

62. Goncz KK, Prokopishyn NL, Chow BL, et al. Application of SFHR to gene therapy of monogenic disorders. Gene Ther 2002;9:691–4.

63. Porteus MH, Baltimore D. Gene targeting in human cells. Science 2003; 300(May):75390.

64. Li L, Krymskaya L, Wang J, et al. Genomic editing of the HIV-1 coreceptor CCR5 in adult hematopoietic stem and progenitor cells using zinc finger nucleases. Mol Ther 2013;21(6):1259–69.

65. Canver MC, Smith EC, Sher F, et al. BCL11A enhancer dissection by Cas9-mediated in situ saturating mutagenesis. Nature 2015;527(7577):192–7.

66. Dever DP, Bak RO, Reinisch A, et al. CRISPR/Cas9 β-globin gene targeting in human haematopoietic stem cells. Nature 2016;539(7629):384–9.

67. Wang J, Exline CM, DeClercq JJ, et al. Homology-driven genome editing in hematopoietic stem and progenitor cells using ZFN mRNA and AAV6 donors. Nat Biotechnol 2015;33(12):1256–63.

68. Hoban MD, Lumaquin D, Kuo CY, et al. CRISPR/Cas9-mediated correction of the sickle mutation in human CD34+ cells. Mol Ther 2016;24(9):1561–9.

69. DeWitt MA, Magis W, Bray NL, et al. Selection-free genome editing of the sickle mutation in human adult hematopoietic stem/progenitor cells. Sci Transl Med 2016;8(360):360ra134.

70. De Ravin SS, Li L, Wu X, et al. CRISPR-Cas9 gene repair of hematopoietic stem cells from patients with X-linked chronic granulomatous disease. Sci Transl Med 2017;9(372) [pii:eaah3480].

71. Komor AC, Kim YB, Packer MS, et al. Programmable editing of a target base in genomic DNA without double-stranded DNA cleavage. Nature 2016;533(7603): 420–4.

72. Boitano AE, Wang J, Romeo R, et al. Aryl hydrocarbon receptor antagonists promote the expansion of human hematopoietic stem cells. Science 2010;329(5997): 1345–8.

73. Fares I, Chagraoui J, Gareau Y, et al. Cord blood expansion. Pyrimidoindole derivatives are agonists of human hematopoietic stem cell self-renewal. Science 2014;345(6203):1509–12.

74. Dravid GG, Crooks GM. The challenges and promises of blood engineered from human pluripotent stem cells. Adv Drug Deliv Rev 2011;63(4–5):331–41.

75. Daniel MG, Pereira CF, Lemischka IR, et al. Making a hematopoietic stem cell. Trends Cell Biol 2016;26(3):202–14.

76. Petrillo C, Cesana D, Piras F, et al. Cyclosporin a and rapamycin relieve distinct lentiviral restriction blocks in hematopoietic stem and progenitor cells. Mol Ther 2015;23(2):352–62.

77. Wang CX, Sather BD, Wang X, et al. Rapamycin relieves lentiviral vector transduction resistance in human and mouse hematopoietic stem cells. Blood 2014; 124(6):913–23.

78. Santoni de Sio FR, Cascio P, Zingale A, et al. Proteasome activity restricts lentiviral gene transfer into hematopoietic stem cells and is down-regulated by cytokines that enhance transduction. Blood 2006;107(11):4257–65.

79. Lisowski L, Sadelain M. Current status of globin gene therapy for the treatment of beta-thalassaemia. Br J Haematol 2008;141(3):335–45.
80. Czechowicz A, Kraft D, Weissman IL, et al. Efficient transplantation via antibody-based clearance of hematopoietic stem cell niches. Science 2007;318(5854): 1296–9.
81. Chhabra A, Ring AM, Weiskopf K, et al. Hematopoietic stem cell transplantation in immunocompetent hosts without radiation or chemotherapy. Sci Transl Med 2016;8(351):351ra105.
82. Palchaudhuri R, Saez B, Hoggatt J, et al. Non-genotoxic conditioning for hematopoietic stem cell transplantation using a hematopoietic-cell-specific internalizing immunotoxin. Nat Biotechnol 2016;34(7):738–45.

Integrating Vectors for Gene Therapy and Clonal Tracking of Engineered Hematopoiesis

Luca Biasco, PhD[a,b], Michael Rothe, PhD[c], Juliane W. Schott, PhD[c],
Axel Schambach, MD, PhD[c,d],*

KEYWORDS

- Retroviral vector • Lentiviral vector • Transposon • Stem cells • Gene therapy
- Clonal tracking • Insertion site analysis • Hematopoietic dynamics

KEY POINTS

- In addition to the integration site preference, vector architecture (SIN vs LTR-driven vectors) and cargo have a major risk-benefit impact.
- The retrovirus- and transposon-based vector toolbox is indispensable for several applications and clinical trials.
- Integrating vectors create an integration site tag, which is used to monitor hematopoietic dynamics in healthy and malignant cells.

Disclosures: Patent holder (A. Schambach); Consultant: Avrobio, Cell Medica (A. Schambach), and GlaxoSmithKline (L. Biasco).
This work was supported by grants from the Deutsche Forschungsgemeinschaft (SFB738 and Cluster of Excellence REBIRTH [EXC 62/1]), the Bundesministerium für Bildung und Forschung (BMBF, IFB-Tx, PidNet), and the European Union (FP7 project CELLPID and SCIDNET). The authors thank M. Morgan for critically reading the article. The work of L. Biasco was supported by the Gene Therapy Program of Dana-Farber/Boston Children's Cancer and Blood Disorders Center, Boston, Massachusetts, and by the UCL Great Ormond Street Institute of Child Health, Faculty of Population Health Sciences, London, UK.
Disclaimer: Because of word limits, only essential references are included.

[a] Gene Therapy Program, Dana-Farber/Boston Children's Cancer and Blood Disorders Center, Harvard Medical School, 1 Jimmy Fund Way, Boston, MA 02115, USA; [b] University College London, UCL Great Ormond Street Institute of Child Health, UCL Faculty of Population Health Sciences, 30 Guilford Street, London WC1N 1EH, UK; [c] Institute of Experimental Hematology, REBIRTH Cluster of Excellence, Hannover Medical School, Carl Neuberg Strasse 1, 30625 Hannover, Germany; [d] Division of Hematology/Oncology, Boston Children's Hospital, Harvard Medical School, 300 Longwood Avenue, Boston, MA 02115, USA
* Corresponding author. Hannover Medical School, I11-01-6070, Carl Neuberg Strasse 1, 30625 Hannover, Germany.
E-mail addresses: schambach.axel@mh-hannover.de; Axel.Schambach@childrens.harvard.edu

Hematol Oncol Clin N Am 31 (2017) 737–752
http://dx.doi.org/10.1016/j.hoc.2017.06.009
0889-8588/17/© 2017 Elsevier Inc. All rights reserved.

hemonc.theclinics.com

INTRODUCTION

After some initial setbacks, gene therapy (GT) has experienced an unquestionable re-naissance over the past decade. The therapeutic efficacy of an increasing number of strategies was demonstrated in clinical trials and some treatments have even recently received market authorization. Generally, the term GT refers to the genetic modification of target cells for therapy for inherited or acquired diseases. Of the various methodologies used for GT (discussed elsewhere in this issue), gene delivery tools are grouped into integrating vectors, such as retrovirus- and transposon-based vectors; and nonintegrating vectors, which do not result in the permanent modification of the genome and often consist of RNA or episomal/extrachromosomal DNA. Approximately 24% of the platforms currently used in GT clinical trials use integrating vectors (http://www.wiley.com/legacy/wileychi/genmed/clinical/), which are the focus of this review. The stable integration into the host cell chromatin offers long-lasting therapeutic possibilities to deliver genes and regulatory RNA and uniquely allows benign and malignant cell behavior to be tracked in healthy or diseased individuals, respectively.

GAMMARETROVIRAL AND LENTIVIRAL VECTORS

Retroviruses have coevolved with their hosts and are thus efficient carriers of genetic information. These viruses have the unique characteristic of reverse transcribing their plus-stranded RNA genome (by the virally encoded enzyme reverse transcriptase) into DNA that is subsequently integrated into the host cell chromatin (catalyzed by the virally encoded integrase).

Although retroviral vectors are derived from wild-type retroviruses, they differ substantially from their natural counterpart in terms of genome content and genetic payload. Indeed, GT vectors are completely, or to the largest degree possible, depleted of original retroviral sequences encoding structural proteins (*gag*), replication enzymes (*pol*), and envelope glycoproteins (*env*). Thus, GT vectors contain only the nucleic acid sequences essential for efficient transfer and expression of the therapeutic information. To improve the biosafety of vector production and to prevent replication-competent retrovirus formation, DNA sequences encoding for *Gag*, *Pol*, and *Env* are provided *in trans* and encoded on separate helper plasmids, a concept that is called split-packaging design.[1,2] Particle production is accomplished with human "packaging cell lines," from which retroviral vector particles (**Fig. 1**A) are harvested after transient or stable transfection of vector and helper plasmids. Modulation of the target cell tropism is possible by modification of the *env* sequences to achieve enforced and/or specific vector entry into the desired cell types or tissues.[3]

Over the past decades, retroviral vectors have been generated from a variety of retroviruses. Exhibiting the highest efficiency, vectors derived from the *Gammaretrovirus* murine leukemia virus (MLV),[4,5] *Lentivirus* human immunodeficiency virus type 1 (HIV1),[2,6,7] Foamy virus[8] and *Alpharetrovirus* avian sarcoma and leukosis virus (ASLV)[9] are most widely used.

The first retrovirus-based gene transfer approaches date back to the 1980s, where gammaretroviral vectors (gRV) were derived from MLV. These experiments provided proof-of-principle for the feasibility of GT in hematopoietic cells. Later work demonstrated that hematopoietic stem and progenitor cells (HSPC) could be genetically modified and could subsequently reconstitute the blood and immune system of transplanted animal models, creating the basis for the translation of GT into clinical trials. Vector improvements included the use of *gag*-free leader regions, intronic sequences, and stronger promoters in the long-terminal repeats (LTRs) to increase transgene expression levels.[10,11] However, gRV are dependent on mitosis for nuclear entry,

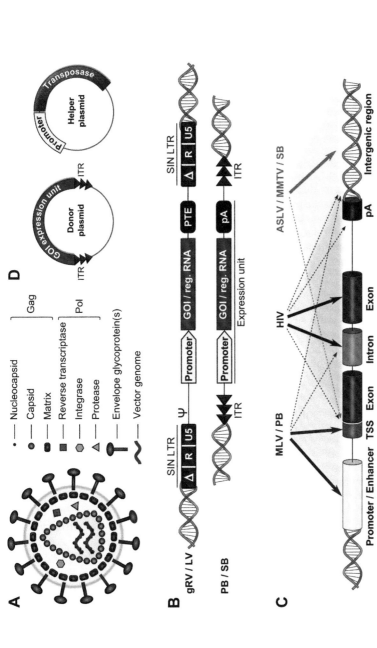

Fig. 1. Integrating vector design and target site preferences. Components for stable genetic modification of target cells through retroviral vectors or transposon-based systems and their integrated configuration and integration site preferences are depicted. (A) HIV1-derived LV particle. (B) Postintegration composition of standard retroviral and transposon vectors. (C) Integration site preferences. (D) ITR-flanked donor plasmid encoding the GOI or regulatory RNA to be integrated into the host cell genome through the activity of transposase transiently expressed from a helper plasmid. Δ, self-inactivating deletion; ψ, viral packaging signal; ASLV, avian sarcoma and leukosis virus; Gag, group-specific antigen; GOI, gene of interest; gRV, gammaretroviral vector; HIV, human immunodeficiency virus; ITR, inverted terminal repeat; LV, lentiviral vector; MLV, murine leukemia virus; MMTV, mouse mammary tumor virus; pA, polyadenylation signal; PB, PiggyBac transposon; Pol, polymerase; PTE, posttranscriptional element; R, repeat region; reg. RNA, regulatory RNA; SB, Sleeping Beauty transposon; SIN LTR, long terminal repeat with self-inactivating design; TSS, transcriptional start site; U5, unique 5' region.

indicating that optimal gene transfer with these vectors can only be achieved in dividing cell populations, such as HSPC and T cells, on in vitro cytokine stimulation.

Because HIV1 exploits an active nuclear import strategy and is thus not reliant on cell cycle status,[12] the lentiviral vectors (LV) derived from HIV1 in 1996 became a logical and promising addition to the retroviral vector toolbox.[2,6,7] Transducing nondividing cell types, including neurons, retina, and liver cells,[13] LV greatly broadened the spectrum of possible target cells. Although the mechanism through which *Lentiviruses* transduce nondividing cells is still not completely understood, the lentiviral capsid and its interaction with nuclear pore components and nuclear import receptors (eg, TNPO3 and RANBP2) are thought to be important.[12,14] In addition, LV contain a so-called self-inactivating (SIN) design (**Fig. 1**B), which refers to the deletion of promoter/enhancer sequences in the U3 region of the LTR (as originally described in an MLV-based vector context).[4] Thus, SIN vectors are devoid of transcriptional activity in the LTRs of integrated vectors and instead use an internal promoter of choice, which allows restriction of transgene expression to desired levels and/or to specific cell types or tissues.

Vector integration is mediated by the retroviral integrase in concert with host cell tethering factors, which results in an insertional preference specific for the individual retroviral vector family members (**Fig. 1**C). For example, gRV (which interact with BET proteins as tethering factors)[15–17] preferentially integrate close to the transcriptional start site and promoter/enhancer regions,[18] whereas LV (which interact with LEDGF) tend to integrate into actively transcribed gene bodies (discussed later).[19] Other retroviral vector types, such as ASLV[9,20] and mouse mammary tumor virus–derived vectors,[21] for which tethering factors have not yet been identified, have a more neutral integration pattern.

In summary, several retrovirus-based vector systems are currently available and the choice of which of these systems is best suited for experimental or clinical use should be made based on the particularities of the intended application. The capacity of these vector systems to efficiently and permanently transduce human primary cells, such as HSPC and T cells, has led to their successful application in several clinical trials.

TRANSPOSON-BASED VECTORS

Transposons represent mobile genetic DNA elements and were first described by McClintock in maize.[22] DNA-transposons are ideally suited for gene transfer and function in a "cut and paste" manner. The uncomplicated natural design of DNA-transposons, which are only composed of a transposase (the enzyme mediating the transposition reaction) and flanking inverted terminal repeats (ITRs), greatly simplified the reconfiguration of these elements into gene transfer vehicles. Analogously to the steps taken to improve the biosafety of retroviral vectors, the transmitted and integrated sequence with the curative transgene information in between the ITRs is delivered on one plasmid, while the transposase is provided *in trans* on a separate helper plasmid (**Fig. 1**D). Mechanistically, the transposase binds to the ITRs, excises the interjacent DNA from the donor plasmid, and reintegrates the excised therapeutic cassette into the host's genome (see **Fig. 1**B).

Because most naturally occurring DNA transposons are not functional, they had to be resurrected from their host genomes and modified to serve as transposon-based vectors for GT purposes. The most widely used systems use the salmon-derived Sleeping Beauty[23] and the insect-derived PiggyBac[24] transposases. Importantly, transposition efficiency of the Sleeping Beauty transposon system was further enhanced by creation of a hyperactive Sleeping Beauty (SB100x) using a systematic molecular evolution approach.[25] Similar strategies were also used to generate hyperactive PiggyBac variants.[26] Noteworthy, Sleeping Beauty transposon–based vectors tend to integrate in an almost random fashion in the host cell genome, whereas PiggyBac-based vectors favor transcriptional start sites and promoter regions (see **Fig. 1**C).[27]

CLINICAL TRIALS WITH INTEGRATING VECTORS AND FURTHER APPLICATIONS

Genetic modification with retrovirus-based and transposon-based vectors has been applied for GT of several inherited and acquired diseases. This article provides an overview of this topic, whereas other articles in this issue cover specific clinical settings and technologies.

HSPC were among the first target cells for GT because their biology is well understood and their genetic modification before hematopoietic stem cell transplantation leads to a constant, long-lived supply of corrected cells of all hematopoietic lineages. In particular, a clear clinical benefit was demonstrated in early trials that used LTR-driven gRV to treat severe combined immunodeficiency (SCID; including the X-linked and the adenosine deaminase [ADA]-deficient SCID forms).[28,29] Unfortunately, severe adverse events (SAE) in the form of leukemia occurred in the Paris[30] and London[31] X-SCID trials, although not in the ADA-SCID trial. Further clinical trials for chronic granulomatous disease[32] and Wiskott-Aldrich syndrome (WAS)[33] also demonstrated a clear benefit of GT, but again SAE were observed[34,35] likely attributable to the LTR-driven architecture and the presence of strong promoter/enhancer sequences (discussed elsewhere in this issue). Subsequent rational modification of vector architecture successfully reduced or even completely eliminated the occurrence of SAE. In a more recent study, a SIN gRV engineered with an internal, cellular EF1a (short) promoter to generate more physiologic expression levels demonstrated clinical efficacy in X-SCID patients without any SAE reported to date.[36] Additional recent clinical trials successfully exploited SIN LV and documented a promising SAE-free clinical track record with clear efficacy and regression or amelioration of disease symptoms in patients affected by leukodystrophies,[37,38] globinopathies,[39] SCID, and WAS.[40]

In addition to treatment of immunodeficiency, successful clinical applications of retroviral vectors include cancer therapy. Here, GT to introduce the chemoresistance gene methylguanine methyltransferase into HSPC mediated induction of tolerance to chemotherapy, which improved the overall outcome in glioblastoma patients.[41] As further attractive targets for genetic modification, autologous T lymphocytes can be easily harvested from the peripheral blood and have become major cellular targets for cancer immunotherapy and prevention of graft-versus-host disease. Genetic retroviral engineering of T cells using chimeric antigen receptors or T-cell receptors (TCR) can induce a potent anticancer response by redirecting these cells to attack cancer cells positive for the selected antigen, as convincingly demonstrated by several clinical trials for CD19[+] leukemias and lymphomas.[42–44]

To control and counteract severe graft-versus-host disease in allogeneic bone marrow transplantation, donor lymphocytes were genetically modified by a retroviral vector expressing the drug-inducible suicide gene herpes simplex virus thymidine kinase.[45,46] For a similar purpose, an inducible caspase 9 suicide switch was retrovirally introduced into donor T cells of patients undergoing haploidentical hematopoietic stem cell transplantation.[47]

Besides in vivo GT, integrating vector technologies have found widespread application in diverse in vitro settings, including (1) reprogramming of somatic cells into induced pluripotent stem cells to create new sources for disease modeling and drug testing[48–50]; (2) transdifferentiation of one cell type into a different, therapeutic cell type[51,52]; and (3) delivery of designer nucleases, such as TALENS and CRISPR-Cas9.[53]

INSERTIONAL MUTAGENESIS AS A DOUBLE-EDGED SWORD: AN IMPORTANT TOOL TO UNDERSTAND GENE FUNCTION AND NETWORKS BUT A GREAT CHALLENGE FOR GENE THERAPY

Integrating vectors are natural insertional mutagens because the genetic payload is placed semirandomly into the host cell genome (see **Fig.** 1C). Gene transfer may therefore either lead to a neutral genetic tag in the chromatin or pose a potential risk by altering the cell's natural genetic program. Specifically, integrating vectors can disrupt tumor suppressor genes, create aberrant isoforms caused by splicing or premature termination of transcripts, and activate neighboring proto-oncogenes.[54] Although the risk of insertional transformation has thus always been a threat for GT applications, it is effectively used as a tool to identify cancer- or stem cell–associated genes and signaling networks,[55,56] which can provide a basis for the discovery of new drug targets. High-throughput integration site analysis and bioinformatics can determine/annotate sites enriched for insertions in tumors and identify cancer-initiating and driver genes (Retroviral Tagged Cancer Gene Database).[57] This knowledge is not only helpful to better understand cancer biology but is also useful as a reference for the longitudinal monitoring of clinical GT trials. Because the natural capacity of retrovirus- and transposon-based elements to dysregulate gene expression profiles of genetically modified cells poses a risk to treated patients, insertion site distribution must be directly monitored in clinical GT trials. This is an especially critical point in the case that potent promoter/enhancer sequences in the LTRs or at internal positions are used to drive transgene expression.

SAFETY OF GENE THERAPY AND INTEGRATION SITE ANALYSIS

The first SAE associated with the use of integrating vectors were reported during the clinical trials for X-linked SCID, where acute T-cell leukemia cases were reported a few years after retroviral-based GT into bone marrow CD34$^+$ HSPC.[30,31,58] These trials used an MLV-derived gRV carrying the common γ-subunit of interleukin-2 receptor under the control of the LTR. The leukemic clones isolated from the individuals who experienced these SAE revealed the presence of common insertion sites (CIS) in proximity of *SPAG6*, *CCND2*, and *LMO2* genes, with a significant *LMO2* overexpression in the transformed cells. The *LMO2* gene is normally expressed in HSPC and early T-cell precursors, whereas it is usually down-regulated on differentiation and its locus is involved in a chromosomal translocation in acute T-cell leukemia.[59] This led to the hypothesis that the leukemic transformation in these patients was triggered via activation of this proto-oncogene by the vector's enhancer sequences present in the LTR.[31] Almost concomitantly, another insertional mutagenesis effect of gRV, which also led to aberrant clonal proliferation, was reported in a GT trial for chronic granulomatous disease.[32,34] This clinical protocol was based on the ex vivo retroviral gene transfer of gp91phox cDNA into mobilized peripheral blood CD34$^+$ cells. The high levels of genetic correction achieved were, unfortunately, related to an unexpected in vivo expansion of vector-positive myeloid cells that exhibited clusters of vector integrations (CIS) in the *MDS-EVI1*, *PRDM16,* and *SETBP1* loci. Soon thereafter, the three treated patients developed a vector-bearing myelodysplastic syndrome with monosomy 7 and one of the patients died of overwhelming sepsis 27 months after GT.[34] It was proposed that the strong enhancer activity of the retroviral spleen focus-forming virus LTR used in the vector construct may have induced the overexpression of the *Evi1* gene to oncogenic levels. On the basis of these unexpected outcomes, safety assessment through integration site (IS) analysis became essential for GT under the assumption that the detection of IS in proximity of proto-oncogenes and of CIS would constitute unfavorable prognostic factors for treated individuals.[60] This view of the role of insertional mutagenesis in generating SAE was further supported by the outcome of a more recent GT trial for WAS, which used an LTR-driven gRV.[33] This clinical trial experienced a high rate of vector-related SAE, with development of *LMO2*- and *MDS-EVI1*-related acute lymphoblastic and myeloid leukemias in 7 out of 10 treated patients.[35]

Despite these observations, some controversial findings arose from other studies that challenged the original view on the predictive value of IS profiling. The strikingly different results observed in a gRV-based GT trial for ADA-SCID raised some doubts on the original interpretation of IS clinical data. Indeed, despite carrying an insertional profile similar to the other LTR-driven gRV trials,[61] ADA-SCID-treated patients did not show any long-term clonal unbalance or vector-related leukemia,[29] and the documented safety of this therapy contributed to its approval for marketing authorization by GlaxoSmithKline as the first commercial ex vivo GT product. Furthermore, original results showed that clusters of integrations in *LMO2* and *MDS-EVI1* were detectable even in event-free GT-treated patients,[62,63] and that these CIS were found already in the infused cell product without any in vivo selection.[64] This suggests that insertional mutagenesis by LTR-driven vectors cannot operate alone for the progression to tumorigenesis in vivo and requires the support of other contributing factors that could be related to the use of a growth-promoting transgene and/or the pre-existence of a tumor-prone disease background. We recently reviewed these aspects and the potential role of cofactors on cellular transformation associated to insertional mutagenesis.[65]

The introduction of gRV or LV with SIN configuration has substantially improved the safety of GT.[66] Several clinical trials based on the use of SIN LV have been conducted over the past decade with no reports of any SAE related to insertional mutagenesis as of today.[37,38,65,67] A recent side-by-side comparison of WAS GT using LTR-driven gRV versus SIN LV gene transfer has unequivocally shown the superior safety profile of the latter vector platform.[40] Despite the detection of LV insertions into the *LMO2* and *MDS-EVI1* loci, the SIN configuration of this platform combined with the different insertional distribution of LV (discussed next) likely contributed to the absence of transformation events driven by insertional mutagenesis. Despite the clear safety improvement of the SIN LV technology, aberrant splicing events led to a growth advantage and benign clonal imbalance in one of the thalassemia GT trials.[39] Hence, the mechanisms of insertional mutagenesis other than enhancer-mediated upregulation of proto-oncogenes should be further investigated in the future.

INSERTIONAL PROPERTIES OF RETROVIRAL VECTORS

The need for safety assessment of GT has encouraged the study of vector-host interactions and the production of an increasing amount of information that widened the view of the molecular biology of viral integration. Crucial findings date back to the early studies on viral insertions, which showed that different viruses have different IS distribution throughout the genome. It was originally described that MLV-derived vectors have a strong tendency to integrate in proximity of the transcription start sites and promoter/regulatory regions (CpG islands) of active genes,[18] whereas HIV1-derived and related vectors display a preference to insert inside coding regions and in gene introns (see **Fig. 1**C).[68] It was later proposed that these biases could be the results of the complex interaction between the LTR-flanked retroviral proviruses and the cellular machinery. It was suggested that gRV are tethered to promoter/enhancer regions via binding with transcription factors[69] and more recently the BET protein family as tethering factors,[15–17] because the HIV-LEDGF/p75 interaction explained the insertional preferences of HIV for transcriptional units.[70]

Adding a new perspective to these studies, Marini and colleagues[71] showed that HIV integration was more likely to occur in regions contained in the outer shell of the nucleus proximal to the routes of entry of HIV proviruses through the nuclear pores. Another level of complexity of retroviral IS selection was related to the cell-specific genomic accessibility of the target cell population. In this regard, we were able to show that gRV integrations were distributed in a different fashion along the genome depending on the cell types hosting the insertional events.[72] This would argue for cell- and tissue-specific risk factors and different risk-benefit assessments for different cell types. While uncovering the genetic and chromatin determinants that led to these preferences, we discovered that *LMO2* and *MDS-EVI1* were specifically targeted by viral IS only in HSPC but not in T cells. Supporting these observations and contrary to the safety outcome of HSPC GT, leukemias or clonal proliferations caused by insertional mutagenesis were not reported in primary cells, animal models,[73] or any of the numerous clinical GT trials based on LTR-driven gRV-mediated T-cell engineering.[74] These findings highlighted that cell-intrinsic features were among the contributing factors impacting the interaction of retroviral vectors with the host genome and in turn potentially affecting the safety of GT. Among the new vector platforms under preclinical tests, *Alpharetrovirus*-based vectors are considered to have a more random insertional profile as compared with gRV or LV (see **Fig. 1**C). Therefore, *Alpharetrovirus*-based vectors have an inherently lower genotoxicity potential,[9,20,75] although the molecular mechanisms driving the insertional preferences and the possible cell-specific influences on *Alpharetrovirus*-based vector accessibility to the host genome have not yet been thoroughly investigated.

METHODS AND EVOLUTION OF INSERTION SITES RETRIEVAL

The advent of high throughput sequencing has greatly enhanced the resolution of IS profiling (**Fig. 2**). The original protocols for IS retrieval were based on the fragmentation of the genome with restriction enzymes followed by inverse polymerase chain reaction (PCR) or linker-mediated PCR, shotgun cloning of the vector-genome amplicons into competent bacteria, and Sanger sequencing of the positive colonies.[61,63,64] Although efficient for detecting major unbalances, this system was expensive and time consuming, which limited the depth of the analysis to only a few hundred IS per patient.

The introduction of a more efficient method for vector-genome junction enrichment, called linear amplification-mediated (LAM) PCR,[76] and its combination with 454 Roche pyrosequencing[77] initially and with Illumina sequencing[38,40] later greatly enhanced the detection of IS, which now reaches several thousand IS per patient, while substantially reducing the costs associated to the analysis. Briefly, the general steps of LAM-PCR are the following: after genomic extraction, two rounds of linear preamplification steps with biotinylated primers are performed to enrich for sequences containing vector LTR. These long genomic segments are then bound to streptavidin beads, magnetically captured, and cleaved by either restriction enzymes or sonication. Ligation of a linker cassette generates DNA fragments with two known sequences at 5′ and 3′ termini flanking an unknown genomic sequence that corresponds to the site where the provirus integrated. The resulting products then undergo two rounds of nested exponential PCR followed by sample tagging with a barcoded adaptor, library preparation, and sequencing. Despite becoming rapidly the gold standard for IS analyses,

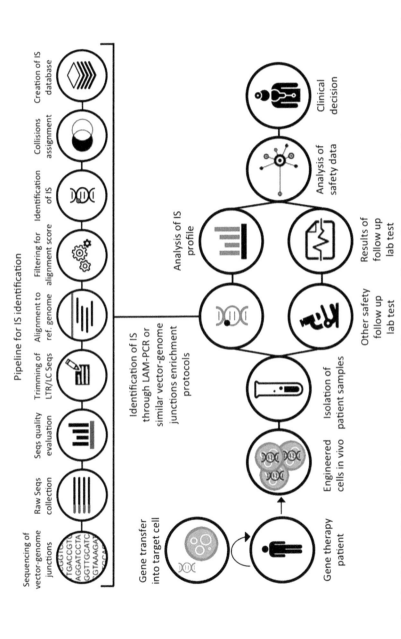

Fig. 2. Flow chart for the identification of IS for safety and clonal tracking studies of human hematopoietic cells in gene therapy–treated patients. LAM, linear amplification-mediated; IS, integration site; LC, linker cassette; PCR, polymerase chain reaction; Seqs, sequences. (*Adapted from* Scala S, Leonardelli L, Biasco L. Current approaches and future perspectives for in vivo clonal tracking of hematopoietic cells. Curr Gene Ther 2016;16(3):189; with permission.)

the current LAM-PCR/Illumina sequencing workflow is not easy to adopt because it requires customized bioinformatics tools to handle sequencing results, to annotate IS on the genome of reference, and to perform proper statistical analysis of the data.[78] The common steps of the current informatics pipelines are (1) raw data quality filtering, LTR and linker cassette trimming, and sample demultiplexing by barcodes; (2) mapping filtered reads to the host reference genome and selecting those characterized by specific features; (3) identifying and annotating the IS, recording them by chromosomal position, strand, name of the closest gene, and amount of reads; and (4) removing/reassigning IS associated to potential cross-contaminations among independent samples.

Most of the pipelines generally return a matrix of incidence containing the list of IS combined with the source, sample, and time points where they were found and with their relative sequence count, shear sites, or other measures of clonal abundance. These raw data serve then as input for higher-level analyses, such as IS distribution, association to genomic features (eg, genes, microRNAs, promoter sequences), clustering discovery, and estimation of clonal diversity.

USE OF INSERTIONAL TAGGING FOR CLONAL TRACKING STUDIES

The ever increasing resolution of IS analyses in the past years allowed the transfer of the method from addressing the safety of GT to a series of new approaches. Given the concept that on genetic engineering with integrating vector each transduced cell becomes unequivocally and permanently marked by a viral IS, which will also be inherited by the progeny of the same cell, the insertion loci can be used as molecular barcodes to track the fate of infused individual cells.[79] In addition, the sequence read counts belonging to each IS could be used as surrogate markers of clonal abundance to allow estimation of diversity and population size of engineered cells.[78] In this regard, new systems based on random genome shearing site counts or on the introduction of random barcodes before PCR amplification steps have been introduced by others and us to further improve the reliability of clonal quantification.[80,81] In contrast to other platforms that involve the use of reporter genes or barcoded vector libraries, IS analysis can be applied for clonal tracking studies not only on animal models but also on GT patients, thus providing a unique source of information on the dynamics of engineered clones directly in vivo in humans. High throughput TCR profiling constitutes an alternative method for performing clonal tracking studies of T cells in humans.[82] However, this approach is based on the concept that TCR specificity is stable in peripheral blood–derived mature lymphocytes, whereas, as recently pointed out, on superantigen exposure a process known as "TCR revisions" might occur in the periphery even after thymic maturation.[83] In this regard, vector insertions constitute more stable and diverse inheritable markers for the tracking of T-cell clones in GT-treated patients. Confirming the potential of this tool, we successfully applied IS-based clonal tracking on blood samples from ADA-SCID patients treated with peripheral blood gRV GT providing the first formal proof that recently described T memory stem cells[84] actively contribute to the long-term graft of infused lymphocytes in humans and constitute a reservoir for the in vivo generation of memory T cells.[85] We recently extended this type of approach on a broader scale to study the whole hematopoietic system in WAS patients treated with HSPC LV GT.[86] Our results were consistent with what has been predicted with similar and alternative tracking approaches in murine models and nonhuman primates,[87] further underlining the potential of IS analyses to provide valuable insights on human healthy physiology and pathophysiology.

SUMMARY

This article provides an overview on composition, generation, and application of retrovirus- and transposon-based vectors, and an introduction into past and ongoing clinical GT trials. Although especially the more recent clinical studies using improved SIN architectures and a more "physiologic" internal promoter gave promising results and had a clearly documented safety track record, there is still room for improvement on various aspects of GT with integrating vectors in the clinical arena.

Recent progress into the tracking of IS and identification of CIS that overlap with cancer signatures enabled a better prediction of "dangerous" IS. However, not every integration into a CIS is harmful and leads to a dysregulation on the RNA or protein level. Here, there is a need to develop better and more robust assays, coupling IS analysis to expression differences. Other forms of genotoxicity should be analyzed, including aberrant splicing[75,88] and effect on the epigenetic level,[89] to develop vectors avoiding these problems.

Exploitation of transcriptional, posttranscriptional, and translational control principles and elements from synthetic biology has allowed better control of phenotoxicity, that is, a toxic gene product, by proper regulation of transgene expression. Furthermore, one should consider that genotoxicity heavily depends on the target cell type of GT, so that T cells and mature hepatocytes may have a lower risk profile.[73,90]

If only a short duration of transgene expression is needed, then retrovirus-derived nonintegrating vector systems may be a possible alternative. Via defined interventions of the retroviral life cycle retroviral "vectors" can be engineered for delivery of proteins, mRNA, and episomal DNA. Because especially the cell modification strategies without DNA do not harbor the risk of integration, their likelihood to contribute to malignant transformation of transduced cells is greatly reduced.[91] However, this would only lead to a transient correction. In addition to generating safer vectors for "semirandom" integration, strategies using designer nucleases and homology-directed repair of mutated sequences, or alternatively the incorporation of curative transgenes into "safe harbor" genomic sites,[92] are promising but need further work to establish better efficacy, analysis of risk factors, and proper vectorization.

Given the general improvements in the risk-benefit assessment of integrating vectors, also broader applications addressing other cell types are within reach. In addition to T cells, other lymphoid cell types may be of interest for cancer therapy, including natural killer cells and natural killer T cells.[93] To provide a better efficacy of immunotherapeutics against solid tumors, combined strategies of chimeric antigen receptors/TCRs and local cytokine administration in so-called TRUCKs may be a way to better attack tumors and their microenvironment.[94] In addition, proper targeting strategies using defined envelope strategies may guide retroviral vectors to cell populations and sites of the body where the GT treatment is needed most.[3]

Taken together, integrating vectors represent promising vector systems for GT and, with the growing safety documentation, will enable more broadly applicable strategies in the near future.

REFERENCES

1. Miller AD, Buttimore C. Redesign of retrovirus packaging cell lines to avoid recombination leading to helper virus production. Mol Cell Biol 1986;6(8):2895–902.
2. Naldini L, Blomer U, Gallay P, et al. In vivo gene delivery and stable transduction of nondividing cells by a lentiviral vector. Science 1996;272(5259):263–7.
3. Buchholz CJ, Friedel T, Buning H. Surface-engineered viral vectors for selective and cell type-specific gene delivery. Trends Biotechnol 2015;33(12):777–90.

4. Yu SF, von Ruden T, Kantoff PW, et al. Self-inactivating retroviral vectors designed for transfer of whole genes into mammalian cells. Proc Natl Acad Sci U S A 1986; 83:3194–8.

5. Schambach A, Mueller D, Galla M, et al. Overcoming promoter competition in packaging cells improves production of self-inactivating retroviral vectors. Gene Ther 2006;13(21):1524–33.

6. Naldini L, Blomer U, Gage FH, et al. Efficient transfer, integration, and sustained long-term expression of the transgene in adult rat brains injected with a lentiviral vector. Proc Natl Acad Sci U S A 1996;93(21):11382–8.

7. Dull T, Zufferey R, Kelly M, et al. A third-generation lentivirus vector with a conditional packaging system. J Virol 1998;72(11):8463–71.

8. Trobridge G, Vassilopoulos G, Josephson N, et al. Gene transfer with foamy virus vectors. Methods Enzymol 2002;346:628–48.

9. Suerth JD, Maetzig T, Brugman MH, et al. Alpharetroviral self-inactivating vectors: long-term transgene expression in murine hematopoietic cells and low genotoxicity. Mol Ther 2012;20(5):1022–32.

10. Baum C, Eckert HG, Stockschlader M, et al. Improved retroviral vectors for hematopoietic stem cell protection and in vivo selection. J Hematother 1996;5(4): 323–9.

11. Baum C, Hegewisch-Becker S, Eckert HG, et al. Novel retroviral vectors for efficient expression of the multidrug-resistance (mdr-1) gene in early hemopoietic cells. J Virol 1995;69:7541–7.

12. Suzuki Y, Craigie R. The road to chromatin - nuclear entry of retroviruses. Nat Rev Microbiol 2007;5(3):187–96.

13. Naldini L. Lentiviruses as gene transfer agents for delivery to non-dividing cells. Curr Opin Biotechnol 1998;9(5):457–63.

14. Bin Hamid F, Kim J, Shin CG. Cellular and viral determinants of retroviral nuclear entry. Can J Microbiol 2016;62(1):1–15.

15. Sharma A, Larue RC, Plumb MR, et al. BET proteins promote efficient murine leukemia virus integration at transcription start sites. Proc Natl Acad Sci U S A 2013; 110(29):12036–41.

16. De Rijck J, de Kogel C, Demeulemeester J, et al. The BET family of proteins targets moloney murine leukemia virus integration near transcription start sites. Cell Rep 2013;5(4):886–94.

17. Gupta SS, Maetzig T, Maertens GN, et al. Bromo- and extraterminal domain chromatin regulators serve as cofactors for murine leukemia virus integration. J Virol 2013;87(23):12721–36.

18. Wu X, Li Y, Crise B, et al. Transcription start regions in the human genome are favored targets for MLV integration. Science 2003;300(5626):1749–51.

19. Schroder AR, Shinn P, Chen H, et al. HIV-1 integration in the human genome favors active genes and local hotspots. Cell 2002;110(4):521–9.

20. Moiani A, Suerth JD, Gandolfi F, et al. Genome-wide analysis of alpharetroviral integration in human hematopoietic stem/progenitor cells. Genes (Basel) 2014; 5(2):415–29.

21. Konstantoulas CJ, Indik S. Mouse mammary tumor virus-based vector transduces non-dividing cells, enters the nucleus via a TNPO3-independent pathway and integrates in a less biased fashion than other retroviruses. Retrovirology 2014;11:34.

22. McClintock B. The origin and behavior of mutable loci in maize. Proc Natl Acad Sci U S A 1950;36(6):344–55.

23. Ivics Z, Hackett PB, Plasterk RH, et al. Molecular reconstruction of Sleeping Beauty, a Tc1-like transposon from fish, and its transposition in human cells. Cell 1997;91(4):501–10.

24. Fraser MJ, Brusca JS, Smith GE, et al. Transposon-mediated mutagenesis of a baculovirus. Virology 1985;145(2):356–61.

25. Mates L, Chuah MK, Belay E, et al. Molecular evolution of a novel hyperactive sleeping beauty transposase enables robust stable gene transfer in vertebrates. Nat Genet 2009;41(6):753–61.

26. Yusa K, Zhou L, Li MA, et al. A hyperactive piggyBac transposase for mammalian applications. Proc Natl Acad Sci U S A 2011;108(4):1531–6.

27. Huang X, Guo H, Tammana S, et al. Gene transfer efficiency and genome-wide integration profiling of sleeping beauty, Tol2, and piggyBac transposons in human primary T cells. Mol Ther 2010;18(10):1803–13.

28. Hacein-Bey-Abina S, Le Deist F, Carlier F, et al. Sustained correction of X-linked severe combined immunodeficiency by ex vivo gene therapy. N Engl J Med 2002;346(16):1185–93.

29. Aiuti A, Cattaneo F, Galimberti S, et al. Gene therapy for immunodeficiency due to adenosine deaminase deficiency. N Engl J Med 2009;360(5):447–58.

30. Hacein-Bey-Abina S, Garrigue A, Wang GP, et al. Insertional oncogenesis in 4 patients after retrovirus-mediated gene therapy of SCID-X1. J Clin Invest 2008; 118(9):3132–42.

31. Howe SJ, Mansour MR, Schwarzwaelder K, et al. Insertional mutagenesis combined with acquired somatic mutations causes leukemogenesis following gene therapy of SCID-X1 patients. J Clin Invest 2008;118(9):3143–50.

32. Ott MG, Schmidt M, Schwarzwaelder K, et al. Correction of X-linked chronic granulomatous disease by gene therapy, augmented by insertional activation of MDS1-EVI1, PRDM16 or SETBP1. Nat Med 2006;12(4):401–9.

33. Boztug K, Schmidt M, Schwarzer A, et al. Stem-cell gene therapy for the Wiskott-Aldrich syndrome. N Engl J Med 2010;363(20):1918–27.

34. Stein S, Ott MG, Schultze-Strasser S, et al. Genomic instability and myelodysplasia with monosomy 7 consequent to EVI1 activation after gene therapy for chronic granulomatous disease. Nat Med 2010;16(2):198–204.

35. Braun CJ, Boztug K, Paruzynski A, et al. Gene therapy for Wiskott-Aldrich syndrome–long-term efficacy and genotoxicity. Sci Transl Med 2014;6(227): 227ra233.

36. Hacein-Bey-Abina S, Pai SY, Gaspar HB, et al. A modified gamma-retrovirus vector for X-linked severe combined immunodeficiency. N Engl J Med 2014;371(15): 1407–17.

37. Cartier N, Hacein-Bey-Abina S, Bartholomae CC, et al. Hematopoietic stem cell gene therapy with a lentiviral vector in X-linked adrenoleukodystrophy. Science 2009;326(5954):818–23.

38. Biffi A, Montini E, Lorioli L, et al. Lentiviral hematopoietic stem cell gene therapy benefits metachromatic leukodystrophy. Science 2013;341(6148):1233158.

39. Cavazzana-Calvo M, Payen E, Negre O, et al. Transfusion independence and HMGA2 activation after gene therapy of human beta-thalassaemia. Nature 2010;467(7313):318–22.

40. Aiuti A, Biasco L, Scaramuzza S, et al. Lentiviral hematopoietic stem cell gene therapy in patients with Wiskott-Aldrich syndrome. Science 2013;341(6148): 1233151.

41. Adair JE, Johnston SK, Mrugala MM, et al. Gene therapy enhances chemotherapy tolerance and efficacy in glioblastoma patients. J Clin Invest 2014; 124(9):4082–92.

42. Kochenderfer JN, Dudley ME, Kassim SH, et al. Chemotherapy-refractory diffuse large B-cell lymphoma and indolent B-cell malignancies can be effectively treated with autologous T cells expressing an anti-CD19 chimeric antigen receptor. J Clin Oncol 2015;33(6):540–9.

43. Maude SL, Frey N, Shaw PA, et al. Chimeric antigen receptor T cells for sustained remissions in leukemia. N Engl J Med 2014;371(16):1507–17.

44. Brentjens RJ, Davila ML, Riviere I, et al. CD19-targeted T cells rapidly induce molecular remissions in adults with chemotherapy-refractory acute lymphoblastic leukemia. Sci Transl Med 2013;5(177):177ra138.

45. Bonini C, Ferrari G, Verzeletti S, et al. HSV-TK gene transfer into donor lymphocytes for control of allogeneic graft-versus-leukemia. Science 1997;276(5319): 1719–24.

46. Bordignon C, Bonini C, Verzeletti S, et al. Transfer of the HSV-tk gene into donor peripheral blood lymphocytes for in vivo modulation of donor anti-tumor immunity after allogeneic bone marrow transplantation. Hum Gene Ther 1995;6(6):813–9.

47. Di Stasi A, Tey SK, Dotti G, et al. Inducible apoptosis as a safety switch for adoptive cell therapy. N Engl J Med 2011;365(18):1673–83.

48. Sommer CA, Stadtfeld M, Murphy GJ, et al. Induced pluripotent stem Cell generation using a single lentiviral stem cell cassette. Stem Cells 2009;27(3):543–9.

49. Warlich E, Kuehle J, Cantz T, et al. Lentiviral vector design and imaging approaches to visualize the early stages of cellular reprogramming. Mol Ther 2011;19(4):782–9.

50. Di Matteo M, Belay E, Chuah MK, et al. Recent developments in transposon-mediated gene therapy. Expert Opin Biol Ther 2012;12(7):841–58.

51. Song G, Pacher M, Balakrishnan A, et al. Direct reprogramming of hepatic myofibroblasts into hepatocytes in vivo attenuates liver fibrosis. Cell Stem Cell 2016; 18(6):797–808.

52. Vo LT, Daley GQ. De novo generation of HSCs from somatic and pluripotent stem cell sources. Blood 2015;125(17):2641–8.

53. Kim H, Kim JS. A guide to genome engineering with programmable nucleases. Nat Rev Genet 2014;15(5):321–34.

54. Uren AG, Kool J, Berns A, et al. Retroviral insertional mutagenesis: past, present and future. Oncogene 2005;24(52):7656–72.

55. Kool J, Berns A. High-throughput insertional mutagenesis screens in mice to identify oncogenic networks. Nat Rev Cancer 2009;9(6):389–99.

56. Copeland NG, Jenkins NA. Harnessing transposons for cancer gene discovery. Nat Rev Cancer 2010;10(10):696–706.

57. Akagi K, Suzuki T, Stephens RM, et al. RTCGD: retroviral tagged cancer gene database. Nucleic Acids Res 2004;32:D523–7.

58. Hacein-Bey-Abina S, Von Kalle C, Schmidt M, et al. LMO2-associated clonal T cell proliferation in two patients after gene therapy for SCID-X1. Science 2003;302(5644):415–9.

59. Chambers J, Rabbitts TH. LMO2 at 25 years: a paradigm of chromosomal translocation proteins. Open Biol 2015;5(6):150062.

60. Biasco L, Baricordi C, Aiuti A. Retroviral integrations in gene therapy trials. Mol Ther 2012;20(4):709–16.

61. Aiuti A, Cassani B, Andolfi G, et al. Multilineage hematopoietic reconstitution without clonal selection in ADA-SCID patients treated with stem cell gene therapy. J Clin Invest 2007;117(8):2233–40.
62. Schwarzwaelder K, Howe SJ, Schmidt M, et al. Gammaretrovirus-mediated correction of SCID-X1 is associated with skewed vector integration site distribution in vivo. J Clin Invest 2007;117(8):2241–9.
63. Deichmann A, Hacein-Bey-Abina S, Schmidt M, et al. Vector integration is nonrandom and clustered and influences the fate of lymphopoiesis in SCID-X1 gene therapy. J Clin Invest 2007;117(8):2225–32.
64. Cattoglio C, Facchini G, Sartori D, et al. Hot spots of retroviral integration in human CD34+ hematopoietic cells. Blood 2007;110(6):1770–8.
65. Rothe M, Schambach A, Biasco L. Safety of gene therapy: new insights to a puzzling case. Curr Gene Ther 2014;14(6):429–36.
66. Montini E, Cesana D, Schmidt M, et al. Hematopoietic stem cell gene transfer in a tumor-prone mouse model uncovers low genotoxicity of lentiviral vector integration. Nat Biotechnol 2006;24(6):687–96.
67. Naldini L. Gene therapy returns to centre stage. Nature 2015;526(7573):351–60.
68. Mitchell RS, Beitzel BF, Schroder AR, et al. Retroviral DNA integration: ASLV, HIV, and MLV show distinct target site preferences. PLoS Biol 2004;2(8):E234.
69. Felice B, Cattoglio C, Cittaro D, et al. Transcription factor binding sites are genetic determinants of retroviral integration in the human genome. PLoS One 2009;4(2): e4571.
70. Maertens G, Cherepanov P, Pluymers W, et al. LEDGF/p75 is essential for nuclear and chromosomal targeting of HIV-1 integrase in human cells. J Biol Chem 2003; 278(35):33528–39.
71. Marini B, Kertesz-Farkas A, Ali H, et al. Nuclear architecture dictates HIV-1 integration site selection. Nature 2015;521(7551):227–31.
72. Biasco L, Ambrosi A, Pellin D, et al. Integration profile of retroviral vector in gene therapy treated patients is cell-specific according to gene expression and chromatin conformation of target cell. EMBO Mol Med 2011;3(2):89–101.
73. Newrzela S, Cornils K, Li Z, et al. Resistance of mature T cells to oncogene transformation. Blood 2008;112(6):2278–86.
74. Gill S, June CH. Going viral: chimeric antigen receptor T-cell therapy for hematological malignancies. Immunol Rev 2015;263(1):68–89.
75. Kaufmann KB, Buning H, Galy A, et al. Gene therapy on the move. EMBO Mol Med 2013;5(11):1642–61.
76. Schmidt M, Hoffmann G, Wissler M, et al. Detection and direct genomic sequencing of multiple rare unknown flanking DNA in highly complex samples. Hum Gene Ther 2001;12(7):743–9.
77. Brugman MH, Suerth JD, Rothe M, et al. Evaluating a ligation-mediated PCR and pyrosequencing method for the detection of clonal contribution in polyclonal retrovirally transduced samples. Hum Gene Ther Methods 2013;24(2):68–79.
78. Scala S, Leonardelli L, Biasco L. Current approaches and future perspectives for in vivo clonal tracking of hematopoietic cells. Curr Gene Ther 2016;16(3):184–93.
79. Wang GP, Berry CC, Malani N, et al. Dynamics of gene-modified progenitor cells analyzed by tracking retroviral integration sites in a human SCID-X1 gene therapy trial. Blood 2010;115(22):4356–66.
80. Berry CC, Gillet NA, Melamed A, et al. Estimating abundances of retroviral insertion sites from DNA fragment length data. Bioinformatics 2012;28(6):755–62.

81. Leonardelli L, Pellin D, Scala S, et al. Computational pipeline for the identification of integration sites and novel method for the quantification of clone sizes in clonal tracking studies. Mol Ther 2016;24(Suppl 1):S212–3.

82. Robins HS, Campregher PV, Srivastava SK, et al. Comprehensive assessment of T-cell receptor beta-chain diversity in alphabeta T cells. Blood 2009;114(19): 4099–107.

83. Wagner DH Jr. Re-shaping the T cell repertoire: TCR editing and TCR revision for good and for bad. Clin Immunol 2007;123(1):1–6.

84. Gattinoni L, Lugli E, Ji Y, et al. A human memory T cell subset with stem cell-like properties. Nat Med 2011;17(10):1290–7.

85. Biasco L, Scala S, Basso Ricci L, et al. In vivo tracking of T cells in humans unveils decade-long survival and activity of genetically modified T memory stem cells. Sci Transl Med 2015;7(273):273ra213.

86. Biasco L, Pellin D, Scala S, et al. In vivo tracking of human hematopoiesis reveals patterns of clonal dynamics during early and steady-state reconstitution phases. Cell Stem Cell 2016;19(1):107–19.

87. Gerrits A, Dykstra B, Kalmykowa OJ, et al. Cellular barcoding tool for clonal analysis in the hematopoietic system. Blood 2010;115(13):2610–8.

88. Cesana D, Sgualdino J, Rudilosso L, et al. Whole transcriptome characterization of aberrant splicing events induced by lentiviral vector integrations. J Clin Invest 2012;122(5):1667–76.

89. Aranyi T, Stockholm D, Yao R, et al. Systemic epigenetic response to recombinant lentiviral vectors independent of proviral integration. Epigenetics Chromatin 2016;9:29.

90. Rittelmeyer I, Rothe M, Brugman MH, et al. Hepatic lentiviral gene transfer is associated with clonal selection, but not with tumor formation in serially transplanted rodents. Hepatology 2013;58(1):397–408.

91. Schott JW, Galla M, Godinho T, et al. Viral and non-viral approaches for transient delivery of mRNA and proteins. Curr Gene Ther 2011;11(5):382–98.

92. Papapetrou EP, Schambach A. Gene insertion into genomic safe harbors for human gene therapy. Mol Ther 2016;24(4):678–84.

93. Vivier E, Ugolini S, Blaise D, et al. Targeting natural killer cells and natural killer T cells in cancer. Nat Rev Immunol 2012;12(4):239–52.

94. Chmielewski M, Abken H. TRUCKs: the fourth generation of CARs. Expert Opin Biol Ther 2015;15(8):1145–54.

Nonintegrating Gene Therapy Vectors

Takis Athanasopoulos, PhD[a], Mustafa M. Munye, PhD[a],
Rafael J. Yáñez-Muñoz, PhD[b],*

KEYWORDS

- Nonintegrating • Gene therapy • Adenovirus vectors
- Adeno-associated virus vectors • Poxvirus vector
- Integration-deficient lentiviral vectors (IDLVs) • Plasmid • Genome editing

KEY POINTS

- Host cell genome integration of first-generation gene therapy vectors may result in various effects on cellular genes (knockout, overexpression, altered splicing), variegated levels of transgene expression, or transcriptional silencing, as well as clonal expansion and oncogenic transformation.
- Nonintegrating gene therapy vectors can be viral and nonviral. Viral vectors can be nonintegrating like their parental organisms (adenovirus, herpesvirus, poxvirus, Sendai) or engineered to minimize integration (adeno-associated virus, retro-lentivirus).
- Nonintegrating vectors can provide stable transgene expression in quiescent cells and transient or stable expression in proliferating cells.
- Variants of nonintegrating vectors carrying suitable payloads (transposons, site-specific recombination cassettes, genome editing cassettes) are suitable platforms for genetic modification of the cellular genome by transposition, site-directed integration, and genome editing.
- Successful clinical trials have already been reported using adenoviral vectors (genome editing of *CCR5* for AIDS), herpesvirus vectors (cancer), and adeno-associated virus vectors (hemophilia).

The authors declare no commercial or financial conflict of interest.
Funding Sources: R.J. Yáñez-Muñoz is the Editor-in-Chief of *Gene Therapy*. Research in the Yáñez-Muñoz laboratory has been funded by Association Française contre les Myopathies (14781) Genoma España, the European Union, the Primary Immunodeficiency Association (2002/13), the Friends of Guy's Hospital (393), the Medical Research Council (G0301182), the SouthWest London Academic Network, Action Medical Research (SP4394), Clinigene (LSBH-CT-2006-018933/Flexibility Funding 200805f and LSBH-CT-2006-018933/Flexibility Funding 200805m), Spinal Research (TR1004_04), The SMA Trust (HMR01140), and Royal Holloway, University of London. T. Athanasopoulos and M. M. Munye are GSK employees. GSK's publication practices are intended to uphold GSK's commitment to the values of patient focus, transparency, and integrity.
Disclaimer: Due to word limits, only essential references are included.
[a] Cell and Gene Therapy Discovery Research, Platform Technology and Sciences, GSK Medicines Research Centre, Gunnels Wood Road, Stevenage, Hertfordshire SG1 2NY, UK; [b] AGCTlab.org, Centre for Biomedical Sciences, School of Biological Sciences, Royal Holloway, University of London, Egham, Surrey TW20 0EX, UK
* Corresponding author.
E-mail address: rafael.yanez@royalholloway.ac.uk

BRIEF HISTORICAL OVERVIEW OF GENE THERAPY

The concept of gene therapy arose during the 1960s and early 1970s. Rogers and Pfuderer[1] carried out the first genetic modification of a virus (Tobacco mosaic virus [TMV]), and proposed in 1970 that so-called good DNA could be used to replace defective DNA in people afflicted by genetic disorders. In 1972, Friedmann and Roblin[2] assessed the requirements and risks and called for a moratorium. An unsuccessful early attempt at gene therapy was reported in the scientific literature in 1975.[3] The first subject with some degree of long-term transgene persistence from a gene therapy clinical trial was in adenosine deaminase severe combined immunodeficiency (ADA-SCID), following an autologous transplant of T-cells treated *ex vivo* with an integration-proficient retroviral vector, initiated in 1990 and reported in 1995.[4] The first clear success was published by the group of Fischer in 2000, describing the treatment of X-linked severe combined immunodeficiency (SCID-X1) patients with autologous hematopoietic stem or progenitor cells (HSPC) genetically modified with similar retroviral technology.[5] Efforts with developing therapies with integrative vectors were ultimately crowned with success in 2016 when Strimvelis was approved in Europe for the treatment of patients with ADA-SCID for whom no suitable human leukocyte antigen (HLA)-matched stem cell donor is available. This represented the first autologous ex vivo stem cell gene therapy. It was developed in collaboration between GSK together with the Telethon Foundation and the Hospital San Raffaele, acting through their joint San Raffaele Telethon Institute for Gene Therapy (SR-TIGET), a world-leading research centre for stem cell gene therapy in Milan, Italy.

Despite the initial success with integrating vectors, nonintegrating viral vectors were the first approved products for cell and gene therapies in China and Europe. Onyx-015[6] (originally named Ad2/5 dl1520), an experimental oncolytic adenoviral (Ad) vector trialed as a possible treatment of head and neck cancer, was the first gene therapy product licensed, in China in 2006, under the name *H101*.[7] An adeno-associated viral (AAV) vector, Glybera (uniQure/Chiesi),[8] was subsequently approved by european medicines agency (EMA) in 2012 as the first gene therapy in Europe, for lipoprotein lipase deficiency. An oncolytic herpes simplex virus (HSV)-1 (IMLYGIC, Amgen),[9] was approved in 2015 for the treatment of advanced melanoma by both the US Food and Drug Administration (US FDA) and EMA.

NONINTEGRATING VECTORS

Optimal vectors for gene delivery should exhibit high payload capacity, cell tropism for specific target cell types, high transduction efficiency, little or no genotoxicity and cytotoxicity, and should elicit minimal or no immune response. Nonintegrating vectors specifically share reduced risk of genotoxicity, offering a safer profile *in vivo* and *in vitro*, and expression can be retained for long periods in postmitotic tissues. However, unless they have been specifically genetically engineered for replication and segregation, nonintegrating vectors will dilute progressively in proliferating cells. If stable expression in dividing cells is required, repeated administration of nonintegrating vectors is an option, provided that an immune response can be avoided or managed.

This article provides an overview of the main nonintegrating viral vectors: Ad, AAV, integration-deficient lentiviral vectors (IDLVs), poxviral, and others. Nonviral vectors (plasmid, artificial chromosomes) are also discussed. The structure of the main nonintegrating viral vectors is illustrated (**Fig. 1**) and the use of nonintegrating vectors in clinical trials is summarized (**Table 1**). Different vector systems provide a variety of advantageous properties and challenges (**Table 2**). Customarily, viral vectors are

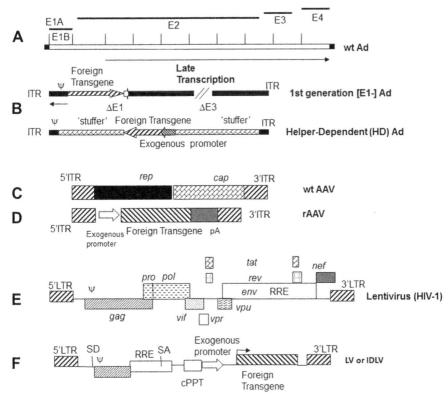

Fig. 1. The basic genome structure of commonly used viruses and derived nonintegrating vector constructs for gene therapy applications. Adenoviral (first-generation and helper-dependent), AAV, and lentiviral vector structures are illustrated. Diagrams are not to scale. (*A, B*) Adenovirus and Ad-based gene transfer vectors. The capacity of [E1-] Ad vectors is further increased by deletion of E3. HD-Ad vectors contain the expression cassette of interest and approximately 500 base pairs of viral sequences required for DNA replication and packaging. The stuffer fragments are important for vector stability. (*C, D*) wt-AAV and recombinant AAV vector with expression transgene cassette flanked by ITRs. (*E, F*) Lentiviral provirus and gene transfer vectors. Integrating lentiviral vectors (LVs) and IDLVs are produced similarly but, for the latter, the packaging plasmid encodes a mutated version of the integrase gene. cPPT, central polypurine tract; ITR, inverted terminal repeat; LTR, long terminal repeat; pA, polyadenylation signal; RRE, rev response element; SA, splice acceptor; SD, splice donor; Ψ, encapsidation sequence.

considered more efficient, whereas nonviral methods have advantages in terms of large-scale production and low immunogenicity.

NONINTEGRATING VIRAL VECTORS
Adenovirus Vectors

Adenovirus vectors key features include

- Efficient delivery to dividing and nondividing cells
- Retained as nonintegrated nuclear linear episomes
- High but transient expression
- High immunogenicity
- Approximately 8 to 30 kilobase (kb) capacity.

Table 1
Clinical trials using nonintegrating viral and nonviral vectors

Vector	Gene Therapy Clinical Trials Worldwide	
	Number	%
Adeno-associated virus	173	7.2
Adenovirus	505	21.0
Adenovirus + Modified vaccinia Ankara virus (MVA)	11	0.5
Adenovirus + Retrovirus[a]	3	0.1
Adenovirus + Sendai virus	1	0.0
Adenovirus + Vaccinia virus	8	0.3
Alphavirus (VEE) Replicon Vaccine	1	0.0
Antisense oligonucleotide	6	0.2
Bifidobacterium longum	1	0.0
Escherichia coli	2	0.1
Flavivirus	8	0.3
Gene gun	5	0.2
Herpes simplex virus	89	3.7
Lactococcus lactis	6	0.2
Lentivirus[a]	144	6.0
Lipofection	115	4.8
Listeria monocytogenes	22	0.9
Measles virus	10	0.4
MVA	7	0.3
mRNA Electroporation	5	0.2
Naked plasmid DNA	414	17.2
Naked plasmid DNA + Adenovirus	4	0.2
Naked plasmid DNA + MVA	2	0.1
Naked plasmid DNA + RNA transfer	1	0.0
Naked plasmid DNA + Vaccinia virus	3	0.1
Naked plasmid DNA + Vesicular stomatitis virus	3	0.1
Newcastle disease virus	1	0.0
Nonviral	2	0.1
Poliovirus	3	0.1
Poxvirus	70	2.9
Poxvirus + Vaccinia virus	36	1.5
Retrovirus[a]	449	18.6
RNA transfer	43	1.8
RNA virus	5	0.2
Saccharomyces cerevisiae	9	0.4
Salmonella typhimurium	4	0.2
Self-adjuvanting RNA	1	0.0
Semliki forest virus	2	0.1
Sendai virus	4	0.2
Shigella dysenteriae	1	0.0
Simian Immunodeficiency Virus (SIVagm)[a]	1	0.0
Simian virus 40	1	0.0
siRNA	5	0.2
Sleeping Beauty transposon[a]	10	0.4
Streptococcus mutans	1	0.0
Vaccinia virus	125	5.2
Venezuelan equine encephalitis virus replicon	3	0.1
Vesicular stomatitis virus	3	0.1
Vibrio cholerae	1	0.0
Unknown	80	3.3
Total	2409	100%

To date at least 71.5% (1722 trials of a total 2409 registered) of the clinical trials reported have used nonintegrating viral and/or nonviral vectors.

Blue, nonintegrating vectors; red, integrating vector or mixture; black, unknown.

[a] Integrating vector.

Adapted from Gene therapy clinical trials worldwide. J Gene Med. Wiley Database. Available at: http://www.abedia.com/wiley/vectors.php. Accessed February 15, 2017; with permission.

Table 2
Properties of nonintegrating gene therapy vectors

Vector	Carrying Capacity (kb)	Features	Advantages	Disadvantages	Initial Applications
Adenovirus	~8–30	Nuclear episome	Efficient delivery to dividing and nondividing cells High, but transient expression	High Immunogenicity	Cancer therapeutics Vaccination
AAV	~4.5	Episomal concatemers	Efficient delivery to dividing and nondividing cells Relatively low immunogenicity	Possible long-term persistence of capsids in vivo Potential for encapsidation of prokaryotic sequences	Efficient and persistent in vivo delivery to postmitotic tissues Delivery of gene-editing components
IDLV	~7.5	Mutations of integrase gene in packaging plasmid	Efficient delivery to dividing and nondividing cells Transient expression in proliferating cells and sustained expression in postmitotic tissues Relatively low immunogenicity	Low expression in proliferating cells	Vaccination Delivery of gene editing templates
Poxvirus	>25	Poxviral RNA pol-based	Large capacity Delivery of substantial cassettes of heterologous antigens Activates innate immune mediators	Potential for adverse events, particularly in immunocompromised patients	Transient expression of immunologically relevant proteins Vaccination
Nonviral	Potentially unlimited	Chemical formulation	Inexpensive to manufacture Can achieve stable expression with replication and segregation capacity Relatively low immunogenicity	Relatively inefficient delivery	Gene delivery to muscle

Adenoviruses are a family of DNA viruses with an icosahedral, 70 to 100 nm in diameter, nonenveloped capsid engulfing a double-stranded (ds) DNA genome. These viruses can infect quiescent and dividing cells and replicate in the cell nucleus. Ad vectors were used early in clinical trials of cystic fibrosis, in various cancer types, and in more recent clinical trials of peripheral vascular and coronary artery disease.[10] Serotypes 2 and 5 are the most extensively characterized human Ad serotypes from a range of greater than 50 Ad subdivisions or clades, with a typical Ad5 vector genome of approximately 36 kb encoding genes that are expressed before (Early [E]) and after (Late [L]) viral replication. Early transcription units encode proteins required for viral transactivation and host-virus interactions. More than 30 novel nonhuman primate adenoviruses from chimpanzees, bonobos, and gorillas, as well as various other species, such as canine, equine, and others, have been isolated and characterized.

Conventional Ad vectors were constructed by substituting the E1 region of the adenovirus genome with the transgene cassette of interest (E1-) (see **Fig. 1**A, B). Thus, first-generation Ad vectors (E1-) had a carrying capacity of less than 8 kb. However, other viral genes are expressed and Ad capsid proteins seem to activate innate host immune responses that within 2 weeks can result in the loss of Ad-transduced cells.[11] Different combinations of early region Ad deletions have been tested providing the Ad vector with modified properties and allowing for enhanced duration of transgene expression. Subsequent generations of adenoviral vectors were characterized by deletions of E1 and E2 and/or E4 genes, although toxicity from an E1/E4 deleted Ad vector led to the first reported fatality in gene therapy.[12] Ad vectors with multiple backbone deletions also reduce the risk of generation of replication competent adenoviral particles. Latest generations of gutless helper-dependent (HD) Ad vectors are devoid of most viral sequences, minimally retaining only the viral inverted terminal repeats (ITRs), and the packaging recognition signal. They can accommodate up to 28 to 32 kb foreign exogenous DNA sequences and have been used in various preclinical animal studies with apparent stable expression and low levels of toxicity.[13] Hence, HD-Ad vectors seem to have significant advantages over first-generation Ad vectors. However, it should be noted that production of HD-Ad is considerably more challenging.

Neutralizing Abs and preexisting immunity (see later discussion) represent a significant barrier to repeated vector administration, a strategy of potential importance with episomally maintained vectors. Low-level expression of viral vector genes in such settings almost always results in the generation of immune responses directed against Ad-transduced cells and ultimately in loss of transgene expression. Latest-generation HD-Ad vectors represent a significant advantage, but it is possible that they may still potentiate cytotoxic T-cell responses even in the absence of de novo viral gene expression. However, repeated administration using HD-Ad vectors of different serotypes has been achieved.[14]

Future directions and hematopoietic application
Current Ad vectors are primarily derived from common serotypes 2 and 5. There are now efforts, however, to exploit other human or nonhuman adenoviral serotypes or mosaic, chimeric, or hybrid[15] adenoviruses to avoid administration problems associated with pre-existing immunity and transduction longevity issues. Approaches targeting uncontrolled blood thrombogenesis by systemically overexpressing prothrombin via Ad vector-mediated gene transfer have been explored.[16] Efficient genome editing of *CCR5* in HSPC with HD-Ad5/35 vectors expressing site-specific endonucleases is mediating positive results in AIDS clinical trials; expression under microRNA regulation can be a useful tool for therapeutic and biotechnology purposes.[17]

Adeno-Associated Virus Vectors

Adeno-associated virus vectors key features include

- Efficient delivery to dividing and nondividing cells
- Approximately 4.5 kb cloning capacity
- Capable of sustained expression as episomal concatemers in postmitotic tissues
- Relatively low immunogenicity.

AAV is a human defective parvovirus whose 4.7 kb single-stranded (ss) genome is flanked by 2 ITRs and comprises 2 genes, *rep* and *cap*. *rep* encodes for nonstructural (replication) proteins, and is also important for site-specific integration into *AAVS1*[18] (see **Fig. 1** C, D). *cap* encodes for structural (encapsidation) proteins, and the accessory assembly-activating protein, essential for serotype-specific assembly. In recombinant AAV vectors, the viral backbone segment, including the *rep* and *cap* genes is removed and supplied in *trans*. The ITRs are the most prominent genomic characteristic of the virus. They consist of a 125 nucleotide-long palindromic hairpin structure and a 20 nucleotide stretch, designated as the D-sequence, which remains single-stranded. The ITRs contain recognition signals for replication, packaging into functional virions and integration. Efficient replication and lytic growth of AAV depends on coinfection by a helper virus. Ads, HSV type I/II, pseudorabies virus and cytomegalovirus can provide complete helper functions for AAV replication.

Wild-type (wt)-AAV2 preferentially integrates into the *AAVS1* site, in the long arm of human chromosome 19 (19q13.3-qter), in a process mediated by rep-binding.[18] In addition, more than 20 alternative integration sites have been identified.[19] The absence of obvious pathogenic effects of AAV integration into *AAVS1* has led to the development of this site as a safe-harbor locus for multiple applications. However, recombinant AAV vectors fail to integrate in the absence of rep protein and instead essentially become nonintegrating vectors, able to impart long-term episomal persistence in postmitotic tissues such as muscle. Mostly, they are maintained as large head-to-tail circularized multimeric concatemer structures, with a common structural element, including a complete ITR flanked by 2 D-region elements. The generation of such concatemers may involve recombination and a possible rolling circle-type DNA replication mechanism.[20]

More than 170 (7.2%) of human trials have used AAV vectors (clinical studies available as of August 2016; see **Table 1**). The low immunologic response to AAV-mediated gene transfer was initially attributed to limited transduction of antigen-presenting dendritic cells, although further data demonstrated the ability of AAV to transduce immature dendritic cell populations[21] and provoke humoral immune responses. At least 12 naturally isolated AAV serotypes have been identified to date. In addition, a wide range of mosaic or hybrid and novel capsids generated by *de novo* shuffling approaches are rapidly expanding the current AAV toolbox.[22] This is important because different serotypes display varying tropism, and because dose-escalation of recombinant AAV-2 in clinical trials may have caused acute inflammatory responses to viral coat proteins similar to the ones encountered in Ad trials. The use and combination of various AAV serotypes provides flexibility, low-immunogenicity, possible differential antigenic display, and lack of antibody cross-reactivity. A detailed understanding of the tropism of AAV serotypes is playing a key role in transduction studies and clinical trials.[23]

Future directions and hematopoietic application

AAV gene therapy has progressed rapidly over the past decade, with the advent of novel capsid serotypes, organ-specific promoters, and an increasing understanding of the immune response to AAV administration.[24] Recently, using nonbiased haploid or knockout genetic screening approaches, AAVR has been identified as a universal host receptor for AAV-2 infections.[25] New AAV isolates, particularly AAV Hematopoietic Stem Cells (AAVHSCs), represent a new class of genetic vectors that may be particularly suited for the manipulation of HSPC.[26]

In a clinical setting, as discussed extensively elsewhere in this issue, peripheral-vein infusion of scAAV2/8-LP1-hFIXco (codon-optimized factor IX gene targeted to the liver) resulted in FIX transgene expression at levels sufficient to improve the bleeding hemophilia B phenotype, with few side effects.[27] Following on from these studies, there are now 3 ongoing trials (with more underway) of AAV-mediated gene transfer in hemophilia B, all aiming to express the factor IX gene from the liver.[28] Additionally, AAV liver expression of the hyperactive variant FIX-Padua prevented and eradicated FIX inhibitor without increasing uncontrolled thrombogenesis in hemophilia B dogs and mice, supporting the potential translation of gene-based strategies using FIX-Padua at lower vector doses.[29] Recently, preliminary data from infused participants in an ongoing phase 1-2 clinical trial of FIX-Padua-containing AAV vector (SPK-9001) for hemophilia B have been released. Following a single administration of 5×10^{11} vector genomes (vg)/kg, all participants experienced consistent and sustained ($\sim$30% in average) increases in factor IX activity.[30] Developments of relevance to other forms of hemophilia are also in the pipeline. Liver-directed gene therapy with AAV-FVIII in 2 outbred dogs with severe hemophilia A resulted in sustained expression of 1% to 2% of normal FVIII levels and prevented 90% of expected bleeding episodes.[31] Engineering of factor VIII to reduce its size and facilitate its delivery with AAV vectors has recently shown success in interim results from a clinical trial. B-domain deleted FVIII construct was administered in an AAV5 vector (BMN 270) to subjects with severe hemophilia A. High-dose (6×10^{13} vg/kg) subjects required no further FVIII prophylactic post-BMN 270 infusion.[32]

Codon optimization of human FVII (hFVIIcoop) improved AAV transgene expression by 37-fold compared with the wt-hFVII complementary DNA (cDNA), whereas in the same study in adult macaques, a single peripheral vein injection of 2×10^{11} vg/kg of the hFVIIcoop AAV vector resulted in therapeutic levels of hFVII expression.[33] Regarding other diseases, AAV has also been used in a murine model of thrombotic thrombocytopenic purpura (TTP), which is caused by severe deficiency of plasma ADAMTS13 activity. Current treatment of hereditary TTP is through plasma infusions. AAV8-hAAT-mdtcs (expressing MDTCS, a C-terminus truncated variant of ADAMTS13, driven by the liver-specific alpha-1 anti-trypsin promoter) at doses greater than 2.6×10^{11} vg/kg body weight (required to achieve therapeutic levels of ADAMTS13 plasma or antigen activity and comparable with those reported for hemophilia B studies) resulted in sustained expression of plasma ADAMTS13 activity at therapeutic levels.[34] Separately, AAV is also a very promising tool for genome editing, both for delivery of chimeric nucleases and repair template in culture and in vivo.[35]

Integration-Deficient Lentiviral Vectors

IDLVs key features include

- Generated through the use of mutations in the integrase gene
- Approximately 7.5 kb capacity for foreign DNA
- Efficient delivery to dividing and nondividing cells
- Transient expression in proliferating cells and sustained expression in postmitotic tissues
- Relatively low immunogenicity.

Retroviruses are ssRNA viruses whose genome is reverse transcribed into dsDNA and integrated into the infected cell genome. Genomic integration leads to stable maintenance and potentially sustained expression. These features are kept in retroviral vectors, which make them particularly appreciated when stable, long-term expression is sought. The lentivirus genus of retroviruses includes species with a more complex genome, which, in addition to genes *gag*, *pol*, and *env*, features a variable array of accessory genes.[36] Lentiviruses offer additional tropism because they are able to infect quiescent as well as dividing cells, the former not being suitable targets for classic gamma retroviruses. Lentiviruses infecting various mammals have been converted into lentiviral vectors, but the most used are those based on HIV-1[37] (see **Fig. 1**E, F). Vectors based on equine infectious anemia virus (EIAV) are also highly engineered and have been developed for commercial use.[38] Both HIV-1 and EIAV vectors have been used successfully for transduction of the central nervous system.[37,38]

Several strategies have been implemented to improve the biosafety of lentiviral vectors. These vectors do not encode any viral product because the viral proteins are provided in *trans* from several packaging plasmids to split the original viral genome. Accessory genes, often responsible for pathogenic features, have been progressively removed from the production system.[39] Vectors have also been made self-inactivating (SIN) by deleting the transcriptional promoter or enhancer from the 3′ long terminal repeat (LTR) in the transfer plasmid; this deletion is copied onto the 5′ end of the vector during the reverse transcription cycle, essentially abolishing expression from the viral LTR. SIN vectors, therefore, depend on an internal promoter to provide transgenic expression.[40]

The theoretic risk from insertional mutagenesis mediated by retroviral vectors unfortunately first materialized in SCID-X1 clinical trials, in which *ex vivo* transduction of HSPC with retroviral vectors led to clinical success but also some cases of leukemia.[41] Lentiviral vectors display a safer integration pattern than gamma-retroviral vectors, and the SIN configuration also contributes to increasing biosafety.[42] Additionally, high-efficiency lentiviral transduction can be achieved with IDLVs, produced through the use of integrase mutations that specifically prevent proviral integration, resulting in the generation of increased levels of circular vector episomes[43] (**Fig. 2**A). Lacking replication signals, lentiviral episomes mediate transient transduction in dividing cells and stable expression in quiescent cells. The authors and others have shown efficient and sustained transgene expression *in vivo* in rodent ocular, cerebral, and spinal cord tissues,[44–46] and substantial rescue of clinically relevant rodent models of retinal degeneration[46] and Parkinson disease.[47] It is also possible to use retroviral vectors for so-called retrovirus particle-mediated messenger RNA (mRNA) transfer, whereby vector mutants unable to start reverse transcription are instead transiently translated,[48] and lentiviral vectors for protein delivery.[49]

Future directions and hematopoietic application

IDLVs have been shown to transiently transduce HSPC.[50] More recently, other applications for IDLVs have emerged (see **Fig. 2**B–D). They can be used as platforms to deliver cassettes and zinc-finger nuclease (ZFN) genes for gene editing by homology-dependent repair in hematopoietic cells and others,[51] for transposition,[52] and for site-specific recombination.[53] Using the latter, IDLVs can yield site-specific recombination of a selectable donor cassette at the safe-harbor *AAVS1* locus previously edited by ZFN to contain an acceptor site.[54] Dendritic cells are of particular interest and have been successfully targeted for transgenic expression with IDLVs.[55] An IDLV-based platform (ID-VP02) that targets and delivers antigen-encoding nucleic acids to human dendritic cells has also been recently developed. It was constructed by incorporating a novel genetic variant of Sindbis virus envelope glycoprotein with posttranslational carbohydrate modifications in combination with Vpx, a SIVmac viral accessory protein.[56] Replicating IDLVs would be of considerable importance, and attempts to develop them have included the incorporation of the simian virus 40 (SV40)

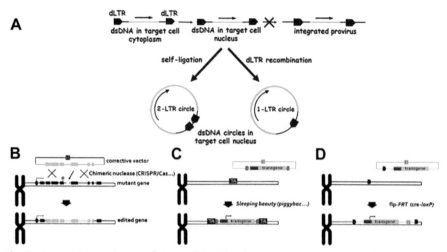

Fig. 2. Generation and uses of IDLVs. (*A*) Following reverse transcription of the lentiviral genome, dsDNA present in the cytoplasm is translocated into the nucleus. In the absence of catalytically active integrase, proviral integration is minimized, and increased levels of transcription-proficient viral episomes are generated by nonhomologous end-joining mediated self-ligation and homologous recombination of 5'-deleted self-inactivating long terminal repeat (dLTR) sequences. (*B*) Genome editing using IDLV-mediated template delivery. In the presence of an engineered chimeric nuclease able to cut the target locus (*thin black arrow*), efficient homology-dependent repair can take place, repairing a mutant gene. The mutation is represented as an orange signpost. (*C*) IDLV-mediated transposon delivery. Cointroduction of a transposase, such as *sleeping beauty* or *piggybac*, and the corresponding transposon allows efficient transposition into the target cell genome. TA: di-nucleotide targeted by *sleeping beauty* and flanking the inserted transposon. Inverted orange arrows head: transposon *cis*-acting sequences. (*D*) IDLV-mediated site-specific integration. An IDLV containing a site-specific recombination cassette can be integrated at the target genomic site in the presence of the relevant integrase. Examples are flippase (flp)-mediated recombination at flp recombination target (*FRT*) sites and cre-mediated recombination at *loxP* sites. The recombination site is represented as a black arrow head. Note that in B–D genes encoding engineering nuclease, transposase, or site-specific recombinase can also be delivered with IDLVs.

promoter or origin of replication in cells expressing SV40 large T-antigen.[57] A version of this vector incorporating HSV thymidine kinase allows suicide gene therapy using ganciclovir.[58] The authors have shown that replicating IDLVs can be established at high frequency by inducing transient cell-cycle arrest at the time of vector transduction, with no requirement for replication sequences.[59]

Poxviral Vectors, Including Vaccinia

Poxviral vectors key features include

- Large-capacity dsDNA viruses (>25 kb of foreign DNA)
- Provide transient expression of immunologically relevant proteins
- Ability to activate appropriate innate immune mediators on vaccination
- Relatively high-level of biological safety but potential for adverse events.

Poxviruses have played an important role in the development of virology, immunology, and vaccinology. In 1796, deliberate inoculation of cowpox virus into humans by Jenner demonstrated protection against the antigenically related smallpox virus (variola).[60] Poxviruses are members of the family Poxviridae. They are dsDNA viruses about 200 to 400 nm in length with a genome of about 190 kb, which is flanked by approximately 10 kb ITRs, and exist in 2 forms: an intracellular naked virion and an extracellular enveloped virion. Transcription and DNA replication occur in the cytoplasm, where the progeny DNA is generated by the synthesis and resolution of large concatemeric molecules.[60] Recombinant forms of the virus (with vaccinia as the prototype vector) are the vectors of choice for transient expression of immunologically relevant proteins[61] and thus serve as an alternative approach to the development of vaccines against a variety of infectious agents.[62] Recombinant poxviruses have the transgene of interest commonly inserted by homologous recombination and driven by a poxviral promoter rather than a constitutive viral or mammalian promoter because they are cytoplasmatic viruses and encode their own RNA polymerase. Classic experiments showed that vaccinia can carry at least 25 kb of foreign DNA.[63] Modified Vaccinia virus Ankara (MVA) is licensed as third-generation vaccine against smallpox. Recombinant MVAs can be used for protein production and as vaccines against infectious diseases, cancer, and other pathologic conditions.[64]

Future directions and hematopoietic application
Airway epithelial cells are the initial replication site of vaccinia virus, before spreading to secondary sites of infection, mainly the draining lymph nodes, spleen, gastrointestinal tract, and reproductive organs.[65] Stimulation of natural killer (NK) cell subsets during the antiviral response occurs through receptors apparently directed at viral products.[66] Understanding of the importance of NK cells in viral infections is improving, and poxviruses have been instrumental to improve this knowledge. After smallpox was eradicated, vaccinia has been used for the development of a variety of therapeutics: recombinant vaccines, immunotherapies, oncolytic therapies, and others.[67]

Other Nonintegrating Viral Vector Systems

No single viral vector is optimal for all potential gene therapy applications. The availability of many vector systems differing in cloning capacity, stability, tropism, immunogenicity, and other properties provides options to target the tissue and strategy of interest. In addition to those previously reviewed, herpesvirus vectors also merit a prominent place, particularly those based on HSV-1 for the purposes of gene transfer for cancer and neurodegenerative disease.[68] Sendai virus, an RNA virus with no risk of genomic integration, which can infect a wide range of cell types including HSPC, has recently attracted significant interest. Sendai vectors have been used for delivery of CRISPR/Cas9 for efficient gene editing,[69] and for the generation of human-induced pluripotent stem cells.[70]

Nonviral Vectors

Nonviral vectors key features include

- Potentially unlimited packaging capacity
- Inexpensive to manufacture at Good Manufacturing Practice
- Can be endowed with replication and segregation capabilities for stable expression in proliferating cells
- Relatively inefficient delivery
- Relatively low immunogenicity.

Nonviral vectors for gene delivery were among the earliest to be developed, starting with plasmids. Wilson and colleagues[71] cloned the β-globin cDNA into a bacterial plasmid in 1978, and Green and colleagues[72] successfully transfected the plasmid into cells by calcium phosphate coprecipitation. A distinctive feature of nonviral gene delivery is the ability to carry and deliver a broad range of nucleic acids. For gene addition studies, plasmids have been the most commonly used. However, more recently, next-generation DNA molecules, including minicircle DNA,[73] mini-intronic plasmids,[74] and closed-ended linear duplex DNA,[75] have been developed that show both enhanced transgene expression and persistence compared with conventional plasmids. In addition to DNA, mRNA, smal interfering RNA (siRNA), and guide RNA (gRNA) can also be delivered using nonviral vectors to provide short-term transgene expression, gene suppression, and CRISPR/Cas genome editing, respectively. In the case of mRNA and siRNA, because they only need to enter the cytoplasm to function, nuclear entry is removed as a significant barrier to function. This can be particularly advantageous in nondividing cells. The transient expression obtained with mRNA delivery is also useful for gene editing applications in which expression and function of nucleases and transposons are needed for only a short period of time and in which constitutive long-term expression could induce off-target mutagenesis.[76]

For large transgenes, or whole genes, human artificial chromosomes (HACs) are an option that can be used with nonviral vectors. HACs can carry entire genes, including their introns, and be maintained in dividing cells as the artificial chromosomes are replicated and segregated with the host chromosomes. Yeast artificial chromosomes with 200-kb to 800-kb inserts of human DNA and first approaches to human mapping were described in the late 1980s.[77] Since those early days, applications of HACs have included development of transgenic mice with megabase-sized transgenes, stable maintenance in human embryonic stem cells, combination of human alpha satellite and single-copy DNAs, and development of therapeutic HACs in preclinical models for Duchenne muscular dystrophy, which is caused by defects in the largest gene, *DMD*.[78] There is little consensus as to what constitutes a true artificial *versus* an engineered human chromosome.[79] However, the low efficiency of chromosome transfer and the relatively complex engineering of artificial chromosomes present significant challenges that have limited their utility as a therapeutic.

Several nonviral methods for nucleic acid delivery have been developed that can be classified as physical or chemical. Physical methods include the use of ultrasound[80] or electrical currents[81] to temporarily increase the permeability of target cells (sonoporation and electroporation, respectively), direct injection of DNA into single cells,[82] ballistic propulsion of DNA-coated particles,[83] and hydrodynamic gene delivery involving the rapid injection of a large volume of DNA solution (8%–10% of body weight).[84] Gene delivery by physical methods is fairly simple but offers no protection from nucleases for the nucleic acid.

In contrast, chemical carriers typically encapsulate nucleic acids, thereby protecting the payload from nucleases. Chemical gene delivery vectors usually use a cationic species to condense the anionic nucleic acids and, in the process, form nanoparticles for delivery. Cationic liposomes have been extensively studied and are among the most widely used nonviral vectors.[85] Later, addition of cationic polymers (producing so-called lipopolyplex) was shown to enhance gene delivery[86] (**Fig. 3**). Mechanistically, the liposome likely provides the mechanism for endosomal escape while the polymer enables efficient condensation and packaging of the nucleic acid, therefore forming small, stable, discrete, and homogenous nanoparticles. Further attempts at improving nonviral formulations have been made with the addition of components to improve bioavailability *in vivo* through shielding of complexes using polyethylene glycols, to enhance cell-specific targeting using targeting moieties, to aid endosomal escape using fusogenic lipids or pH-sensitive

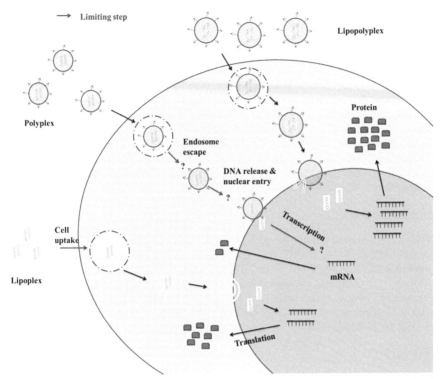

Fig. 3. Barriers to nonviral transfection. Red arrows show limiting steps for lipoplex and pol-yplex technologies, potentially overcome by the use of lipopolyplex complexes. *Black arrows* indicate non-rate limiting steps.

polymers, and to improve nuclear entry using nuclear targeting sequences or nuclear localization signal-containing peptides.

Future directions and hematopoietic application

The application of nonviral vectors to the hematopoietic system has been limited, but recent technologies are promising. T-cells can be genetically engineered to express a chimeric antigen receptor (CAR) using electroporation for sleeping beauty (SB) trans-position, in which SB was delivered as an mRNA or minicircle, and the SB donor (con-sisting of the CAR sequences, flanked by SB inverted repeats) was provided as a minicircle.[87] Of importance, the integration pattern observed was considered safer than that present in CAR T-cells obtained with integrating lentiviral vector. Given the ease of scaling up production of mRNA and minicircles and the close-to-random inte-gration profile of SB transposition, there may be significant advantages to using nonviral methods for generating functional CAR T-cells. Novel electroporation tech-nologies, such as nucleofection, have also been reported to mediate efficient delivery of DNA, mRNA, and siRNA to various hematopoietic cell lineages.[88]

SUMMARY

HSPC have great therapeutic potential because of their ability to self-renew, differen-tiate, and accomplish corrective reconstitution of the hematopoietic system in patients with various hematologic disorders. Specialized blood lineages are of relevance to specific strategies, such as dendritic cells for immunization or engineered CAR T-cells for lymphoma and leukemia treatment. Gene addition therapies targeted to HSPC and using integrating retroviral vectors have shown clear clinical benefits and potential in multiple diseases, among them immune deficiencies, storage disorders, and hemoglobinopathies. However, the potential for insertional mutagenesis remains a risk. Gene editing technologies are also undergoing massive expansion and optimized, transient delivery is of clear benefit. The development of nonintegrating nucleic acid delivery methods that combine low or no genotoxicity and high efficiency in hematopoietic cells is, therefore, highly desirable. This article has described several such methods using Ad, AAV, IDLV, poxviral, and nonviral vector technologies. The authors are optimistic regarding the potential of nonintegrating vectors in gene and stem cell therapy-based regenerative medicine.

ACKNOWLEDGMENTS

R.J. Yáñez-Muñoz would like to thank the European Union (PERSIST, FP7 grant agreement 222878; NEUGENE, FP7 grant agreement 222925; CLINIGENE, FP6 grant agreement 18933), The SMA Trust (The UK SMA Research Consortium) and Royal Holloway, University of London for financial support. The authors would like to thank Christopher Herring, Director CGT DR; Tim Kim, Pattern Attorney; Amy Altshul, VP Legal & Compliance; and Laurent Jespers, VP Head of Discovery Research, CGT DR GSK for critically reading and commenting on the article.

REFERENCES

1. Rogers S, Pfuderer P. Use of viruses as carriers of added genetic information. Nature 1968;219(5155):749–51.
2. Friedmann T, Roblin R. Gene therapy for human genetic disease? Science 1972; 175(4025):949–55.
3. Terheggen HG, Lowenthal A, Lavinha F, et al. Unsuccessful trial of gene replacement in arginase deficiency. Z Kinderheilkd 1975;119(1):1–3.
4. Blaese RM, Culver KW, Miller AD, et al. T lymphocyte-directed gene therapy for ADA- SCID: initial trial results after 4 years. Science 1995;270(5235):475–80.
5. Cavazzana-Calvo M, Hacein-Bey S, de Saint Basile G, et al. Gene therapy of human severe combined immunodeficiency (SCID)-X1 disease. Science 2000; 288(5466):669–72.
6. Heise C, Sampson-Johannes A, Williams A, et al. ONYX-015, an E1B gene-attenuated adenovirus, causes tumor-specific cytolysis and antitumoral efficacy that can be augmented by standard chemotherapeutic agents. Nat Med 1997; 3(6):639–45.
7. Yu W, Fang H. Clinical trials with oncolytic adenovirus in China. Curr Cancer Drug Targets 2007;7(2):141–8.
8. Miller N. Glybera and the future of gene therapy in the European Union. Nat Rev Drug Discov 2012;11(5):419.
9. Pol J, Kroemer G, Galluzzi L. First oncolytic virus approved for melanoma immunotherapy. Oncoimmunology 2016;5(1):e1115641.
10. Laakkonen JP, Yla-Herttuala S. Recent advancements in cardiovascular gene therapy and vascular biology. Hum Gene Ther 2015;26(8):518–24.
11. Cianciola NL, Chung S, Manor D, et al. Adenovirus Modulates Toll-Like Receptor 4 Signaling by Reprogramming ORP1L-VAP Protein Contacts for Cholesterol

Transport from Endosomes to the Endoplasmic Reticulum. J Virol 2017;91(6) [pii: e01904-16].

12. Carmen IH. A death in the laboratory: the politics of the Gelsinger aftermath. Mol Ther 2001;3(4):425–8.

13. Cots D, Bosch A, Chillon M. Helper dependent adenovirus vectors: progress and future prospects. Curr Gene Ther 2013;13(5):370–81.

14. Parks R, Evelegh C, Graham F. Use of helper-dependent adenoviral vectors of alternative serotypes permits repeat vector administration. Gene Ther 1999; 6(9):1565–73.

15. Smith RP, Riordan JD, Feddersen CR, et al. A hybrid adenoviral vector system achieves efficient long-term gene expression in the Liver via piggyBac Transposition. Hum Gene Ther 2015;26(6):377–85.

16. Liu X, Ni M, Ma L, et al. Targeting blood thrombogenicity precipitates atherothrombotic events in a mouse model of plaque destabilization. Scientific Rep 2015;5:10225.

17. Saydaminova K, Ye X, Wang H, et al. Efficient genome editing in hematopoietic stem cells with helper-dependent Ad5/35 vectors expressing site-specific endonucleases under microRNA regulation. Mol Ther Methods Clin Dev 2015;1:14057.

18. Musayev FN, Zarate-Perez F, Bishop C, et al. Structural Insights into the Assembly of the Adeno-associated Virus Type 2 Rep68 Protein on the Integration Site AAVS1. J Biol Chem 2015;290(46):27487–99.

19. Huser D, Gogol-Doring A, Lutter T, et al. Integration preferences of wildtype AAV-2 for consensus rep-binding sites at numerous loci in the human genome. PLoS Pathog 2010;6(7):e1000985.

20. Athanasopoulos T, Fabb S, Dickson G. Gene therapy vectors based on adeno-associated virus: characteristics and applications to acquired and inherited diseases (review). Int J Mol Med 2000;6(4):363–75.

21. Wilde B, van Paassen P, Damoiseaux J, et al. Dendritic cells in renal biopsies of patients with ANCA-associated vasculitis. Nephrol Dial Transplant 2009;24(7):2151–6.

22. Zinn E, Pacouret S, Khaychuk V, et al. In silico reconstruction of the viral evolutionary lineage yields a potent gene therapy vector. Cell Rep 2015;12(6):1056–68.

23. Srivastava A. In vivo tissue-tropism of adeno-associated viral vectors. Curr Opin Virol 2016;21:75–80.

24. Kotterman MA, Schaffer DV. Engineering adeno-associated viruses for clinical gene therapy. Nat Rev Genet 2014;15(7):445–51.

25. Pillay S, Meyer NL, Puschnik AS, et al. An essential receptor for adeno-associated virus infection. Nature 2016;530(7588):108–12.

26. Smith LJ, Ul-Hasan T, Carvaines SK, et al. Gene transfer properties and structural modeling of human stem cell-derived AAV. Mol Ther 2014;22(9):1625–34.

27. Nathwani AC, Tuddenham EG, Rangarajan S, et al. Adenovirus-associated virus vector-mediated gene transfer in hemophilia B. N Engl J Med 2011;365(25): 2357–65.

28. High KH, Nathwani A, Spencer T, et al. Current status of haemophilia gene therapy. Haemophilia 2014;20(Suppl 4):43–9.

29. Crudele JM, Finn JD, Siner JI, et al. AAV liver expression of FIX-Padua prevents and eradicates FIX inhibitor without increasing thrombogenicity in hemophilia B dogs and mice. Blood 2015;125(10):1553–61.

30. George L, Sullivan S, Giermasz A, et al. Initiation of Oral Steroid Therapy Produced Rapid Normalization of Transaminase Levels and Stabilization of FIX Activity in Subjects Who Developed T-Cell Responses in the SPK-9001: AAV Gene Transfer for Hemophilia B Phase 1/2 Trial. Haemophilia 2017;23(S3):15–6.

31. Callan MB, Haskins ME, Wang P, et al. Successful phenotype improvement following gene therapy for severe hemophilia a in privately owned dogs. PLoS One 2016;11(3):e0151800.

32. Pasi J, Wong W, Rangarajan S, et al. Interim results of an open-label, phase 1/2 study of BMN 270, an AAV5-FVIII gene transfer in severe hemophilia A. Haemophilia 2016;22(S4):151.

33. Binny C, McIntosh J, Della Peruta M, et al. AAV-mediated gene transfer in the perinatal period results in expression of FVII at levels that protect against fatal spontaneous hemorrhage. Blood 2012;119(4):957–66.

34. Jin SY, Xiao J, Bao J, et al. AAV-mediated expression of an ADAMTS13 variant prevents shigatoxin-induced thrombotic thrombocytopenic purpura. Blood 2013;121(19):3825–9. S3821–3.

35. Sharma R, Anguela XM, Doyon Y, et al. In vivo genome editing of the albumin locus as a platform for protein replacement therapy. Blood 2015;126(15):1777–84.

36. Delenda C. Lentiviral vectors: optimization of packaging, transduction and gene expression. J Gene Med 2004;6(Suppl 1):S125–38.

37. Naldini L, Blömer U, Gallay P, et al. In vivo gene delivery and stable transduction of nondividing cells by a lentiviral vector. Science 1996;272:263–7.

38. Mitrophanous K, Yoon S, Rohll J, et al. Stable gene transfer to the nervous system using a non-primate lentiviral vector. Gene Ther 1999;6(11):1808–18.

39. Vigna E, Naldini L. Lentiviral vectors: excellent tools for experimental gene transfer and promising candidates for gene therapy. J Gene Med 2000;2(5):308–16.

40. Zufferey R, Dull T, Mandel RJ, et al. Self-inactivating lentivirus vector for safe and efficient in vivo gene delivery. J Virol 1998;72:9873–80.

41. Hacein-Bey-Abina S, von Kalle C, Schmidt M, et al. A serious adverse event after successful gene therapy for X-linked severe combined immunodeficiency. N Engl J Med 2003;348(3):255–6.

42. Montini E, Cesana D, Schmidt M, et al. The genotoxic potential of retroviral vectors is strongly modulated by vector design and integration site selection in a mouse model of HSC gene therapy. J Clin Invest 2009;119(4):964–75.

43. Wanisch K, Yáñez-Muñoz RJ. Integration-deficient lentiviral vectors: a slow coming of age. Mol Ther 2009;17(8):1316–32.

44. Peluffo H, Foster E, Ahmed SG, et al. Efficient gene expression from integration-deficient lentiviral vectors in the spinal cord. Gene Ther 2013;20(6):645–57.

45. Philippe S, Sarkis C, Barkats M, et al. Lentiviral vectors with a defective integrase allow efficient and sustained transgene expression in vitro and in vivo. Proc Natl Acad Sci U S A 2006;103(47):17684–9.

46. Yáñez-Muñoz RJ, Balaggan KS, MacNeil A, et al. Effective gene therapy with nonintegrating lentiviral vectors. Nat Med 2006;12(3):348–53.

47. Lu-Nguyen NB, Broadstock M, Schliesser MG, et al. Transgenic expression of human glial cell line-derived neurotrophic factor from integration-deficient lentiviral vectors is neuroprotective in a rodent model of Parkinson's Disease. Hum Gene Ther 2014;25(7):631–41.

48. Galla M, Will E, Kraunus J, et al. Retroviral pseudotransduction for targeted cell manipulation. Mol Cell 2004;16(2):309–15.

49. Cai Y, Bak RO, Mikkelsen JG. Targeted genome editing by lentiviral protein transduction of zinc-finger and TAL-effector nucleases. eLife 2014;3:e01911.

50. Nightingale SJ, Hollis RP, Pepper KA, et al. Transient gene expression by nonintegrating lentiviral vectors. Mol Ther 2006;13(6):1121–32.

51. Joglekar AV, Hollis RP, Kuftinec G, et al. Integrase-defective lentiviral vectors as a delivery platform for targeted modification of adenosine deaminase locus. Mol Ther 2013;21(9):1705–17.

52. Staunstrup NH, Moldt B, Mates L, et al. Hybrid lentivirus-transposon vectors with a random integration profile in human cells. Mol Ther 2009;17(7):1205–14.

53. Moldt B, Staunstrup NH, Jakobsen M, et al. Genomic insertion of lentiviral DNA circles directed by the yeast Flp recombinase. BMC Biotechnol 2008;8:60.

54. Torres R, Garcia A, Jimenez M, et al. An integration-defective lentivirus-based resource for site-specific targeting of an edited safe-harbour locus in the human genome. Gene Ther 2014;21(4):343–52.

55. Daenthanasanmak A, Salguero G, Borchers S, et al. Integrase-defective lentiviral vectors encoding cytokines induce differentiation of human dendritic cells and stimulate multivalent immune responses in vitro and in vivo. Vaccine 2012; 30(34):5118–31.

56. Tareen SU, Kelley-Clarke B, Nicolai CJ, et al. Design of a novel integration-deficient lentivector technology that incorporates genetic and posttranslational elements to target human dendritic cells. Mol Ther 2014;22(3):575–87.

57. Vargas J Jr, Gusella GL, Najfeld V, et al. Novel integrase-defective lentiviral episomal vectors for gene transfer. Hum Gene Ther 2004;15(4):361–72.

58. Vargas J Jr, Klotman ME, Cara A. Conditionally replicating lentiviral-hybrid episomal vectors for suicide gene therapy. Antiviral Res 2008;80(3):288–94.

59. Kymäläinen H, Appelt JU, Giordano FA, et al. Long-term episomal transgene expression from mitotically stable integration-deficient lentiviral vectors. Hum Gene Ther 2014;25(5):428–42.

60. Vanderplasschen A, Pastoret PP. The uses of poxviruses as vectors. Curr Gene Ther 2003;3(6):583–95.

61. Moroziewicz D, Kaufman HL. Gene therapy with poxvirus vectors. Curr Opin Mol Ther 2005;7(4):317–25.

62. Moss B. Poxviridae. In: Knipe DM, Howley PM, editors. Fields virology. 6th edition. Philadelphia: Lippincott Williams & Wilkins; 2013. p. 2129–59.

63. Smith GL, Moss B. Infectious poxvirus vectors have capacity for at least 25 000 base pairs of foreign DNA. Gene 1983;25(1):21–8.

64. Volz A, Sutter G. Modified Vaccinia Virus Ankara: History, Value in Basic Research, and Current Perspectives for Vaccine Development. Adv Virus Res 2017;97:187–243.

65. Abboud G, Tahiliani V, Desai P, et al. Natural killer cells and innate interferon gamma participate in the host defense against respiratory vaccinia virus infection. J Virol 2015;90(1):129–41.

66. Burshtyn DN. NK cells and poxvirus infection. Front Immunol 2013;4:7.

67. Verardi PH, Titong A, Hagen CJ. A vaccinia virus renaissance: new vaccine and immunotherapeutic uses after smallpox eradication. Hum Vaccin Immunother 2012;8(7):961–70.

68. Latchman DS. Herpes simplex virus-based vectors for the treatment of cancer and neurodegenerative disease. Curr Opin Mol Ther 2005;7(5):415–8.

69. Park A, Hong P, Won ST, et al. Sendai virus, an RNA virus with no risk of genomic integration, delivers CRISPR/Cas9 for efficient gene editing. Mol Ther Methods Clin Dev 2016;3:16057.

70. Ban H, Nishishita N, Fusaki N, et al. Efficient generation of transgene-free human induced pluripotent stem cells (iPSCs) by temperature-sensitive Sendai virus vectors. Proc Natl Acad Sci U S A 2011;108(34):14234–9.

71. Wilson JT, Wilson LB, deRiel JK, et al. Insertion of synthetic copies of human globin genes into bacterial plasmids. Nucleic Acids Res 1978;5(2):563–81.
72. Green MR, Treisman R, Maniatis T. Transcriptional activation of cloned human beta-globin genes by viral immediate-early gene products. Cell 1983;35(1):137–48.
73. Munye MM, Tagalakis AD, Barnes JL, et al. Minicircle DNA provides enhanced and prolonged transgene expression following airway gene transfer. Scientific Rep 2016;6:23125.
74. Lu J, Zhang F, Kay MA. A mini-intronic plasmid (MIP): a novel robust transgene expression vector in vivo and in vitro. Mol Ther 2013;21(5):954–63.
75. Li L, Dimitriadis EK, Yang Y, et al. Production and characterization of novel recombinant adeno-associated virus replicative-form genomes: a eukaryotic source of DNA for gene transfer. PLoS One 2013;8(8):e69879.
76. Fu Y, Foden JA, Khayter C, et al. High-frequency off-target mutagenesis induced by CRISPR-Cas nucleases in human cells. Nat Biotechnol 2013;31(9):822–6.
77. Little RD, Porta G, Carle GF, et al. Yeast artificial chromosomes with 200- to 800-kilobase inserts of human DNA containing HLA, V kappa, 5S, and Xq24-Xq28 sequences. Proc Natl Acad Sci U S A 1989;86(5):1598–602.
78. Tedesco FS. Human artificial chromosomes for Duchenne muscular dystrophy and beyond: challenges and hopes. Chromosome Res 2015;23(1):135–41.
79. Basu J, Willard HF. Artificial and engineered chromosomes: non-integrating vectors for gene therapy. Trends Mol Med 2005;11(5):251–8.
80. Fechheimer M, Boylan JF, Parker S, et al. Transfection of mammalian cells with plasmid DNA by scrape loading and sonication loading. Proc Natl Acad Sci U S A 1987;84(23):8463–7.
81. Neumann E, Schaefer-Ridder M, Wang Y, et al. Gene transfer into mouse lyoma cells by electroporation in high electric fields. EMBO J 1982;1(7):841–5.
82. Capecchi MR. High efficiency transformation by direct microinjection of DNA into cultured mammalian cells. Cell 1980;22(2 Pt 2):479–88.
83. Klein TM, Wolf ED, Wu R, et al. High-velocity microprojectiles for delivering nucleic acids into living cells. Nature 1987;327(6117):70–3.
84. Budker V, Zhang G, Danko I, et al. The efficient expression of intravascularly delivered DNA in rat muscle. Gene Ther 1998;5(2):272–6.
85. Fraley R, Subramani S, Berg P, et al. Introduction of liposome-encapsulated SV40 DNA into cells. J Biol Chem 1980;255(21):10431–5.
86. Gao X, Huang L. Potentiation of cationic liposome-mediated gene delivery by polycations. Biochemistry 1996;35(3):1027–36.
87. Monjezi R, Miskey C, Gogishvili T, et al. Enhanced CAR T-cell engineering using non-viral Sleeping Beauty transposition from minicircle vectors. Leukemia 2017;31(1):186–94.
88. Scherer O, Maess MB, Lindner S, et al. A procedure for efficient non-viral siRNA transfection of primary human monocytes using nucleofection. J Immunol Methods 2015;422:118–24.

In Vivo Hematopoietic Stem Cell Transduction

Maximilian Richter, PhD[a,1], Daniel Stone, PhD[b,1], Carol Miao, PhD[c,d],
Olivier Humbert, PhD[e], Hans-Peter Kiem, MD, PhD[e,f],
Thalia Papayannopoulou, MD[g], André Lieber, MD, PhD[a,h,*]

KEYWORDS

• Intravenous • Intraosseal • Viral vectors • Mobilization

KEY POINTS

- Current protocols for hematopoietic stem gene therapy, involving the transplantation of ex vivo genetically modified hematopoietic stem cell (HSC), are complex and not without risk for the patient.
- HSCs in the bone marrow are intricately connected with the bone marrow stroma, which creates a physical barrier to transduction with intravenously injected gene transfer vectors.
- Intraosseal injection of viral vectors has been shown to result in in vivo transduction of HSCs in mice. It might be more feasible and efficient in large animals and humans.
- A new approach that involves the mobilization of HSCs from the bone marrow, their transduction in the periphery, and return to the bone marrow has shown first promising results.

INTRODUCTION
Hematopoietic Stem Cells in the Bone Marrow

Most hematopoietic stem cells (HSCs) reside in so-called stem cell niches regions of the bone marrow in which nonhematopoietic cells interact with HSCs and regulate their dormancy and self-renewal or their differentiation and expansion.[1] However, a

The authors declare no commercial or financial interest.
[a] Division of Medical Genetics, University of Washington, 1705 NE Pacific Street, Seattle, WA 98195, USA; [b] Vaccine and Infectious Disease Division, Fred Hutchinson Cancer Research Center, 1100 Fairview Avenue N, Seattle, WA 98109, USA; [c] Department of Pediatrics, University of Washington, 1705 NE Pacific Street, Seattle, WA 98195, USA; [d] Center for Immunity and Immunotherapy, Research Institute, Seattle Children's Hospital, 1900 9th Avenue, Seattle, WA 98101, USA; [e] Clinical Research Division, Fred Hutchinson Cancer Research Center, 1100 Fairview Aveune N, Seattle, WA 98109, USA; [f] Department of Medicine, University of Washington School of Medicine, 1705 NE Pacific Street, Seattle, WA 98195, USA; [g] Division of Hematology, University of Washington, 1705 NE Pacific Street, Seattle, WA 98195, USA; [h] Department of Pathology, University of Washington, 1705 NE Pacific Street, Seattle, WA 98195, USA
[1] Equal contribution.
* Corresponding author. Division of Medical Genetics, University of Washington, Box 357720, Seattle, WA 98195.
E-mail address: lieber00@uw.edu

small fraction of HSCs circulate in the peripheral blood under steady-state conditions.[2] HSCs that leave the bone marrow under steady-state conditions provide a means of exchange between different stem cell niches as well as a way to react to local damage within hematopoietic tissues. Even under normal conditions, circulating HSCs appear to be able to rapidly re-engraft in bone marrow so that there is a cycle of constant egress and re-engraftment of HSCs.[3] HSC regulation and retention within the bone marrow stem cell niche are mediated through multiple interactions between HSC surface receptors and their respective ligands expressed or secreted by surrounding cells, including osteoblasts and sinusoidal endothelial and perivascular cells.

Hematopoietic Stem Cell Mobilization

The induced egress of HSCs is referred to as stem cell mobilization. Although egress of HSCs from the bone marrow can be observed in response to stress, for example, following injury of hematopoietic organs, stimulated mobilization is commonly achieved through drug administration. The most commonly used mobilizing agent is recombinant human granulocyte colony-stimulating factor (G-CSF), which is given in the form of subcutaneous injections for 5 days and leads to efficient mobilization of both HSCs and more differentiated cells.[2] Another class of mobilizing agents is CXCR4 antagonists, most prominently the US Food and Drug Administration–approved drug Plerixafor/AMD3100. CXCR4 antagonists lead to more rapid mobilization of HSCs than G-CSF[4] and are thought to cause mobilization solely through disruption of the SDF-1-CXCR4 axis. AMD3100 has been shown to synergize with G-CSF mobilization. Because of its higher mobilization power, the combination of G-CSF and AMD3100 is used as a regimen in poor HSC mobilizers such as chemotherapy patients.[5] In a similar manner, soluble stem cell factor (SCF) is able to interrupt the connection between membrane-bound SCF and c-kit, even though SCF is considered to be a slow mobilizing agent and has to be administered for several days.[6] Another class of mobilizing agents target VLA-4, and both VLA-4 binding antibodies[7] and small molecules[8] are able to rapidly mobilize HSCs. VLA-4 binding agents are also thought to have a synergistic or additive effect when used together with G-CSF and AMD3100.[9] One VLA-4 inhibitor, the small molecule BIO5192, was shown to efficiently and rapidly mobilize HSCs. Furthermore, BIO5192 can be combined with G-CSF alone or with AMD31000 to increase levels of mobilized HSCs. BOP (N-(benzenesulfonyl)-L-prolyl-L-O-(1-pyrrolidinylcarbonyl)tyrosine), a small molecule targeting $\alpha9\beta1/\alpha4\beta1$ integrins, also rapidly mobilizes long-term multilineage reconstituting HSC.[10] Synergistic engraftment augmentation is observed when BOP is coadministered with AMD3100.

EXAMPLES FOR IN VIVO HEMATOPOIETIC STEM CELL GENE THERAPY
Example 1: Intravenous Injection of Triplex-Forming Peptide Nucleic Acids

Peptide nucleic acids (PNAs) are designed to bind site-specifically to genomic DNA via strand invasion and formation of PNA/DNA/PNA triplexes with a displaced DNA strand. PNAs consist of a charge-neutral peptide-like backbone and nucleobases enabling high-affinity hybridization with DNA (**Fig. 1**). PNA/DNA/PNA triplexes can be used to modify DNA by recruiting endogenous DNA repair proteins to initiate site-specific modification of the genome when single-stranded "donor DNAs" are codelivered as templates containing the desired sequence modification.[11]

A recent study reported in vivo HSC gene editing in mice using intravenously (IV) injected triplex-forming PNAs in combination with SCF given intraperitoneally 3 hours before the PNAs.[12] Treatment of transgenic mice carrying a β-globin/GFP reporter transgene with PNAs and single-stranded donor DNA yielded gene editing in mouse

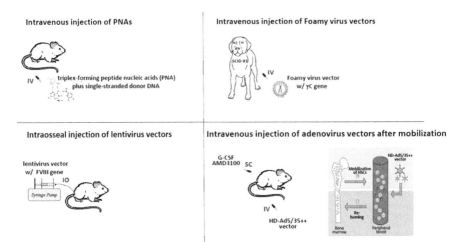

Fig. 1. Schematic representation of 4 approaches for in vivo HSC gene therapy. The upper left panel shows an example of in vivo HSC gene editing using nonviral nanoparticles injected IV into mice. Site-specific triplex-forming PNA interact site-specifically with genomic DNA via strand invasion resulting in the displacement of a DNA strand. This recruits endogenous DNA repair proteins to initiate site-specific modification of the genome when single-stranded donor DNAs are codelivered. The upper right panel shows a study in dogs with a mutation causing SCID-X1. An FV vector carrying the γC gene capable of phenotypic correction of the disease is delivered IV. The lower left panel depicts an IO approach of gene delivery into bone marrow HSCs. In this example, a lentivirus vector carrying a human FVIII clotting factor expression cassette is injected via a syringe pump into the femurs of mice. The lower right panel shows an in vivo HSC gene transfer approach that involves the mobilization of HSCs from the bone marrow by subcutaneous (SC) injections of G-CSF/AMD3100. Although HSC are in the peripheral blood, a capsid-modified, integrating HDAd5/35^{++} is injected IV. HSC is transduced in the periphery home back to the bone marrow where they persist long term.

CD117$^+$ cells at frequencies up to 1% with a single treatment. In a thalassemic mouse model, in vivo treatment resulted in a gene-editing frequency of almost 4% in total bone marrow mononuclear cells and 6.9% in HSCs, resulting in amelioration of the disease phenotype. The investigators reported that, based on their ex vivo studies, SCF could enhance PNA-mediated gene editing in vivo. The authors speculate that SCF treatment might also have resulted in HSC mobilization and thus caused better gene transfer. A nonviral PNA-based platform for in vivo HSC gene editing has the advantage of circumventing host immune responses and, if it can be scaled up, has great potential over designer nucleases–based approaches for gene editing that introduce an active nuclease into cells, which can lead to off-target cleavage in the genome and can affect the viability and function of HSCs.

Example 2: Intravenous Injection of Foamy Virus Vectors in Dogs

Current Vesicular Stomatitis Virus G-protein (VSV-G) pseudotyped lentivirus vectors are not suitable for direct in vivo injection, because VSVG is rapidly inactivated by human complement.[13] In this respect, several pseudotyping partners have emerged in the field, such as the complement-resistant gibbon ape leukemia virus or the endogenous feline leukemia virus RD114 glycoproteins. The authors have used foamy virus (FV) vectors, which are nonpathogenic integrating retroviruses

with properties that distinguish them from other viral vectors. Unlike VSV-G pseudotyped lentiviral vectors (LVs), FV vectors are resistant to human serum inactivation,[14] which gives them a specific advantage in the context of in vivo delivery. FV
vector integrations are less frequent near transcriptional start sites when compared
with γ-retrovirus vectors, and FV vectors also do not show a preference for integrating within highly expressed genes, as has been observed for lentivirus vectors.[15] Importantly, Hendrie and colleagues[16] also showed that FV vector
proviruses are less likely to activate nearby genes even if they do integrate close
to them. Several groups demonstrated that FV vectors are highly proficient in
gene transfer to HSCs from both human and large animals, such that promising
therapeutic constructs can be efficiently evaluated under preclinical settings.
Safety of FV vectors for gene therapy applications has also been established in
dogs[17] and in human severe combined immunodeficiency (SCID) repopulating
cells.[18] FV vectors thus offer a unique combination of properties that makes
them a potentially superior choice for retrovirus gene therapy and for therapeutic
gene corrections with diseases such as SCID-X1. The authors have used the canine
SCID-X1 model, which is a naturally occurring genetic disease caused by inactivat-
ing mutations in the IL2RG gene that encodes the shared common gamma chain
(γC) signaling component of the interleukin-2 (IL-2), IL-4, IL-7, IL-9, and IL-15 receptors.[19] Canine SCID-X1 provides an excellent preclinical model because it man-
ifests nearly identical characteristics compared with human SCID-X1. Both
disorders are characterized by absent thymic T-cell development leading to an
absence of mature peripheral T cells, resulting in the lack of T-cell–mediated immune responses and dysregulated B-cell germinal center responses that, in
turn, lead to low immunoglobulin A (IgA), IgM, and IgG levels, absence of lymph
nodes, failure to thrive, and early infant mortality due to viral and/or bacterial
infection.[20]

The authors and others have explored in vivo gene therapy.[21] In collaboration with
Dr Peter Felsburg, the authors investigated in vivo delivery using FV vectors in
SCID-X1 dogs. IV injection of an FV vector expressing a codon-optimized human
γC gene in newborn SCID-X1 dogs resulted in expansion of corrected CD3 T lymphocytes that expressed the CD4 or CD8 coreceptors, underwent antigen receptor
gene rearrangement, and were functionally mature enough to respond to T-cell mi-
togens. Furthermore, FV integration site analysis demonstrated that the provirus did
not integrate near known proto-oncogenes, and there was no evidence of clonal
expansion that indicated a leukemic transformation.[21] The authors also evaluated
generation of specific antibody responses and immunoglobulin class-switching in
treated animals after immunization with the T-cell–dependent neoantigen bacteriophage, phiX174. This neoantigen has been used to evaluate dogs and humans with
SCID-X1 before and after bone marrow transplantation and gene therapy. The authors found that treated animals showed a primary and secondary antibody
response that is very similar to that seen in normal human controls, indicating
that the authors' treatment restored both the B- and the T-cell cytokine signaling
that is required for class switching and memory responses to this neoantigen. Alto-
gether, the authors' results demonstrate that in vivo gene therapy using FV vectors
is safe. In vivo delivery of γC-expressing FV vector to dogs resulted in immune
reconstitution with gene-corrected T cells, but the treated animals still developed infections and had low immunoglobulin levels, and marking levels in granulocytes and
monocytes were very low (0.6%), indicating that further increase in the efficacy of
HSC transduction is required to achieve long-term phenotypic correction. There
are several ways in which this type of in vivo gene therapy can be further optimized.

The kinetics of immune reconstitution may be enhanced by modifying FV vector design, for example, by using a stronger promoter in place of the currently used human elongation factor-1 alpha promoter (EF1α) to drive expression of γC. In addition, gene marking in other cell lineages that do not have a selective advantage like T lymphocytes may be increased by more efficiently targeting HSCs. More efficient HSC transduction could be accomplished by using mobilizing agents to increase the number of circulating HSCs in peripheral blood or by the in vivo selection of gene-modified HSCs. Importantly, the in vivo gene therapy procedure developed here for SCID-X1 is highly portable and could be disseminated worldwide for the treatment of additional genetic blood disorders.

Example 3: Intraosseal Lentivirus Injection in Mice

Although LVs have traditionally been used in ex vivo HSC gene therapy, recent advances showed that LVs can have utility for in vivo gene therapy. As an example, the authors discuss LV-mediated FVIII gene transfer by intrafemoral injection in mice. LV-mediated gene transfer into HSCs resulted in stable integration of FVIII gene into the host genome, leading to a persistent therapeutic effect.[22-24] This intraosseous (IO) infusion method was improved by using a syringe pump to slowly infuse LVs into the bone marrow so that more vectors can be retained for longer in the marrow cavity in order to achieve high levels of transduction of bone marrow cells.[22] In another study, a single infusion of GFP-LV achieved persistent GFP expression in 10% to 50% of HSCs for up to 160 days, indicating that IO LV delivery mediates sustained transduction of hematopoietic stem/progenitor cells.[22,25] Furthermore, IO delivery of E-F8-LVs encoding the FVIII gene driven by a ubiquitous EF1α promoter produced FVIII expression in various types of cells, including antigen-presenting cells, and high levels of FVIII were initially secreted into the circulation. However, a high-titer inhibitory antibody response to FVIII was rapidly induced, which completely eliminated functional FVIII activity. In contrast, a single IO infusion of G-F8-LVs driven by a megakaryocyte-specific promoter produced long-term stable expression of FVIII in platelets and initiated a long-term corrected hemophilia phenotype.[22] Most importantly, this strategy was also proven successful in hemophilia A mice with preexisting inhibitory antibodies.[22] This is because FVIII stored in α-granules of platelets is protected from high-titer anti-FVIII antibodies, and the locally excreted FVIII following platelet activation that participates directly in clot formation is functionally more potent than plasma FVIII.

Another example of IO injection was described by Frecha and colleagues.[13] They used LVs displaying stem cell factor and thrombopoietin, which allows for targeting of the vector particles to HSCs expressing c-Kit and c-Mpl. These vectors were more efficient in transducing CD34+ cells after intrafemural injection into mice with engrafted human CD34+ cells. However, the overall percentage of GFP+ cells in human CD45+ cells in the BM was only 0.7%.

Although IO LV injection in mice is technically difficult and challenging to standardize due to limited space for the injected virus in the bone, IO injection could be more feasible in large animals and humans. This is supported by studies with IO transplantation of HSCs. IO delivery of donor hematopoietic cells has been tested to mitigate the inevitable early loss of cells given IV to high blood volume organs, like liver and lung. It was first attempted in mice using different approaches[26-28] and later in larger animals, canines,[29] nonhuman primates,[30] and patients with cancer.[31,32] The source of cells was bone marrow, cord blood, or mobilized peripheral blood, and recipients either were myeloablated or received reduced intensity or no conditioning. Regarding the mouse, the overall assessment is that, despite multiple efforts, the outcome has not been better than the IV infusion, most likely because of anatomic constraints. In larger animals, the results differ depending on the number of cells used or the conditioning. The effort of using cord blood via the IO route is in its early stages, and many variables influencing the outcome need to be firmly ascertained; these include the optimum volume to be injected, the cell concentration, the number of injection sites, and the optimum conditioning.

Example 4: Hematopoietic Stem Cell Transduction Using Adeno-Associated Virus Vectors

Although the authors are not aware of published data describing direct in vivo HSC transduction following IV adeno-associated virus (AAV) vector delivery, this vector system has potential for in vivo HSC gene addition and targeting. Furthermore, AAV has proved highly promising in both preclinical and clinical safety and efficacy studies for hepatocyte-targeted gene therapy.[33,34] Several ex vivo studies with AAV and HSCs demonstrate their potential utility for in vivo HSC transduction, although HSCs from some but not all species can be efficiently transduced by AAV when the best serotype and culture conditions are used. AAV1 vectors, for example, can transduce mouse $Lin^-Sca1^+Kit^+$ (LSK) cells, whereas $CD34^+$ cells from cynomolgus monkeys are poorly transduced by AAV vectors derived from serotypes 1 to 10.[35] Several groups have shown that human HSCs can be readily transduced with AAV6-based vectors,[35,36] and vectors with AAV6 capsids containing surface-exposed tyrosine-to-phenylalanine mutations transduce human HSCs with the highest efficiency.[35,37]

The ability of AAV vectors to efficiently deliver their genomes to the nucleus of HSCs has led to the development of gene-targeting strategies, because their single-stranded vector genomes can be efficiently used as donor templates during the process of homologous recombination-directed targeted integration.[38] Two recent studies demonstrated that codelivery of an AAV6 donor template in combination with a target site–directed endonuclease leads to efficient ex vivo gene editing in human HSCs that retain the ability to engraft in NSG mice and differentiate into multiple hematopoietic lineages.[38] In vivo engraftment studies have also successfully been performed in mice using self-complementary AAV1 (scAAV) vector-transduced LSK cells. Unlike classical AAV vectors, scAAV vectors do not require second-strand synthesis or intermolecular annealing of their genomes to initiate transgene expression, so typically provide more efficient gene marking. Both primary and secondary transplant recipients showed up to 7% transgene expression in peripheral blood.[39] More recently, gene-edited HSCs that were engineered using ZFN endonucleases and AAV6-derived targeting vectors showed long-term engraftment and differentiation in NSG mice.[36] A similar ZFN plus AAV6–based ex vivo approach to HSC gene editing has subsequently been used for the treatment of X-linked chronic granulomatous disease, with up to 11% of bone marrow cells in primary recipients containing an introduced copy of the gp91phox subunit of the NADPH oxidase.[40]

AAV does have some potential disadvantages for direct in vivo use such as the relatively high cost of production and limited knowledge of the in vivo tropism for AAV serotypes that can transduce HSCs ex vivo. For example, AAV6 shows high affinity for skeletal muscle upon IV administration,[41] which will likely impede attempts to target HSCs in situ. Furthermore, although efficient gene expression in the liver can theoretically be achieved from episomal AAV vector genomes, HSC gene therapy requires vector integration, a process that is not well studied in HSCs.

Example 5: In Vivo Transduction of Primitive Hematopoietic Stem Cells After Mobilization and Intravenous Injection of Integrating Helper-Dependent Adenovirus Vectors

Human adenovirus (Ad) has long been used as a gene transfer vector to various tissues. However, early studies showed that the most commonly used serotype, Ad5, was incapable of efficiently transducing HSCs. In contrast, other less studied Ad serotypes, especially those belonging to human species B, showed much more promise in their ability to transduce HSCs. Several species of B Ads, including serotypes 11, 16, 21, 34, 35, and 50, use CD46 as a receptor,[42] a membrane protein expressed on all nucleated cells in humans. Its main function is to protect self-tissue from inadvertent killing by the complement system, but it also has important signaling functions, for example, in the regulation of T-cell activity.[43] The authors and others have found that CD46 is uniformly expressed on all CD34$^+$ cells.[42,44]

In order to harness the well-understood biology of Ad5, the tools to manipulate and vectorize Ad, as well as the enhanced HSC transduction capabilities of species B Ads, fiber-chimeric vectors containing species B fibers on an Ad5 capsid were developed. Vectors carrying the fiber of CD46-tropic adenovirus type 35 (Ad5/35) were subsequently shown to efficiently transduce human HSCs.[44–48] Importantly, after IV injection into mice and nonhuman primates, first-generation Ad5/35 vectors did not cause liver toxicity,[49–51] a problem seen with serotype 5 (Ad5) -based vectors.[52] Moreover, the authors' group introduced mutations in the Ad35 fiber knob to further increase its affinity toward the Ad35 cellular receptor CD46, leading to increased transduction capabilities when targeting HSCs.[53]

To further increase the suitability as a gene transfer vector for HSCs, helper-dependent adenovirus vectors (HDAds) have been developed.[54–57] These vectors are devoid of all viral genes and only contain minimal amounts of viral DNA. This completely abolishes the leaky expression of adenoviral genes that had been shown to lead to cytotoxicity in HSCs that have been transduced with earlier Ad vectors that still encoded these genes.[56,57]

The goal of HSC gene therapy is the lifelong correction of an underlying genetic disease. To fulfill this requirement, integration of the therapeutic transgene is generally required so that gene-corrected HSCs are able to give rise to gene corrected progeny cells. Ad5, however, does not actively integrate its genetic material into the genome of infected cells. To counteract this shortcoming, HDAd vectors can be armed with transposon-based transgene integration systems. Multiple class II DNA transposons display activity in human cells, including Tol2, piggyBac, and Sleeping Beauty (SB). Tol2 and piggyBac have the propensity to integrate transposons in and around actively transcribed genes.[58] In the authors' studies, they have used a hyperactive Sleeping Beauty (SB100x) transposase system.[59,60] The SB transposase, when coexpressed in trans from a second vector, recognizes specific DNA sequences (inverted repeats, "IRs") flanking the transgene cassette and triggers its integration into thymidine-adenosine (TA) dinucleotides of chromosomal DNA. Unlike retrovirus integration, SB-mediated integration does not depend on the transcriptional status of the targeted genes nor on cellular DNA repair proteins.[61] Studies with human cell lines and mouse hepatocytes in vitro and in vivo showed that SB-mediated transgene integration is random and has not been associated with the activation of protooncogenes.[60]

In the authors' experience, IV injection of Ad vectors in mice and nonhuman primates does not lead to transduction of HSCs in the bone marrow, even if the vector is capable of efficiently transducing HSCs in vitro.[49,50] They therefore decided to mobilize HSCs from the bone marrow and transduced them in the periphery with integrating HDAd5/35^{++} vectors.

In the authors' studies, they used the SB100x vector platform in the context of HSC gene therapy and a human CD46 transgenic mouse model to study stable transfer a reporter gene cassette into HSCs in vivo.[62] HSCs were mobilized from the bone marrow of mice into the peripheral blood through administration of G-CSF and AMD3100, after which integrating HDAd5/35 vectors were injected IV. The authors were able to show in vivo transduction following this regimen as reporter gene–positive LSK cells could be detected in the bone marrow of mice (**Fig. 2**A). The authors saw that 6.5% of bone marrow LSK cells expressed a reporter transgene at 20 weeks after in vivo transduction. Furthermore, HSCs transduced in this way could give rise to progenitor colonies consisting of reporter gene-positive progeny cells (**Fig. 2**B), and at 20 weeks after in vivo transduction, 9% of CFU progenitor colonies were positive for the transgene. This showed that the reporter gene had been integrated into the HSC genome and that the gene-modified cells were still functional stem cells capable of proliferation and differentiation. Importantly, CFU assays showed an increase in GFP-positive colonies over time, indicating transduction of long-term surviving and potentially self-renewing cells capable of reconstitution of hematopoiesis in lethally irradiated transplant recipients. Moreover, the authors demonstrated that HSCs modified after in vivo transduction could rescue lethally irradiated mice upon transplantation and that the recipients of these transplants showed reporter gene expression in all hematopoietic lineages up to 16 weeks after transplantation. In addition, successful

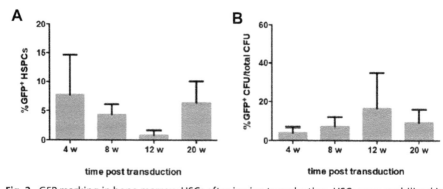

Fig. 2. GFP marking in bone marrow HSCs after in vivo transduction. HSCs were mobilized in human CD46 transgenic mice by SC injections of human recombinant G-CSF (5 μg per mouse per day, 4 days) followed by an SC injection of AMD3100 (5 mg/kg) 18 hours after the last G-CSF injection. Two integrating HD-Ad5/35^{++} vectors at a total dose of 8×10^{10} viral particles were injected IV 1 hour after AMD3100. One Ad (HDAd-GFP) contains a GFP gene under the control of the EF1α promoter, and the transgene cassette is flanked by inverted repeats that are recognized by the SB transposase. The second Ad vector (HDAd-SB) expresses the hyperactive SB transposase SB100x in trans. Animals were sacrificed 4, 8, 12, or 20 weeks after Ad transduction and bone marrow cells were isolated ($n \geq 10$). (A) Shown is the percentage of GFP-positive HSCs (LSK) present in the bone marrow. (B) GFP expression in colony forming units. Bone marrow cells were lineage depleted via magnetic-activated cell sorting (MACS) followed by collection of GFP-positive cells via FACS. Cells were then plated in CFU assays, and colonies were scored 12 days after plating. HSPC, hematopoietic stem and progenitor cell. (*Data from* Richter M, Saydaminova K, Yumul R, et al. In vivo transduction of primitive mobilized hematopoietic stem cells after intravenous injection of integrating adenovirus vectors. Blood 2016;128(18):2206–17).

HSC transduction could be shown in a humanized mouse model when using a similar in vivo transduction regimen.

In addition to the general advantages of in vivo HSC gene therapy, the use of adeno-viral vectors for this application provides several additional advantages. HDAd vectors have a relatively large cloning capacity of up to 34 kb. However, it has to be noted that when using the SB transposase, efficient transposition is only observed for cassettes of up to 10 kb in size. Nevertheless, the adenoviral in vivo delivery approach could also be used in the context of a targeted nuclease approach in which the large cloning ca-pacity of Ad vectors could be exploited to deliver both a nuclease and a homologous recombination template for a gene of interest using the same vector.

Another major advantage of the use of adenoviral gene transfer vectors is their ease of production. HDAd vectors can be easily produced to high titers and scale up is usu-ally uncomplicated because the production of these vectors does not rely on large-scale transfection of genetic material. These advantages also result in a relatively low-vector production cost, often orders of magnitude lower than those encountered for lentiviral or AAV vectors. A further advantage of an Ad vector platform is the ability to lyophilize vector preparations to ensure long-term stability even when stored at 4°C.[63]

DISCUSSION

In vivo HSC gene transfer achieved using a minimally invasive manner and without the need for stem cell harvest or transplantation should simplify HSC gene therapy. Further-more, by avoiding ex vivo HSC manipulation, the risk of cell differentiation or loss of homing/engraftment capability is avoided, because there is no need for the extraction and purification of target cells. In vivo gene delivery also bypasses the issue concerning the markers that enable the isolation of true primitive HSCs. In vivo gene transfer could target all HSCs, including those that are missed by different purification criteria. Finally, in vivo HSC transduction should eliminate the need for myelo-conditioning with chemo-therapy drugs. Preconditioning results in considerable early morbidity owing to transi-tory blood-cell depletion, immunodeficiency, and mucosal damage, which place the recipient at risk of severe infection.[64] It also causes delayed morbidity owing to the risk of developing chemotherapy-induced secondary tumors and infertility. Several HSC gene-therapy trials have attempted to alleviate the morbidity associated with pre-conditioning by lowering the dosage and combination of chemotherapeutic drugs. However, the impact of changing these drug regimens on the risks and benefits of the therapy is yet to be determined in broader comparative studies and through long-term patient follow-up. Finally, the technical complexity and high cost of current ex vivo HSC gene therapy are barriers to a widespread application for common dis-eases. As an example, Strimvelis, an HSC gene therapy for ADA-SCID that has been approved for marketing in the European Union earlier this year, comes at a price of close to $700,000 per treatment, and the regimen is only available at a single center in Europe, making access to it difficult even within the developed countries of Europe.

In vivo HSC gene transfer approaches do pose several potential problems, with the most important ones being due to direct contact between the gene transfer vector and the patient, which can trigger innate and adaptive immune responses. This problem is specifically pronounced for approaches involving IV vector injection. Viral vectors and nonviral nanoparticles are taken up by monocytes and macrophages in various tis-sues, specifically within the liver and spleen, and the incoming particle and DNA or RNA is sensed by innate immune mechanism. This results in release and activation of proinflammatory cytokines.[65] It is thought that AAV vectors provoke weaker innate immune responses than other viral vectors such as Ad or LV[66]; however, at this point no direct comparisons of these vector systems with regards to innate toxicity have been made following IV injection. In the authors' studies with HDAd5/35[++] vectors, they found that the release of proinflammatory cytokines upon vector administration is increased by mobilization. Mobilization, specifically regimens that involve G-CSF, triggers acute leukocytosis so that more monocytes in the circulation can come into contact with the IV-injected vector. Acute cytokine release however can be prevented by pretreatment with glucocorticoids,[67] or anti-IL-6/anti-IL-6–receptor antibodies.[68]

Another problem, specifically when using Ad and AAV vectors, is preexisting B- and T-cell responses against capsid proteins that can target infected cells or neutralize IV-injected particles before they transduce HSCs and prevent readministration. For example, the serum prevalence of neutralizing antibodies against AAV6 is 46%,[69] and most people have serum antibodies against Ad5 and specifically against the part of Ad5 that is present in Ad5/35.[70] One alternative would be to use vectors derived from Ad35, because it is one of the rarest human serotypes, with a seroprevalence of less than 7%.[71] After IV injection of Ad35 vectors, there is only minimal transduction (only detectable by PCR) of tissues, including the liver, in human CD46 transgenic mice[72] and nonhuman primates.[73] Ad35 vectors have been used in clinical trials as vaccine vectors. Should preexisting immunity remain a problem, transient immunosuppression has been effective when countering humoral immunity in liver gene therapy trials that used AAV8 vectors.[34]

Another potential drawback for IV HSC gene transfer is the requirement for higher doses of gene therapy vectors when compared with ex vivo approaches due to vector sequestration by the reticuloendothelial system and the transduction of cells other than HSCs. Also, most mobilization treatments do not specifically mobilize HSCs into the bloodstream. In the authors' studies, they have shown transduction of lineage-positive cells at day 3 after HDAd5/35[++] injection.[62] Even though these non-HSCs could express the transgene, their half-life, compared with HSCs, is short, and the potential harm of them expressing the transgene would soon be lost. As a potential solution to this problem, vectors specifically targeted to HSCs could be generated. Some work has been done in this respect,[74] whereby a LV retargeted toward CD133 efficiently transduced cells with high multilineage reconstituting potential. Vector sequestration by macrophages of the liver, lung, and spleen also remains a major unsolved obstacle to lowering IV-injected vector doses, although the impact of the requirement of higher vector titers is highly dependent on the vector platform that is being used. For example, although Ad vectors are relatively inexpensive and easy to produce in large amounts, this will be more challenging for lentivirus and AAV vectors.

Another group of potential problems could be associated with the mobilization process that results in a significant increase in white blood cell counts. In the authors' mouse studies, they observed up to 20-fold higher white blood cells 1 hour after G-CSF/AMD3100 mobilization. A significant fraction of mobilized cells might resettle in the spleen, and this has, in rare cases, led to splenic ruptures in patients.

In summary, in vivo HSC gene therapy has the potential to move HSC-directed gene therapy out of a few very specialized centers and may enable applications for common diseases at more affordable prices. However, before a widespread application of this approach can become a reality, more rigorous efficacy and safety studies are required.

REFERENCES

1. Zhang J, Niu C, Ye L, et al. Identification of the haematopoietic stem cell niche and control of the niche size. Nature 2003;425(6960):836–41.

2. Bonig H, Papayannopoulou T. Mobilization of hematopoietic stem/progenitor cells: general principles and molecular mechanisms. Methods Mol Biol 2012; 904:1–14.
3. Trumpp A, Essers M, Wilson A. Awakening dormant haematopoietic stem cells. Nat Rev Immunol 2010;10(3):201–9.
4. Broxmeyer HE, Orschell CM, Clapp DW, et al. Rapid mobilization of murine and human hematopoietic stem and progenitor cells with AMD3100, a CXCR4 antagonist. J Exp Med 2005;201(8):1307–18.
5. Calandra G, McCarty J, McGuirk J, et al. AMD3100 plus G-CSF can successfully mobilize CD34+ cells from non-Hodgkin's lymphoma, Hodgkin's disease and multiple myeloma patients previously failing mobilization with chemotherapy and/or cytokine treatment: compassionate use data. Bone Marrow Transplant 2008;41(4):331–8.
6. Andrews RG, Bartelmez SH, Knitter GH, et al. A c-kit ligand, recombinant human stem cell factor, mediates reversible expansion of multiple CD34+ colony-forming cell types in blood and marrow of baboons. Blood 1992;80(4):920–7.
7. Craddock CF, Nakamoto B, Andrews RG, et al. Antibodies to VLA4 integrin mobilize long-term repopulating cells and augment cytokine-induced mobilization in primates and mice. Blood 1997;90(12):4779–88.
8. Ramirez P, Rettig MP, Uy GL, et al. BIO5192, a small molecule inhibitor of VLA-4, mobilizes hematopoietic stem and progenitor cells. Blood 2009;114(7):1340–3.
9. Bonig H, Watts KL, Chang KH, et al. Concurrent blockade of alpha4-integrin and CXCR4 in hematopoietic stem/progenitor cell mobilization. Stem Cells 2009; 27(4):836–7.
10. Cao B, Zhang Z, Grassinger J, et al. Therapeutic targeting and rapid mobilization of endosteal HSC using a small molecule integrin antagonist. Nat Commun 2016; 7:11007.
11. Rogers FA, Vasquez KM, Egholm M, et al. Site-directed recombination via bifunctional PNA-DNA conjugates. Proc Natl Acad Sci U S A 2002;99(26):16695–700.
12. Bahal R, Ali McNeer N, Quijano E, et al. In vivo correction of anaemia in beta-thalassemic mice by gammaPNA-mediated gene editing with nanoparticle delivery. Nat Commun 2016;7:13304.
13. Frecha C, Fusil F, Cosset FL, et al. In vivo gene delivery into hCD34+ cells in a humanized mouse model. Methods Mol Biol 2011;737:367–90.
14. Russell DW, Miller AD. Foamy virus vectors. J Virol 1996;70(1):217–22.
15. Trobridge GD, Miller DG, Jacobs MA, et al. Foamy virus vector integration sites in normal human cells. Proc Natl Acad Sci 2006;103(5):1498–503.
16. Hendrie PC, Huo Y, Stolitenko RB, et al. A rapid and quantitative assay for measuring neighboring gene activation by vector proviruses. Mol Ther 2008; 16(3):534–40.
17. Kiem HP, Allen J, Trobridge G, et al. Foamy-virus-mediated gene transfer to canine repopulating cells. Blood 2007;109(1):65–70.
18. Everson EM, Olzsko ME, Leap DJ, et al. A comparison of foamy and lentiviral vector genotoxicity in SCID-repopulating cells shows foamy vectors are less prone to clonal dominance. Mol Ther Methods Clin Dev 2016;3:16048.
19. Henthorn PS, Somberg RL, Fimiani VM, et al. IL-2R gamma gene microdeletion demonstrates that canine X-linked severe combined immunodeficiency is a homologue of the human disease. Genomics 1994;23(1):69–74.
20. Gougeon ML, Drean G, Le Deist F, et al. Human severe combined immunodeficiency disease: phenotypic and functional characteristics of peripheral B lymphocytes. J Immunol 1990;145(9):2873–9.

21. Burtner CR, Beard BC, Kennedy DR, et al. Intravenous injection of a foamy virus vector to correct canine SCID-X1. Blood 2014;123(23):3578–84.

22. Wang X, Shin SC, Chiang AF, et al. Intraosseous delivery of lentiviral vectors targeting factor VIII expression in platelets corrects murine hemophilia A. Mol Ther 2015;23(4):617–26.

23. Ide LM, Gangadharan B, Chiang KY, et al. Hematopoietic stem-cell gene therapy of hemophilia A incorporating a porcine factor VIII transgene and nonmyeloablative conditioning regimens. Blood 2007;110(8):2855–63.

24. Kuether EL, Schroeder JA, Fahs SA, et al. Lentivirus-mediated platelet gene therapy of murine hemophilia A with pre-existing anti-factor VIII immunity. J Thromb Haemost 2012;10(8):1570–80.

25. Wang CX, Sather BD, Wang X, et al. Rapamycin relieves lentiviral vector transduction resistance in human and mouse hematopoietic stem cells. Blood 2014; 124(6):913–23.

26. Mazurier F, Doedens M, Gan OI, et al. Rapid myeloerythroid repopulation after intrafemoral transplantation of NOD-SCID mice reveals a new class of human stem cells. Nat Med 2003;9(7):959–63.

27. Wang J, Kimura T, Asada R, et al. SCID-repopulating cell activity of human cord blood-derived CD34- cells assured by intra-bone marrow injection. Blood 2003; 101(8):2924–31.

28. van Os R, Ausema A, Dontje B, et al. Engraftment of syngeneic bone marrow is not more efficient after intrafemoral transplantation than after traditional intravenous administration. Exp Hematol 2010;38(11):1115–23.

29. Lange S, Steder A, Killian D, et al. Engraftment efficiency after intra-bone marrow versus intravenous transplantation of bone marrow cells in a canine nonmyeloablative dog nucleoside antigen-identical transplantation model. Biol Blood Marrow Transplant 2017;23(2):247–54.

30. Feng Q, Chow PK, Frassoni F, et al. Nonhuman primate allogeneic hematopoietic stem cell transplantation by intraosseus vs intravenous injection: engraftment, donor cell distribution, and mechanistic basis. Exp Hematol 2008;36(11): 1556–66.

31. Rocha V, Labopin M, Ruggeri A, et al. Unrelated cord blood transplantation: outcomes after single-unit intrabone injection compared with double-unit intravenous injection in patients with hematological malignancies. Transplantation 2013;95(10):1284–91.

32. Massollo M, Podesta M, Marini C, et al. Contact with the bone marrow microenvironment readdresses the fate of transplanted hematopoietic stem cells. Exp Hematol 2010;38(10):968–77.

33. Kay MA, Manno CS, Ragni MV, et al. Evidence for gene transfer and expression of factor IX in haemophilia B patients treated with an AAV vector. Nat Genet 2000; 24(3):257–61.

34. Nathwani AC, Reiss UM, Tuddenham EG, et al. Long-term safety and efficacy of factor IX gene therapy in hemophilia B. N Engl J Med 2014;371(21):1994–2004.

35. Song L, Kauss MA, Kopin E, et al. Optimizing the transduction efficiency of capsid-modified AAV6 serotype vectors in primary human hematopoietic stem cells in vitro and in a xenograft mouse model in vivo. Cytotherapy 2013;15(8): 986–98.

36. Wang J, Exline CM, DeClercq JJ, et al. Homology-driven genome editing in hematopoietic stem and progenitor cells using ZFN mRNA and AAV6 donors. Nat Biotechnol 2015;33(12):1256–63.

37. Song L, Li X, Jayandharan GR, et al. High-efficiency transduction of primary human hematopoietic stem cells and erythroid lineage-restricted expression by optimized AAV6 serotype vectors in vitro and in a murine xenograft model in vivo. PLoS One 2013;8(3):e58757.
38. Khan IF, Hirata RK, Russell DW. AAV-mediated gene targeting methods for human cells. Nat Protoc 2011;6(4):482–501.
39. Maina N, Han Z, Li X, et al. Recombinant self-complementary adeno-associated virus serotype vector-mediated hematopoietic stem cell transduction and lineage-restricted, long-term transgene expression in a murine serial bone marrow transplantation model. Hum Gene Ther 2008;19(4):376–83.
40. De Ravin SS, Reik A, Liu PQ, et al. Targeted gene addition in human CD34(+) hematopoietic cells for correction of X-linked chronic granulomatous disease. Nat Biotechnol 2016;34(4):424–9.
41. Gregorevic P, Blankinship MJ, Allen JM, et al. Systemic delivery of genes to striated muscles using adeno-associated viral vectors. Nat Med 2004;10(8):828–34.
42. Gaggar A, Shayakhmetov D, Lieber A. CD46 is a cellular receptor for group B adenoviruses. Nat Med 2003;9:1408–12.
43. Marie JC, Astier AL, Rivailler P, et al. Linking innate and acquired immunity: divergent role of CD46 cytoplasmic domains in T cell induced inflammation. Nat Immunol 2002;3(7):659–66.
44. Li L, Krymskaya L, Wang J, et al. Genomic editing of the HIV-1 coreceptor CCR5 in adult hematopoietic stem and progenitor cells using zinc finger nucleases. Mol Ther 2013;21(6):1259–69.
45. Shayakhmetov DM, Papayannopoulou T, Stamatoyannopoulos G, et al. Efficient gene transfer into human CD34(+) cells by a retargeted adenovirus vector. J Virol 2000;74(6):2567–83.
46. Yotnda P, Onishi H, Heslop HE, et al. Efficient infection of primitive hematopoietic stem cells by modified adenovirus. Gene Ther 2001;8(12):930–7.
47. Lu ZZ, Ni F, Hu ZB, et al. Efficient gene transfer into hematopoietic cells by a retargeting adenoviral vector system with a chimeric fiber of adenovirus serotype 5 and 11p. Exp Hematol 2006;34(9):1171–82.
48. Nilsson M, Karlsson S, Fan X. Functionally distinct subpopulations of cord blood CD34+ cells are transduced by adenoviral vectors with serotype 5 or 35 tropism. Mol Ther 2004;9(3):377–88.
49. Di Paolo N, Ni S, Gaggar A, et al. Evaluation of adenovirus vectors containing serotype 35 fibers for tumor targeting. Cancer Gene Ther 2006;13:1072–81.
50. Ni S, Bernt K, Gaggar A, et al. Evaluation of biodistribution and safety of adenovirus vectors containing group B fibers after intravenous injection into baboons. Hum Gene Ther 2005;16(6):664–77.
51. Kalyuzhniy O, Di Paolo NC, Silvestry M, et al. Adenovirus serotype 5 hexon is critical for virus infection of hepatocytes in vivo. Proc Natl Acad Sci U S A 2008;105(14):5483–8.
52. Brunetti-Pierri N, Palmer DJ, Beaudet AL, et al. Acute toxicity after high-dose systemic injection of helper-dependent adenoviral vectors into non-human primates. Hum Gene Ther 2004;15:35–46.
53. Wang H, Liu Y, Li Z, et al. In vitro and in vivo properties of adenovirus vectors with increased affinity to CD46. J Virol 2008;82(21):10567–79.
54. Morral N, Parks RJ, Zhou H, et al. High doses of a helper-dependent adenoviral vector yield supraphysiological levels of alpha1-antitrypsin with negligible toxicity. Hum Gene Ther 1998;9(18):2709–16.

55. Balamotis MA, Huang K, Mitani K. Efficient delivery and stable gene expression in a hematopoietic cell line using a chimeric serotype 35 fiber pseudotyped helper-dependent adenoviral vector. Virology 2004;324(1):229–37.

56. Wang H, Cao H, Wohlfahrt M, et al. Tightly regulated gene expression in human hematopoietic stem cells after transduction with helper-dependent Ad5/35 vectors. Exp Hematol 2008;36(7):823–31.

57. Wang H, Shayakhmetov DM, Leege T, et al. A capsid-modified helper-dependent adenovirus vector containing the beta-globin locus control region displays a nonrandom integration pattern and allows stable, erythroid-specific gene expression. J Virol 2005;79(17):10999–1013.

58. Guerrero AD, Moyes JS, Cooper LJ. The human application of gene therapy to reprogram T-cell specificity using chimeric antigen receptors. Chin J Cancer 2014; 33(9):421–33.

59. Hausl MA, Zhang W, Muther N, et al. Hyperactive sleeping beauty transposase enables persistent phenotypic correction in mice and a canine model for hemophilia B. Mol Ther 2010;18(11):1896–906.

60. Yant SR, Ehrhardt A, Mikkelsen JG, et al. Transposition from a gutless adeno-transposon vector stabilizes transgene expression in vivo. Nat Biotechnol 2002; 20(10):999–1005.

61. Yant SR, Wu X, Huang Y, et al. High-resolution genome-wide mapping of transposon integration in mammals. Mol Cell Biol 2005;25(6):2085–94.

62. Richter M, Saydaminova K, Yumul R, et al. In vivo transduction of primitive mobilized hematopoietic stem cells after intravenous injection of integrating adenovirus vectors. Blood 2016;128(18):2206–17.

63. Croyle MA, Cheng X, Wilson JM. Development of formulations that enhance physical stability of viral vectors for gene therapy. Gene Ther 2001;8(17):1281–90.

64. Copelan EA. Hematopoietic stem-cell transplantation. N Engl J Med 2006; 354(17):1813–26.

65. Atasheva S, Shayakhmetov DM. Adenovirus sensing by the immune system. Curr Opin Virol 2016;21:109–13.

66. Suzuki M, Bertin TK, Rogers GL, et al. Differential type I interferon-dependent transgene silencing of helper-dependent adenoviral vs. adeno-associated viral vectors in vivo. Mol Ther 2013;21(4):796–805.

67. Seregin SS, Appledorn DM, McBride AJ, et al. Transient pretreatment with glucocorticoid ablates innate toxicity of systemically delivered adenoviral vectors without reducing efficacy. Mol Ther 2009;17(4):685–96.

68. Chen F, Teachey DT, Pequignot E, et al. Measuring IL-6 and sIL-6R in serum from patients treated with tocilizumab and/or siltuximab following CAR T cell therapy. J Immunol Methods 2016;434:1–8.

69. Boutin S, Monteilhet V, Veron P, et al. Prevalence of serum IgG and neutralizing factors against adeno-associated virus (AAV) types 1, 2, 5, 6, 8, and 9 in the healthy population: implications for gene therapy using AAV vectors. Hum Gene Ther 2010;21(6):704–12.

70. Bradley RR, Maxfield LF, Lynch DM, et al. Adenovirus serotype 5-specific neutralizing antibodies target multiple hexon hypervariable regions. J Virol 2012;86(2): 1267–72.

71. Barouch DH, Kik SV, Weverling GJ, et al. International seroepidemiology of adenovirus serotypes 5, 26, 35, and 48 in pediatric and adult populations. Vaccine 2011;29(32):5203–9.

72. Sakurai F, Kawabata K, Koizumi N, et al. Adenovirus serotype 35 vector-mediated transduction into human CD46-transgenic mice. Gene Ther 2006;13(14): 1118–26.
73. Sakurai F, Nakamura S, Akitomo K, et al. Transduction properties of adenovirus serotype 35 vectors after intravenous administration into nonhuman primates. Mol Ther 2008;16(4):726–33.
74. Brendel C, Goebel B, Daniela A, et al. CD133-targeted gene transfer into long-term repopulating hematopoietic stem cells. Mol Ther 2015;23(1):63–70.

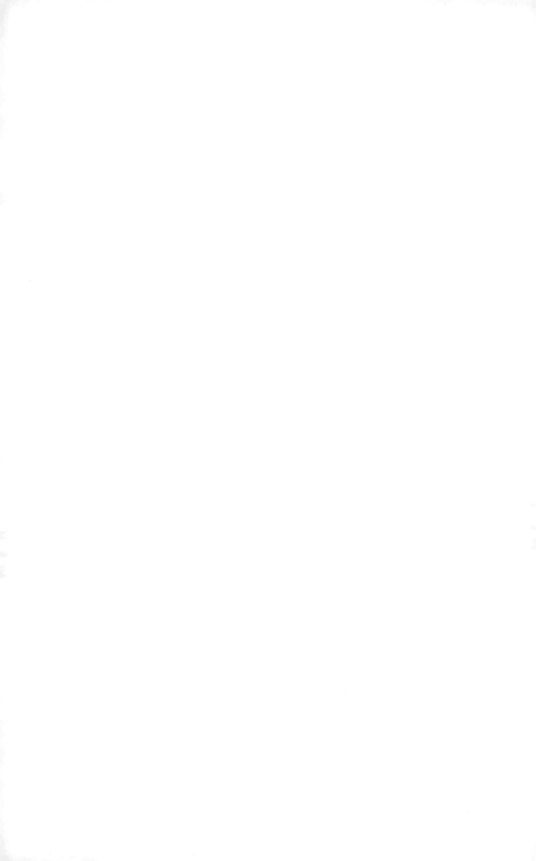

Therapeutic Gene Editing Safety and Specificity

Christopher T. Lux, MD, PhD[a],*, Andrew M. Scharenberg, MD[b,c]

KEYWORDS

• Gene therapy • Safety • Specific • Gene editing • Off-target

KEY POINTS

- Safety of gene editing is closely tied to specificity.
- Careful design of gene editing tools can improve specificity and thus safety.
- A high degree of specificity is possible with the new generation of targeted nucleases.
- Assessing the impact of gene therapy tools during their design, study, and clinical use is essential.

INTRODUCTION

Therapeutic gene editing is advancing at an ever-increasing pace. As the list of diseases that can be treated or potentially cured with gene editing grows, it is imperative to dedicate time and energy to the topics of the safety and specificity of these technologies. This article is dedicated to a discussion of this topic in a broad sense with examples to detail how these issues affect various aspects of modifying the genetic code of patients.

As discussed in the opening article of this issue, expectations have always been high for the potential of gene therapy but early forays into its clinical application had unexpected consequences. (See Kohn DB's article, "Historical Perspective on the Current Renaissance for Hematopoietic Stem Cell Gene Therapy," in this issue.) These early setbacks in the implementation of gene therapy caused the research community and the public at large to take pause and consider the safety of this fledgling field. All involved realized that this was new and unexplored territory. Unexpected consequences can and do occur with new medical technologies. It is important to remember that expectations today may be higher for these pursuits than previous eras of medical exploration. Modifying genetic code is fundamentally different from the study of chemicals to kill a particular bacterial strain or slow the growth of a tumor. Rather than externally manipulating the biology of organisms or aberrant cells, the aim is to alter the

[a] Department of Pediatrics, Cancer and Blood Disorders Center, Seattle Children's Hospital, 4800 Sand Point Way NE, Seattle, WA 98105, USA; [b] Department of Pediatrics, Seattle Children's Hospital, 4800 Sand Point Way NE, Seattle, WA 98105, USA; [c] Department of Immunology, Seattle Children's Hospital, 4800 Sand Point Way NE, Seattle, WA 98105, USA
* Corresponding author.
E-mail address: Christopher.Lux@seattlechildrens.org

Hematol Oncol Clin N Am 31 (2017) 787–795
http://dx.doi.org/10.1016/j.hoc.2017.05.002
0889-8588/17/© 2017 Elsevier Inc. All rights reserved.

hemonc.theclinics.com

blueprint of the disease-associated cells to restore or modify their function. Like a surgeon pinpoints a physical defect based on accepted anatomical function and makes repairs, so too are oncologists starting with a map (the normal genome) and working to correct errors. Precision and safety will be expected and demanded. Trial and error will only be acceptable to a point.

Before proceeding, a brief discussion of the stewardship of the human genome is prudent. The most fundamental elements of what defines being human are beginning to be modified. This requires an enormous amount of public support and trust. Although there is clearly support for the treatment and cure of genetic diseases, history shows that these technologies can also be misused. Part of safely developing these tools is considering the consequences of their misapplication. The pursuit or even the perception of the application of gene therapy for eugenics or genetic discrimination could be devastating. Care should be taken in the selection of disease targets and even in the words chosen to describe the diseases to be treated. Respect should be given to historic and cultural diversity. Maintaining a sense of transparency and being open to discussion of the practical impacts of genetic modifications are important elements to maintaining the integrity of gene therapy.

SAFETY

Safe manipulation of the human genome is paramount to gene therapy because the intended effect of gene therapy is a permanent modification of cell function. Thus, unintended modifications that alter cell function may have long-lasting consequences.

The last decade has seen the rapid introduction of new tools, including zinc finger nucleases, homing endonucleases, transcription activator-like effector nucleases (TALENs), and RNA-guided nucleases that allow for the targeted modification of cellular genomes. The unifying activity for all of these tools is their nuclease activity, which is the ability to bind a specific sequence anywhere in the genome and introduce a DNA double-strand break (DSB). Once a DSB is generated, repair occurs through one of two basic types of mechanisms: nonhomologous end joining (NHEJ) or homology-directed repair, such as homologous recombination (HR). With enzymatically generated DSBs, NHEJ will typically lead to seamless religation of the break. However, NHEJ may introduce insertions or deletions at the DSB at appreciable frequencies, which can be useful for disrupting gene expression or function, or modifying regulatory functions mediated by the targeted sequences. HR involves the repair of a DSB using a repair template with homology to the sequences flanking the cut site. This template can either be endogenous, such as from a sister chromatid, or may be exogenously introduced. Thus, in addition to simple disruption of the targeted region, HR can be used to introduce complex engineered genetic elements.

When the genome is edited with therapeutic intent, it is an attempt to generate controlled genetic damage and the native repair mechanisms of the cell are relied on to repair the damage. In the safe translation of gene editing to a patient population, it is worth considering that induced genetic damage in the form of chemotherapy and radiation for has been used for decades. The underlying principle of cancer treatment is inducing genetic damage in a fashion that is toxic to cancer cells but does not overwhelm the repair mechanisms of healthy cells. An assessment of chromosomal instability has recently been shown to help predict the survival of a patient receiving chemotherapy and/or radiation.[1] Attempts to concentrate the genetic damage to sites of disease, such as administering intrathecal chemotherapy for central nervous system malignancies or using proton beam therapy to narrow the radiation window are steps toward tissue-level specificity but the impact on treated cells is genome wide.

Side effects, both short term and long term, do occur and are well known to the oncologist. Thankfully, although secondary malignancies can occur as a result of chemotherapy and radiation treatment, most patients do not develop treatment-related tumors. The cells either repair their genetic damage or undergo cell death in the presence of excessive damage. By comparison, the risk posed by introducing a transiently expressed, targeted endonuclease that has passed through extensive screening for off-target cutting should be significantly less dangerous. Although the introduction of synthetic genetic elements by HR raises the potential for unintended consequences, the editing process and integration are similarly designed for specificity and would not be predicted to approach the magnitude of risk seen with already accepted treatments for cancer therapy.

Among potential safety concerns of gene editing, the most fundamental is the potential for the nuclease to introduce DSBs at unintended sites in the genome. If the precise targeted sequence or sequence sufficiently similar exists elsewhere in the genome, that site has the potential to be cleaved in addition to the intended site. When designing a targeted endonuclease, it is critical to anticipate potential off-target cleavage sites and select sequences that minimize this potential. This is most commonly carried out initially in silico using tools such as the Predicted Report Of Genome-wide Nuclease Off-target Sites tool for zinc fingers and TALENS (designed and maintained by the Gang Bao Laboratory of Rice University; http://bao.rice.edu/Research/BioinformaticTools/prognos.html) and the clustered regularly-interspaced short palindromic repeats (CRISPR) Design tool (designed and maintained by the Feng Zhang Laboratory of MIT; http://crispr.mit.edu/).[2,3] Unlike basic primer design or sequence alignment tools, these algorithms take into account the nature of the endonuclease platform, such as spacer length for TALENS and Protospacer Adjacent Motif sites for CRISPR, and are better suited for identifying accurate off-target sites within the genome.[4] These tools offer rapid results to aid in the selection and design of potential nucleases. Once an endonuclease has been generated, in vitro screening has been made possible by means of Systematic Evolution of Ligands by eXponential Enrichment (SELEX).[5] SELEX queries the propensity of the endonuclease to cleave a library of various oligonucleotides. The genome can then be probed for the presence of sequences with the highest rates of in vitro cleavage. Matching sequences are an excellent starting point for the search of off-target cleavage postediting in target cells.

Screening for off-target activity is also necessarily performed following the genetic modification of target cells using the intended manufacturing process for cells to be engrafted in patients. Sequencing at in silico predicted off-target cut sites can reveal if mutation has occurred at these specific loci. Mutation events at sites not included in the in silico prediction, as well as nonmutational on-target cleavage repairs, will be missed by this technique. Genome-wide off-target editing analysis has been analyzed either by detection of repair template integration or chromatin immunoprecipitation followed by high-throughput sequencing (ChIP-seq) analysis. Repair templates delivered by nonintegrating viruses should only be detectable at sites of endonuclease activity, therefore primers specific to the repair template but not present in the genome at large can be used to map sites of nuclease activity.[6] ChIP-seq can be used to demonstrate sites of nuclease binding to the genome but does not necessarily indicate cleavage events have occurred.[7] Although both methods offer insight into potential off-target cleavage sites, neither offers comprehensive coverage of the genome or quantification of the likelihood of such events occurring. A hybrid approach called Genome-wide, Unbiased Identification of DSBs Enabled by sequencing has also been described that uses blunt ended double-stranded oligodeoxynucleotide (dsODN) integration at cut sites, followed by next-generation sequencing.[8] DNA DSBs, either on-target or off-target, also have the potential to result in translocation events that can be difficult to detect. A high-throughput genome-wide translocation sequencing (HTGTS) technique has been described that aims to both predict and monitor for these events at specific on-target or off-target sites.[9]

Care should also be taken to consider the anticipated and unanticipated biological impact of the intended gene modification when designing a targeted endonuclease. Unintended impacts can range from decreased cell survival and function to clonal proliferation and oncologic transformation. Gene therapies have been proposed that target intronic sequence, repressor as well as promoter and enhancer elements, transcription factors, and the insertion of synthetic constructs, to name a few.[10] Therapies that rely on the targeted disruption of a transcription factor must consider not just the impact on the gene causing the undesirable phenotype but genes in other pathways as well. The introduction of synthetic gene elements by HR requires further scrutiny to monitor for correct insertion and the potential impact on nearby genes both at the intended and off-target integration sites. One approach to mitigate the potential risk of oncologic transformation is the introduction of a suicide gene that can be activated to eradicate the offending population if needed.[11]

Safety considerations should also extend beyond the direct safety of the patient and include laboratory staff, clinical staff, and direct contacts of the patient. Laboratory staff safety starts with the proper handling of cells and reagents based on appropriate biosafety level assignment to the reagents being used. Transfection of messenger RNA (mRNA) or DNA constructs by electroporation poses little risk to the laboratory staff member. The use of viral elements such as adeno-associated virus (AAV), Integrase-Deficient Lentivirus, or others increases the required safety precautions. Both the nature of the virus and the payload being delivered should be evaluated for the potential to cause harm if laboratory staff members are exposed. Viral carriers that introduce HR templates alone are arguably less dangerous than those containing nuclease elements. Viruses with the potential to integrate into the genome or infect epithelial cells should be handled with greater care. The risk to clinical staff, including nurses and doctors, should be relatively minimal in most cases. Certainly, if the gene therapy takes place in the laboratory (eg, editing hematopoietic stem and progenitor cells), the cells that are infused into the patient are isolated from the clinical staff and pose little risk if an exposure should occur. The risk posed by gene therapy involving the intravenous or direct tissue inoculation with an engineered virus will need to be considered for each protocol. Aerosolization or unintentional needle sticks of infectious elements have the potential to harm clinical staff and a plan to respond to such exposures will need to be part of any gene therapy protocol. Family and close contacts of the patient will need to be aware of any potential shedding of engineered virus by the patient. Fortunately, in almost all cases, the risk will be minimal.

An important topic of debate concerning therapeutic gene editing is the potential modification of germline cells. For families in which one or more members carry a pathogenic genetic trait, ridding their lineage of that trait, even if they would not be able to change their own clinical outcome, is a reasonable aspiration. At the current level of understanding of gene editing, there are both known and unknown risks that render attempts at germline gene editing ethically questionable even for the elimination of traits with unequivocal clinical benefit. First and foremost, genetic tools are not currently understand well enough to know that they can be wielded for a beneficial outcome without unknowingly causing damage. Off-target cleavage events are known potential sequelae of gene editing and, even with current sequencing technology, it is not possible to know that an attempt at beneficial editing has not also resulted in accompanying detrimental genetic alterations. Further issues would arise from any attempt at nontherapeutic genetic enhancement in which the clinical benefit of modifying a genetic trait is less clear. Although modifying a trait or combination of genetic traits in a patient may achieve a desirable phenotypic outcome, it is not known with certainty that the impact will be the same in the genetic milieu of their offspring. With these uncertainties, although a patient can consent to undertake the risk of modifying their own genome, it is not yet clear that those decisions can or should be propagated to their progeny through germline editing. Based in part on these issues, the National Institutes of Health guidelines currently prohibit the use of federal funds for research that aims to alter the germline in either mature adults or human embryos, although it is worth noting that a recent report from the National Academy of Sciences seems leave the door open for such a possibility in the future.[12,13] Due to the technical and ethical issues associated with germline modification, current practice is that any potential modification of germline cells must be carefully considered and arguably avoided.

Medical monitoring in both the short and long term following a gene therapy procedure must also be carefully planned in advance. The concept of the medical home for gene therapy patients has not yet been well established. It is unlikely that there will be a gene therapy division in most hospital settings but care will instead be carried out by the specialty service caring for the underlying diagnosis. A patient with SCID (severe combined immuno-deficiency) will likely be treated by an immunology department, a sickle cell patient by hematology, and so on. The challenge is that if the curative treatment hoped for is achieved, the patient may be lost to follow-up as their symptoms resolve. This is a particularly important issue in the near future because, due to relative inexperience with gene therapy and gene editing, it is advisable (and currently a US Food and Drug Administration requirement) to monitor gene therapy patients over long periods of time for the development of therapy-related complications. Ensuring that detailed information on the exact genetic manipulation the patient undergoes follows them later in life in some form of medical record will be essential so that any adverse events could be related to general or specific aspects of gene therapy or gene editing. If the potential for germline modification exists, multigenerational access to these data may also be advisable but adds a high degree of medicolegal complexity.

SPECIFICITY

Critical to the success and safety of targeted endonucleases and other forms of gene therapy is the degree of specificity that can be achieved. The random integration events that occur with retroviral gene delivery demonstrate the danger of gene therapy in the absence of high degrees of specificity. New generations of targeted endonucleases, including zinc finger nucleases, TALENs, and CRISPR/CRISPR-associated endonuclease (Cas) 9, each have unique mechanisms for binding to specific genomic sequences to induce targeted cleavage events. Zinc fingers and TALENs use nucleotide specific protein motifs and CRISPR/Cas9 relies on Watson-Crick base pairing of an RNA guide to recognize specific genomic targets. The unique features of each of these approaches for engineered specificity are considered here.

Zinc fingers were some of the first sequence specific tools used for gene editing.[14] Zinc fingers are protein motifs that function as transcriptional regulators by recognizing 3–base pair (bp) sequences. Libraries of zinc fingers have been generated that target a wide array of 3-bp sequences. Series of zinc fingers (typically 3–6 per monomer) can be connected to yield sequence specificity of 9 to 18 bp.[15] Additional specificity is achieved by nature of linking the obligate heterodimer restriction enzyme *Fok*I to 2 zinc finger constructs flanking the intended cut site. Because individual zinc finger-*Fok*I monomers are not capable of cleaving without a partner, the target sequence must match not only the sequences encoded by both zinc finger constructs but also be in the correct orientation and separated by roughly the same number of bases required to align the *Fok*I elements. The chance of all elements being present in regions of the genome other than the intended cleavage site becomes exceedingly rare.

Not long after the first reported use of zinc finger–based constructs for gene editing, TALENs were developed as an alternative mechanism for targeting specific sequences. Transcription activator-like effectors (TALEs) were identified as DNA-binding proteins expressed by plant pathogens as a means of avoiding host defenses via genetic manipulation.[16] Unlike zinc fingers that recognize 3-bp sequences, an individual TALE subunit (referred to as a repeat variable diresidue [RVD]) recognizes a single-DNA bp. The TALE subunit is a 34 amino acid protein element that is identical except for amino acids 12 and 13 that impart specific recognition of different DNA bases (ie, A, T, C, or G). Individual TALE subunits can be combined in series (typically of 15–20 subunits) to create a helical structure that traces the major groove of a specific DNA sequence.[17] Like zinc fingers, TALENs are generated by linking TALE subunits to the *Fok*I endonuclease and are also used in heterodimeric pairs, which further increases specificity.[18]

More recently, the CRISPR/Cas9 system has become a major focus of the therapeutic gene editing field. The system is based on a prokaryotic immune defense system that stores short segments of invading virus or plasmid DNA in a form of molecular memory. These sequences are expressed as guide RNA molecules that target the Cas to the same sequence in the offending virus and introduce DSBs.[19] The sequence specificity is imparted by Watson-Crick base pairing of the guide RNA to the target DNA sequence. This mechanism has been adapted for use in eukaryotic cells primarily using an optimized Cas9 endonuclease.[20] What makes the CRISPR/Cas9 system so appealing is the relative ease of generating approximately 20-bp guide RNA sequences. Unlike zinc finger nucleases or TALENs, CRISPR/Cas9 functions as a monomer, thus the specificity relies on the guide sequence binding. The ability to rapidly design and generate guide RNA to test potential target cleavage sites make the CRISPR/Cas9 system particularly appealing for screening guides toward multiple targets, or for editing procedures that require cleavage of multiple targets.

Each of these techniques is based on the specific binding of a targeted genomic sequence. Multiple attempts are underway to improve the specificity of each platform to minimize off-target cleavage and improve safety. One technique involves the directed mutagenesis of *Fok*I to generate obligate heterodimers, which reduces the incidence of homodimer cleavage events.[21] Altering the linker sequence between the *Fok*I and the zinc finger has also been shown to increase the specificity of zinc finger pairs.[22] Further specificity can be gained by joining the TALE subunits to a site-specific meganuclease in place of the *Fok*I to form megaTALs, but only in sites with favorable characteristics.[23] An expanded set of RVDs has been generated and analyzed to achieve improved TALEN specificity.[24] The specificity of the CRISPR/Cas9 system has been a topic of much debate. Some investigators report evidence of decreased specificity resulting in DSBs at sites with only 15 of 20 bp matches or large chromosomal deletions.[25,26] Others report little or no off-target cleavage using CRISPR/Cas9 at other sites, leaving open the possibility of site or sequence-dependent specificity. A recent effort to overcome this potential limitation is the re-engineering of *Streptococcus pyogenes* Cas9 (SpCas9) to reduce off-target cleavage events,[27] although an unintended effect of many types of specificity engineering may be an associated reduction in on-target cleavage efficiency, which may limit utility.

Although the specificity of various targeted endonuclease technologies is based largely on sequence targeting motifs within the construct, there are other factors that contribute to the generation of off-target cleavage. Two important factors are the level and duration of time the genome is exposed to the endonuclease. Even a highly specific cutting tool has the potential for a low rate of off-target editing that can be compounded by particularly high level or prolonged expression. As the field has moved away from lentiviral vectors due to the risk of genomic integration, viral delivery with AAV and other nonintegrating viral vectors has emerged as a mechanism for delivering endonucleases to target cells. Depending on the infectivity of the virus, the activity of the expression cassette delivered, and the rate of clearance of each from the cell, endonuclease activity can persist for days. Although this may increase overall cutting efficiency at the target site, it also has the potential to increase off-target genomic damage. One means of limiting the exposure time of the genome to an engineered endonuclease is to deliver it in RNA form. The transfection of mRNA directly into target cells is possible ex vivo in cells such as hematopoietic stem cells. Zinc fingers, TALENs, and Cas9 can all be delivered in mRNA form.[28] This limits the nuclease exposure time to the persistence of the mRNA and translated protein.[18,29] CRISPR guide RNA and Cas9 protein can also be complexed as a ribonucleoprotein for direct electroporation, which similarly achieves limited duration.

Another aspect of specificity relates to the viral delivery of the engineered nuclease, particularly if delivered as a systemic infusion for in vivo genome editing applications. As described in other articles, AAV has become a major player in the implementation of gene therapy as a means to deliver genes as well as editing components. At least 13 naturally occurring AAV serotypes have been studied and found to have at least partial affinity for various organs. AAV2 has been found to exert natural tropism for skeletal and vascular smooth muscle, hepatocytes, and neurons and AAV8 has a high affinity for hepatocytes as well.[30] Work is also underway to conduct directed evolution of the AAV virus to decrease immunogenicity, increase tissue specific tropism, overcome cellular barriers, and increase packaging capacity.[31] Modified AAV plasmids and vectors have been generated that codeliver Cas9 and guide RNA, and can also preferentially target specific cell types.[32] Tissue specificity of a viral vector delivery system only adds to the overall specificity of a gene editing strategy.

One of the two major endogenous repair mechanisms following the introduction of a DSB (see prior discussion) is template-guided HR. Repair templates contain homology arms on both the 5′ and 3′ ends of the construct that correspond to the sequence flanking the endonuclease cut site. Additional genetic content can be encoded between the arms and incorporated into the cut site. The homology arms are typically hundreds of bps long, making it unlikely that the template will insert anywhere but on-target cut sites. Editing strategies that rely on HR template integration must plan for a subset of cells to undergo NHEJ without template integration and the impact of these events should be reviewed for potential deleterious effects. Worth mentioning here is the importance of ensuring that repair templates do not share homology with the full target site, rendering them cleavable. An analysis of the frequency and impact of SNPs, both at the putative cut site as well as within the homology arm recognition site, is an important aspect to applying an HR-based gene therapy to a patient population. HR template integration is a powerful component of targeted gene editing and further adds to the specificity of these approaches.

SUMMARY

Learning from the challenges of the first gene therapy trials, a large emphasis has been placed on improved specificity to achieve safety. The new generation of targeted nucleases has made the possibility of precise genetic manipulation a reality. The purpose of this article is not to endorse a particular platform over another. Each has their merits and all have the potential for safe and effective therapeutic application. Importantly, large-scale cross-platform comparisons of safety and specificity are of limited utility. Rather, safety and specificity must be assessed for each individual editing process due to multiple potential variables, including target site characteristics, nuclease manufacturing and delivery, editing procedure, and cell handling. Ideally, specificity and safety of each new therapy should be addressed early in the design phase and reassessed as implementation proceeds. It is important to remember gene therapy and gene editing are still in the early stages and prudence is warranted to diligently pursue the highest possible standards of safety. The ability to sequence and modify the human genome will help shape the legacy of modern medical science. How this incredible new ability is studied and implemented has long-ranging implications for the integrity and public trust for both the practice of science and medicine.

ACKNOWLEDGMENT

The authors would like to thank Jackie Morton, Seattle Children's Hospital Librarian, for her assistance in conducting a literature search for this submission.

REFERENCES

1. Blaese RM, Culver KW, Miller AD, et al. T lymphocyte-directed gene therapy for ADA– SCID: initial trial results after 4 years. Science 1995;270(5235):475–80.
2. Fine EJ, Cradick TJ, Zhao CL, et al. An online bioinformatics tool predicts zinc finger and TALE nuclease off-target cleavage. Nucleic Acids Res 2014;42(6):e42.
3. Optimized CRISPR design. Available at: http://crispr.mit.edu/.
4. Hsu PD, Scott DA, Weinstein JA, et al. DNA targeting specificity of RNA-guided Cas9 nucleases. Nat Biotechnol 2013;31(9):827–32.
5. Tuerk C, Gold L. Systematic evolution of ligands by exponential enrichment: RNA ligands to bacteriophage T4 DNA polymerase. Science 1990;249(4968):505–10.
6. Petek LM, Russell DW, Miller DG. Frequent endonuclease cleavage at off-target locations in vivo. Mol Ther 2010;18(5):983–6.
7. O'Geen H, Henry IM, Bhakta MS, et al. A genome-wide analysis of Cas9 binding specificity using ChIP-seq and targeted sequence capture. Nucleic Acids Res 2015;43(6):3389–404.
8. Tsai SQ, Zheng Z, Nguyen NT, et al. GUIDE-seq enables genome-wide profiling of off-target cleavage by CRISPR-Cas nucleases. Nat Biotechnol 2015;33(2):187–97.
9. Chiarle R, Zhang Y, Frock RL, et al. Genome-wide translocation sequencing reveals mechanisms of chromosome breaks and rearrangements in B cells. Cell 2011;147(1):107–19.
10. Maeder ML, Gersbach CA. Genome-editing technologies for gene and cell therapy. Mol Ther J Am Soc Gene Ther 2016;24(3):430–46.
11. Jones BS, Lamb LS, Goldman F, et al. Improving the safety of cell therapy products by suicide gene transfer. Front Pharmacol 2014;5:254.
12. Collins FS. Statement on NIH funding of research using gene-editing technologies in human embryos. Natl Inst Health NIH 2015. Available at: https://www.nih.gov/about-nih/who-we-are/nih-director/statements/statement-nih-funding-research-using-gene-editing-technologies-human-embryos.
13. Committee on Human Gene Editing: Scientific, Medical, and Ethical Considerations, National Academy of Sciences, National Academy of Medicine, National Academies of Sciences, Engineering, and Medicine. Human genome

editing: science, ethics, and governance. Washington, DC: National Academies Press; 2017.

14. Bibikova M, Golic M, Golic KG, et al. Targeted chromosomal cleavage and mutagenesis in *Drosophila* using zinc-finger nucleases. Genetics 2002;161(3): 1169–75.

15. Urnov FD, Rebar EJ, Holmes MC, et al. Genome editing with engineered zinc finger nucleases. Nat Rev Genet 2010;11(9):636–46.

16. Fujikawa T, Ishihara H, Leach JE, et al. Suppression of defense response in plants by the avrBs3/pthA gene family of *Xanthomonas* spp. Mol Plant Microbe Interact 2006;19(3):342–9.

17. Cermak T, Doyle EL, Christian M, et al. Efficient design and assembly of custom TALEN and other TAL effector-based constructs for DNA targeting. Nucleic Acids Res 2011;39(12):e82.

18. Wright DA, Li T, Yang B, et al. TALEN-mediated genome editing: prospects and perspectives. Biochem J 2014;462(1):15–24.

19. van der Oost J, Jore MM, Westra ER, et al. CRISPR-based adaptive and heritable immunity in prokaryotes. Trends Biochem Sci 2009;34(8):401–7.

20. Mali P, Yang L, Esvelt KM, et al. RNA-guided human genome engineering via Cas9. Science 2013;339(6121):823–6.

21. Miller JC, Holmes MC, Wang J, et al. An improved zinc-finger nuclease architecture for highly specific genome editing. Nat Biotechnol 2007;25(7):778–85.

22. Händel EM, Alwin S, Cathomen T. Expanding or restricting the target site repertoire of zinc-finger nucleases: the inter-domain linker as a major determinant of target site selectivity. Mol Ther 2008;17(1):104–11.

23. Boissel S, Jarjour J, Astrakhan A, et al. megaTALs: a rare-cleaving nuclease architecture for therapeutic genome engineering. Nucleic Acids Res 2014;42(4): 2591–601.

24. Miller JC, Zhang L, Xia DF, et al. Improved specificity of TALE-based genome editing using an expanded RVD repertoire. Nat Methods 2015;12(5):465–71.

25. Fu Y, Foden JA, Khayter C, et al. High-frequency off-target mutagenesis induced by CRISPR-Cas nucleases in human cells. Nat Biotechnol 2013;31(9):822–6.

26. Cradick TJ, Fine EJ, Antico CJ, et al. CRISPR/Cas9 systems targeting β-globin and CCR5 genes have substantial off-target activity. Nucleic Acids Res 2013; 41(20):9584–92.

27. Slaymaker IM, Gao L, Zetsche B, et al. Rationally engineered Cas9 nucleases with improved specificity. Science 2016;351(6268):84–8.

28. Hendel A, Bak RO, Clark JT, et al. Chemically modified guide RNAs enhance CRISPR-Cas genome editing in human primary cells. Nat Biotechnol 2015;33: 985–9.

29. Pruett-Miller SM, Reading DW, Porter SN, et al. Attenuation of zinc finger nuclease toxicity by small-molecule regulation of protein levels. PLoS Genet 2009;5(2):e1000376.

30. Srivastava A. In vivo tissue-tropism of adeno-associated viral vectors. Curr Opin Virol 2016;21:75–80.

31. Kotterman MA, Schaffer DV. Engineering adeno-associated viruses for clinical gene therapy. Nat Rev Genet 2014;15(7):445–51.

32. Senís E, Fatouros C, Große S, et al. CRISPR/Cas9-mediated genome engineering: an adeno-associated viral (AAV) vector toolbox. Biotechnol J 2014;9(11): 1402–12.

Gene Editing

Regulatory and Translation to Clinic

Dale Ando, MD[a],*, Kathleen Meyer, MPH, PhD[b],*

KEYWORDS

- Genome editing • Zinc finger nucleases • Hematopoietic stem and progenitor cells
- CCR5 • Genotoxicity • Safety assessment

KEY POINTS

- This review covers the regulatory and translational preclinical activities needed for a CCR5 zinc finger nuclease genome editing clinical trial modifying hematopoietic stem cells.
- CD34[+] HSPC manufacturing and clinical administration considerations are discussed.
- Preclinical evaluations supporting the FIH study include on- and off-target genome editing assessment, in vitro differentiation, in vivo stem cell engraftment, karyotype analysis, 53BP1 assay, soft agar transformation, and an NSG mouse tumorigenicity study.

INTRODUCTION

The clinical application and regulatory strategy of genome editing for ex vivo cell therapy is derived from the intersection of two fields of study: viral vector gene therapy trials (initially retroviral gene therapy[1]), and clinical trials of therapeutics based on ex vivo purification and engraftment of CD34[+] hematopoietic stem cells and T cells and tumor cell vaccines.[1–3] This review covers the regulatory and translational preclinical activities needed for a genome editing clinical trial modifying hematopoietic stem and progenitor cells (HSPCs) and the genesis of this current strategy based on previous clinical trials using genome-edited T cells. The SB-728 zinc finger nuclease (ZFN) platform is discussed because this is the most clinically advanced genome editing technology with completed or ongoing clinical studies evaluating the safety and efficacy of ZFN-modified T cells[4] or CD34[+] HSPCs in human immunodeficiency virus (HIV)-infected human subjects. The ZFNs used in these studies (SB-728) were designed to target and disrupt the CCR5 locus, which encodes the CCR5 cell

Disclosure Statement: Dr D. Ando is President of Gene Editing and Gene Therapy Consulting and is a former Sangamo Therapeutics employee. Dr K. Meyer is currently employed by Sangamo Therapeutics.
a Gene Editing and Gene Therapy Consulting, 159 Venado Corte, Walnut Creek, CA 94598, USA; b Nonclinical Development, Sangamo Therapeutics, 501 Canal Boulevard, Suite A100, Richmond, CA 94804, USA
* Corresponding authors.
E-mail addresses: dgando@aol.com (D.A.); kmeyer@sangamo.com (K.M.)

surface protein used by HIV-1 to gain entry and infect CD4$^+$ T cells. The first clinical studies in 2009 used adenoviral transduction to deliver the genes encoding the CCR5 ZFNs to autologous T cells (SB-728-T) (NCT01044654@clintrials.gov and NCT00842634@clintrials.gov).[4] In a follow-on study, electroporation was used to deliver CCR5 ZFN mRNA to autologous T cells, resulting in the investigational product SB-728mR-T (NCT02388594@clintrials.gov). As stem cell technology advanced, an Investigational New Drug and clinical protocol were developed where the CCR5 ZFN mRNA was delivered via electroporation to autologous HSPCs (referred to as SB-728mR-HSPC) and a clinical trial was initiated in 2015 (NCT02500849@clintrials. gov). This review describes the preclinical studies conducted to support advancing these investigational genome-editing products into phase 1 clinical studies, with focus on the SB-728mR-HSPC program. An advantage of this autologous stem cell therapy is the ability to modify a subject's own HSPCs and circumvent challenges associated with allogeneic transplantation.

OVERVIEW OF ZINC FINGER NUCLEASES FOR GENOME EDITING

ZFNs consist of a zinc finger DNA binding domain (ZFP) fused to the catalytic domain of the type II Fok1 endonuclease, yielding a designer restriction enzyme capable of cleaving DNA specifically at a unique and predetermined site in the human genome.[5–7] The binding domain contains a tandem array of Cys2-His2 fingers, each recognizing approximately three base pairs of DNA (**Fig. 1**). Each Cys2-His2 zinc finger consists

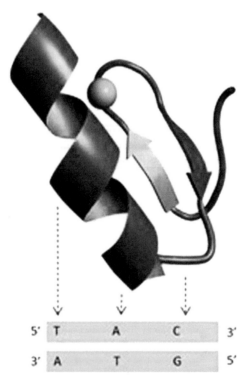

Fig. 1. The zinc finger protein is composed of ~30 residues that fold into a ββα-structure via coordination of a zinc ion, and each finger recognizes approximately three base pairs of DNA. (*Courtesy of* Sangamo Therapeutics, Richmond, CA.)

of approximately 30 residues that fold into a ββα-structure via coordination of a zinc ion. The Fok1 endonuclease domain possesses inherent characteristics that further enforce site-specific cleavage within the genome, including the necessity for dimerization to occur for DNA cleavage (**Fig. 2**). Thus, for double-stranded DNA cleavage to occur, two ZFNs must bind to the targeted DNA in the correct orientation and spacing to enable Fok1 dimerization. Use of engineered Fok1 heterodimers also enforces highly specific nuclease function because cleavage only occurs on the formation of a Fok1 heterodimeric complex.[8] Homodimer complexes of these engineered heterodimers cannot form, and thus the use of the obligate heterodimer Fok1 domains prevent off-target cleavage at potential homodimer sites, further enhancing ZFN specificity. The ZFN-induced site-specific double-strand breaks (DSB) are repaired via nonhomologous end joining (NHEJ) or homology-directed repair,[9,10] resulting in a knockout of the *CCR5* gene. In the absence of a donor template to carry out homology-directed repair, the ZFN-induced DSB are repaired by the error-prone NHEJ repair process, often leading to the insertion and deletions of base pairs (indels), resulting in truncated or nonfunctional gene products that would fail to be expressed on the cell surface. This results in modified cells that are analogous to cells comprising the naturally occurring *CCR5*-delta 32 mutant allele that is associated with HIV resistance (Perez 2013[11]; Liu 1996[12]; Samson 1996[13]).

GENOME EDITING USING CCR5 ZINC FINGER NUCLEASE mRNA; mRNA PRODUCTION

Ex vivo delivery of SB-728 CCR5 ZFN constructs to patient T cells, was evaluated using adenoviral 35/5 vectors and electroporation of mRNA; however, the cytotoxicity of adenoviral vectors with HSPC precluded their use in HSPC and the intended clinical study.[14] Delivery of mRNAs via electroporation is an increasingly popular method for genome editing, especially if transgene addition is not needed. Electroporation of capped mRNA for expression of nucleases avoids prolonged nuclease expression and obviates risk of genomic integration of foreign DNA. The availability of efficient research grade and clinical scale electroporators also makes mRNA delivery practical for translation into the clinic. Accordingly, we chose this method to move forward with the SB-728mR-HSPC study. GMP mRNA production for SB-728mR-HSPC has been well described.[14] For our process, once the clinical lead ZFN gene construct was selected, a highly purified research gold standard plasmid was produced, sequenced,

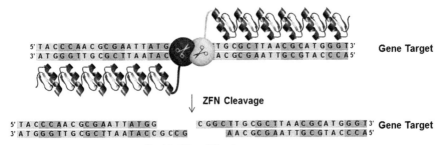

Fig. 2. For DNA cleavage, two zinc finger nucleases must bind in the correct orientation and spacing to enable Fok1 dimerization. The requirement for two heterodimeric ZFNs to bind results in the specific targeting of long and potentially unique recognition sites. These obligate heterodimer Fok1 domains prevent off-target cleavage at potential homodimer sites, thus further enhancing ZFN specificity. (*Courtesy of* Sangamo Therapeutics, Richmond, CA.)

and archived. This research gold standard plasmid was used to generate the plasmid master cell bank DNA. In today's industry, plasmid production and purification are now supported by many contract manufacturing organizations as are mRNA production, capping, and storage. One strategic regulatory consideration is that the plasmid DNA and mRNA can be regarded as accessory products, whereas the modified cell was considered the final drug product. With good quality control of DNA and mRNA manufacturing processes with respect to identity, purity, and potency, GMP manufacturing may not be necessary for these components. This can be discussed with the US Food and Drug Administration (FDA).

CD34$^+$ CELL PURIFICATION AND MODIFICATION

HSPC were isolated from granulocyte colony–stimulating factor/plerixafor-mobilized peripheral blood of HIV-1 infected individuals based on the expression of the CD34 antigen. To prepare the final CD34$^+$ HSPC cell dose (>5 $\times$ 10^6 CD34$^+$ HSPC/kg) after purification and electroporation, two apheresis treatments with granulocyte colony–stimulating factor/plerixafor were conducted from each individual.[15] CD34$^+$ HSPC purification commonly uses CD34$^+$ Miltenyi magnetic bead purification, a process that has been used in autotransplantation in oncology[2] and CD34$^+$ retroviral or lentiviral transplant clinical studies. Research-grade and clinical scale electroporation procedures were optimized using mRNAs encoding the SB-728 CCR5 ZFNs. Because of the limited availability of clinical-grade electroporation equipment, the MaxCyte GT Transfection System (Gaithersburg, MD, USA) was used to develop the clinical process, and used for in vitro toxicology studies, NSG (NOD SCID gamma [NOD.Cg-$Prkdc^{scid}$ $Il2rg^{tm1Wjl}$/SzJ]) mouse CD34$^+$ HPSC engraftment studies, and the 5-month NSG mouse tumorigenicity study.[14]

CD34$^+$ HEMATOPOIETIC STEM AND PROGENITOR CELLS ADMINISTRATION TO HUMAN SUBJECTS

Autologous SB-728mR-HSPC were infused into subjects who had been preconditioned with busulfan, which has known toxicity/engraftment profiles because it has been used in autologous hematopoietic cell transplants for blood malignancies, and also has been used successfully at low doses in combination with gene transfer approaches for nonmalignant diseases.[16,17] Successful autologous engraftment of SB-728mR-HSPC results in stable mixed bone marrow chimerism with modified CD34$^+$ HSPC, a percentage of which have both CCR5 alleles modified and whose progeny express no surface CCR5 receptors. These progeny cells, of which CD4$^+$ T helper cells are most important, are protected from infection and/or destruction by HIV-1, and show preferential survival in the face of HIV-1 viremia.

After exposure to HIV-1 and classical class II major histocompatibility complex processing of HIV-1 antigens, the fully protected CD4$^+$ cell progeny may be able to activate, expand, and provide CD4$^+$ T helper function to CD8$^+$ cytotoxic T and other immunologically active cells sufficient to successfully clear active HIV-1 infection in a way that cannot occur when CD4$^+$ T cells are not protected from HIV-1 entry. This effect may extend to clearance of the HIV-1 reservoir, but absence of CCR5 expression on cell lineages, such as monocytes and macrophages, known to harbor a percentage of the HIV reservoir, may also contribute to reservoir clearance.

REGULATORY STRATEGY FOR PRECLINICAL DEVELOPMENT

The regulatory strategy guiding the SB-728-T, SB-728mR-T, and SB-728mR-HSPC preclinical safety evaluation programs included a literature-based risk assessment; in silico, in vitro, and in vivo studies; and was built on experience gained from the preceding development programs. The main objectives for safety evaluation associated with modification of T cells and/or CD34[+] HSPC were assessment of ZFN specificity (on- and off-target activity) and effectiveness with focus on successful engraftment and potential genotoxicity (**Table 1**). For transplanted CD34[+] HSPC cells, engraftment and survival of ZFN-modified cells were assessed in NSG mice, and the tumorigenic potential of modified cells was evaluated using several in vitro assays and in a 5-month NSG mouse model. The FDA specifically requested evaluation of the tumorigenic potential of a total human dose, made up of T cells or HSPC from three healthy donors, delivered to immunodeficient mice. For SB-728mR-HSPC administered to a 70-kg subject and with dose levels ranging from 2 million to 10 million CD34[+] HSPC/kg, the total human clinical dose ranged from 140 million to 700 million CD34[+] HSPC cells.

LITERATURE-BASED RISK ASSESSMENT OF *CCR5* KNOCK-OUT

A literature-based assessment was conducted to evaluate the risk of *CCR5* knock-out in humans. The data available in mice and humans do not indicate significant safety concerns associated with knockout of *CCR5* in human cells, which is supported by the natural history of individuals who are homozygous for the *CCR5*-delta 32 allele and comprise up to 10% of the populations of European descent.[18] In fact, an HIV-positive subject was successfully transplanted with CD34[+] HSPC from a matched unrelated donor carrying two copies of this same *CCR5*-delta 32 allele, which led to the successful eradication of HIV in this patient.[19,20] In previous studies using ZFNs to disrupt *CCR5* in CD34[+] HSPC from umbilical cord blood, CCR5 ZFN-modified HSPC have been shown to support multilineage engraftment in immunodeficient mice and confer resistance to HIV-1.[21,22] Taken together, the human health risk associated with *CCR5* knock-out was believed to be low.

ASSESSING ON-TARGET CCR5 ZINC FINGER NUCLEASE ACTIVITY

The on-target genome editing activity of the ZFNs at the target *CCR5* locus was evaluated using the Surveyor nuclease assay (Cel-1) and deep sequencing technology (MiSeq, Illumina, San Diego, CA),[14] allowing evaluation of the NHEJ-driven insertion

Table 1
Outline of the in vitro and in vivo studies that provided support for a genome-modified CD34[+] HSPC protocol

Evaluation	Endpoint
On-target editing	Targeted deep sequencing
HSPC function in vitro	Colony formation assays
HSPC function in vivo	Engraftment of immunodeficient mice after 20 wk
Off-target editing	Genome-wide oligonucleotide capture and targeted deep sequencing
Genotoxicity	53BP1 immunofluorescence and karyotype
Transformation in vitro	Soft agar colony assay
Tumorigenicity in vivo (one full human dose)	Histopathology for tumors in xenografted immunodeficient mice after 5 mo

and/or deletion of nucleotides at the predetermined CCR5 nuclease target in the genome. This assessment was conducted post genome editing treatment (before cell administration to animals or human subjects) and then blood samples were collected and evaluated at various times postadministration.

IN VITRO AND IN VIVO STEM CELL FUNCTIONAL ASSAYS

The ability of *CCR5* modification of stem cells to protect against HIV-1 infection in vivo has been published.[21] The novel use of electroporation of mRNA to highly modify CD34$^+$ HSPC made it important to study stem cell functions in vitro and in vivo. Analysis of modified CD34$^+$ HPSC function is complicated by the fact that the phenotype and function of the "true pluripotent stem cell" is not known. In vitro differentiation assays for colony-forming units (CFU)-GM, CFU-GEMM, and CFU-E may not measure true stem cell effects but can enable a comparison of differentiation cell profiles between modified CD34$^+$ HPSC and control unmodified cells. For novel methods of genome editing, this is likely a minimal requirement for in vitro assessment of CD34$^+$ HSPC differentiation. In addition, a limited amount of genetic data, such as the efficiency of monoallelic and biallelic modification, can be gained because clonal cells can be isolated in methylcellulose. Interassay variation, precision of quantification, and donor-to-donor variability are significant limitations for using these CFU assays to determine lot potency.

In vivo assessment of engraftment and lineage differentiation was evaluated in a 20-week study in NSG mice, and has been described by DiGiusto and colleagues.[14] Briefly, animals were intravenously administered 1 million control (nonelectroporated) or SB-728mR-electroporated CD34$^+$ HSPC collected from each of three healthy donors. At 20 weeks, spleen and bone marrow cells were harvested and evaluated for engraftment and differentiation into hematopoietic cell lineages. The results demonstrated that the modified HSPC were able to generate the full assortment of cell lineages in vivo.

ASSESSING OFF-TARGET CCR5 ZINC FINGER NUCLEASE ACTIVITY

Assessment of off-target cleavage activity is important for assessing safety and risk. However, factors in the manufacturing process, mRNA concentrations, and donor variability can influence on- and off-target measurements. Initially in the development of genome editing technology, only bioinformatics approaches were used to select potential off-target sites. Polymerase chain reaction amplification and sequencing were then used for on- and off-target assessments[4] in the modified cells. An alternate approach involving the sequencing of integrated lentivirus at off-target nuclease cleavage sites after integrase-deficient lentiviral vector (IDLV) transduction was also used.[23] This system can be adapted to an oligonucleotide (oligo) duplex capture technique rather than using a lentivirus as the capture template where deep sequencing is used to identify the oligo capture sites in a tumor cell line.[24] This process generates a list of potential candidate sites for off-target cleavage, which then can be used for follow-up indel analysis in the modified CD34$^+$ HSPC (electroporated with the ZFN-encoding mRNAs using the clinical manufacturing process).

It is important to set up on- and off-target deep sequencing analysis as discussed previously to evaluate the clinical materials made for Good Laboratory Practice (GLP) toxicology studies and to assess clinical process. Assessment of these critical parameters is essential for translation of genome editing into the clinic.

ASSESSING POTENTIAL GENOTOXICITY OF CCR5 ZINC FINGER NUCLEASE

Additional orthogonal assays for evaluating the potential for in vitro transformation and DSB induction and repair were used to assess potential CCR5 ZFN genotoxicity. As discussed later, these assays include p53 binding protein 1 (53BP1) staining of untransfected and transfected CD34$^+$ HSPC, karyotyping of untransfected and trans-fected CD34$^+$ HSPC, and a soft agar transformation assay using a human fibroblast cell line. The SB-728mR-HSPC in vivo safety assessment included evaluation of trans-planted cell engraftment, cell differentiation, and potential tumorigenicity in the NSG mouse. Initial studies with modified T cells (SB-728-T or SB-728mR-T) additionally used the NOD/SCID/$\gamma c^{-/-}$ (NOG) mouse and an in vitro cytokine independent growth or transformation assay.

53BP1 STAINING OF SB-728mR-HSPC

Induction of a DSB triggers the recruitment of cellular factors involved in DNA repair to the site of the break. One such protein, 53BP1, is recruited (within 24 hours) to the sites of DSBs.[25] These sites may be visualized as intensely stained and distinct foci within the nucleus of fixed cells using immunofluorescence microscopy with antibodies that recognize 53BP1.[25–29] Importantly, the number of 53BP1 foci per nucleus is an accu-rate measure of the number of DSBs that occurred in the cell.

53BP1 is recruited to any DSB, including those naturally present, and those induced by ZFNs; it plays an important role in DSB repair via NHEJ, the major repair pathway used to repair ZFN-induced DSBs.[30] Immunohistochemical staining of 53BP1 was used to assess repair of ZFN-induced DSB in target cells, including SB-728 T cells and SB-728mR-HPSC. This method is a useful assessment of ZFN-induced DSBs in cells that can be viewed microscopically. The number of 53BP1 foci was quantified in ZFN-treated T cells or CD34$^+$ HSPC and compared with control cells, as part of a general evaluation of off-target ZFN activity following SB-728 mRNA transfection for the SB-728, SB-728mR, and SB-728mR-HSPC pro-grams. Results showed background levels of staining 5 days post ZFN treatment.

This method also requires no prior knowledge of ZFN specificity and is unbiased by off-target site predictions based on homology to the ZFN target sequences. The strength of the 53BP1 approach is therefore that it provides an alternative method for unbiased assessment of general off-target activity across the nucleus (albeit at un-identified locations). Thus, the studies described here complement the bioinformatics- and SELEX-based approaches.

Random DNA DSBs are an expected and frequent occurrence in cells maintained ex vivo. Studies examining normal human fibroblasts and transformed human cell lines show that cells in culture typically contain 1 to 30 DSBs per nucleus principally because of oxidative damage or replication fork collapse.[26,31,32] In contrast, cells treated with etoposide, a DNA-damaging drug used in cancer chemotherapy, can display greater than 50 DSBs per nucleus.[31] Even without drug treatment actively dividing cells display 2 to 50 DSBs per cell cycle. Importantly, although DSBs occur naturally and ubiquitously, they do not result in transformation, in part because of the robust DNA repair pathways present in human cells.

KARYOTYPING OF SB-728mR-HSPC

ZFNs are designed to induce double-stranded DNA breaks in the genome at a spec-ified target locus. Given their mechanism of action, there is concern that possible off-target activity of ZFNs could result in deleterious genetic changes. To detect any large-scale changes created by ZFN treatment, a GLP karyotype analysis was performed to search for changes in chromosome number or structure for all CCR5 ZFN-related investigational therapies.

The visual examination of spread chromosomes from individual cells provides a global view of genetic integrity, and can detect genetic abnormalities that might be missed by other, more targeted molecular tests that have been used to evaluate on- and off-target ZFN activity. Chromosomal translocations or aberrant chromosome numbers are detected by karyotype analysis. Nonclonal technical and culture-related artifacts may result, respectively, in whole chromosome gains or losses (most likely related to chromosome overspreading during slide preparation) and single-cell aberrations related to culture conditions that are usually eliminated from the cell population in subsequent divisions.

The same manufacturing process used in the clinic was used to prepare the various investigational cell products (SB-728, SB-728 mR, and SB-728mR-HSPC) that were subjected to karyotype analysis. The control cells were processed in the same way as the investigational cell products with the exception that control cells were not electroporated or exposed to *CCR5*-targeting ZFNs. In parallel to karyotype analysis, samples from the same cell cultures were evaluated using deep sequencing (MiSeq) to evaluate the on- and off-target ZFN activity. A normal karytoype was seen following ZFN-treatment, and no gross chromosome or clonal aberrations were present in any cell evaluated, even at high levels of CCR5 gene modification (> 50%) by Cel-1 or deep sequencing.

SOFT AGAR TRANSFORMATION ASSAY

Fibroblast transformation and the development of nonanchorage dependent fibroblast growth is a classical transformation assay.[33] An in vitro GLP soft agar transformation assay was conducted to evaluate potential CCR5 ZFN carcinogenicity using human WI-38 cells, an adherent human diploid fibroblast cell line that shows anchorage-dependent growth.

Transformed cells are easily differentiated from normal cells in vitro because growth of normal cells is anchorage-dependent, whereas transformed cells lose this constraint and grow in an anchorage-independent manner. This property may be demonstrated by the clonal growth of cells suspended in semisolid media (eg, soft agar). The soft agar transformation assay is a conventional test of cellular transformation that has been used extensively to study the transformation potential of chemotherapeutic agents.[33]

In parallel to the soft agar transformation assay, samples from the untransfected and CCR5 ZFN-modified WI-38 cultures were analyzed using next-generation deep sequencing to ensure that the level of ZFN-mediated genome modification in WI-38 cells was within or greater than the approximate range anticipated for clinical application. The soft agar transformation assay showed no anchorage-independent growth of ZFN-modified cells, demonstrating a lack of in vitro tumorigenicity potential.

FIVE-MONTH NSG MOUSE STUDY TO EVALUATE POTENTIAL CCR5 ZINC FINGER NUCLEASE TUMORIGENICITY OF SB-728mR-HSPC

For in vivo studies, genetically engineered immunodeficient mice were used to evaluate the potential for carcinogenicity risk. Initial studies for the adenovirus-delivered ZFNs to autologous T cells used the NOG mouse model. Later studies with SB-728mR-HSPC used an improved NSG mouse model that allowed evaluation over 5 months. Recommendations from the FDA were to conduct the study in compliance with GLP if possible, to evaluate cells from three different donors, and to evaluate one full human dose in mice.

The immunodeficient NSG mouse model was selected for evaluation of potential tumorigenicity of SB-728mR-HSPC over a 5 month duration, and has been previously described.[14] NSG mice lack a functional common interleukin (IL)-2 receptor (R) γ-chain, which is indispensible for IL-1, IL-4, IL-7, IL-9, IL-15, and IL-21 high-affinity binding and signaling (reviewed Ref.[34]). IL-2 R γ-chain deficiency blocks natural killer cell development and results in additional defects in innate immunity.[35] NSG mice have impaired signaling through multiple cytokine receptors, resulting in blocked natural killer cell development and severely decreased immune response, providing a unique environment for growth and development of human cells.[36] NSG mice also lack functional T and B cells, natural killer cells, and also have impaired dendritic cell function, so that they are able to accept transplantations of human hematopoietic cells and to establish long-lived grafts of human HSPC and their progeny.

Although immunodeficient rodent models are not able to fully recapitulate the human hematopoietic and immune systems, the NSG mouse model supports the development of multiple human hematopoietic cell lineages (eg, monocytes, B cells, CD4+ T cells, and CD8+ T cells). Moreover, these human cell lineages undergo significant replication and expansion in the peripheral blood and tissues of NSG mice. This makes the engraftment, differentiation, and expansion of the human CD34+ HSPC in NSG mice a useful model to assess the tumorigenic potential of SB-728mR-modified and control CD34+ HSPC. In addition, this model has been shown previously to be a sensitive xenograft model for evaluating leukemogenesis and tumorigenicity compared with other immunodeficient mouse strains (eg, NOD/SCID and NOD/SCID/β2), with a more rapid onset of malignant disease-related symptoms using patient-derived or transformed human cells.[36–38]

To evaluate the potential tumorigenicity of ex vivo–modified SB-728mR-HSPC, and to evaluate general safety and tolerability, a non-GLP quality-controlled 5-month tumorigenicity study with SB-728mR-HSPC was conducted in NSG mice. Mice were subjected to nonlethal radiation (250 cGy) up to 6 hours before HSPC injection to promote engraftment. HSPC were derived from three healthy donors and underwent manufacturing in a manner similar to HSPC intended for the phase 1 clinical study. At the time of treatment, the on-target *CCR5* gene modification profile ranged from 54% to 67% indels. A single dose administration of 1×10^6 CD34+ SB-728mR-transfected HSPC per mouse was given by retro-orbital injection to 158 (75 females; 83 males) animals; 60 control animals (30 females; 30 males) received the same dose of untransfected HSPC. This cell dose was approximately 5×10^7 cells/kg (20-g mouse), which was approximately 20-fold higher than the intended clinical dose ($\geq 2 \times 10^6$ cells/kg; 1.5×10^8 cells; 70-kg subject) in human patients scaled by body weight. At the time of injection, the on-target and off-target gene modification profiles of *CCR5*-modified or control HSPC were assessed by deep sequencing. Study evaluations included clinical observations, body weight, HSPC engraftment, gene modification, and gross and microscopic pathology.

The results from this study demonstrated that control cells and SB-728mR-HSPCs were well tolerated, with no evidence of adverse effects on clinical observations, body weight, or findings at necropsy. The HSPCs showed successful engraftment in mice, with hematopoietic progeny measured in blood and bone marrow in all animals during the course of the study. Gene modification analysis in blood was followed over 5 months, and in bone marrow at the end of the study. Four additional loci (*CCR2*, *CHR.12/KRR1*, *FBXL11*, and *ZCCHC14*) were evaluated for off-target gene modification. Histopathologic analysis resulted in no test-article-related toxicologic findings.

There was no immunohistochemistry evidence of clonality or neoplastic transformation of any of the engrafted human cells. Immunohistochemistry staining (human CD45) and fluorescence in situ hybridization demonstrated that no tumors were of human origin or originated from the engrafted human HSPC. In addition, evaluation of blood smears revealed no unusual findings and no evidence of hematogenous neoplasia. Based on the results of this study, SB-728mR-HSPC modified at the *CCR5* locus were well tolerated, showed successful engraftment, and no evidence of neoplastic transformation of the engrafted human stem cells in the NSG mouse model. Therefore, SB-728mR-HSPC did not demonstrate potential for tumorigenesis or leukemogenesis in NSG mice.

SUMMARY

The recent advances in gene therapy and ex vivo manipulation of hematopoietic stem cells provide the opportunity to edit the genome in a highly targeted manner using ZFNs to disable the *CCR5* gene in subjects infected with HIV-1, with the eventual goal of producing hematopoietic stem cells and $CD4^+$ T cell progeny resistant to HIV-1 infection. The studies described herein were the first using mRNA and electroporation-mediated genome editing in T cells and $CD34^+$ HSPCs in support of a review by the Recombinant DNA Advisory Committee, and for subsequent filing with the FDA for a clinical trial in human subjects. The preclinical and regulatory strategy to assess the safety of these CCR5 ZFN-modified $CD34^+$ HPSC included in silico, in vitro, and in vivo studies and should provide a framework for future studies in the rapidly expanding field of genome editing. In addition, the rapidly advancing technologies of deep sequencing, whole genome sequencing and off-target analysis will further enable evaluation of the effects of genome editing on the cell.

REFERENCES

1. Nemunaitis J, Fong T, Robbins JM, et al. Phase I trial of interferon-gamma (IFN-gamma) retroviral vector administered intratumorally to patients with metastatic melanoma. Cancer Gene Ther 1999;6(4):322–30.
2. Jansen J, Hanks S, Thompson JM, et al. Transplantation of hematopoietic stem cells from the peripheral blood. J Cell Mol Med 2005;9(1):37–50.
3. Deeks SG, Wagner B, Anton PA. A phase II randomized study of HIV-specific T-cell gene therapy in subjects with undetectable plasma viremia on combination antiretroviral therapy. Mol Ther 2002;5(6):788–97.
4. Tebas P, Stein D, Tang WW, et al. Gene editing of CCR5 in autologous CD4 T cells of persons infected with HIV. N Engl J Med 2014;370(10):901–10.
5. Kim YG, Cha J, Chandrasegaran S. Hybrid restriction enzymes: zinc finger fusions to Fok 1 cleavage domain. Proc Natl Acad Sci U S A 1996;93(3):1156–60.
6. Smith J, Berg JM, Chandrasegaran S. A detailed study of the substrate specificity of a chimeric restriction enzyme. Nucleic Acids Res 1999;27(2):674–81.
7. Urnov FD, Miller JC, Lee YL, et al. Highly efficient endogenous human gene correction using designer zinc-finger nucleases. Nature 2005;435(7042):646–51.
8. Miller JC, Holmes MC, Wang J, et al. An improved zinc-finger nuclease architecture for highly specific genome editing. Nat Biotechnol 2007;25(7):778–85.
9. Gaj T, Gersbach CA, Barbas CF. ZFN, TALEN, and CRISPR/Cas-based methods for genome engineering. Trends Biotechnol 2013;31(7):397–405.
10. Sung P, Klein H. Mechanism of homologous recombination: mediators and helicases take on regulatory functions. Nat Rev Mol Cell Biol 2006;7(10):739–50.

11. Perez EE, Wang J, Miller JC, et al. Efficient clinical scale gene modification via zinc finger nuclease-targeted disruption of the HIV co-receptor CCR5. Hum Gene Ther 2013;24(3):245–58.

12. Liu R, Paxton WA, Choe S, et al. Homozygous defect in HIV-1 coreceptor accounts for resistance of some multiply-exposed individuals to HIV-1 infection. Cell 1996;86(3):367–77.

13. Samson M, Libert F, Benjamin J, et al. Resistance to HIV-1 infection in caucasian individuals bearing mutant alleles of the CCR-5 chemokine receptor gene. Nature 1996;382(6593):722–5.

14. DiGiusto DL, Cannon PM, Holmes MC, et al. Preclinical development and qualification of ZFN-mediated CCR5 disruption in human hematopoietic stem/progenitor cells. Mol Ther Methods Clin Dev 2016;3:1–12.

15. Yannaki E, Karponi G, Zervou F, et al. Hematopoietic stem cell mobilization for gene therapy: superior mobilization by the combination of granulocyte-colony stimulating factor plus plerixafor in patients with beta-thalassemia major. Hum Gene Ther 2013;24(10):852–60.

16. Kuramoto K, Follman D, Hematti P, et al. The impact of low-dose busulfan on clonal dynamics in nonhuman primates. Blood 2004;104(5):1273–80.

17. Slavin S, Nagler A, Naparstek E, et al. Nonmyeloablative stem cell transplantation and cell therapy as an alternative to conventional bone marrow transplantation with lethal cytoreduction for the treatment of malignant and nonmalignant hematologic diseases. Blood 1998;91(3):756–63.

18. Martinson JJ, Chapman NH, Rees DC, et al. Global distribution of the CCR5 gene 32-basepair deletion. Nat Genet 1997;16(1):100–3.

19. Allers K, Hutter G, Hofmann J, et al. Evidence for the cure of HIV infection by CCR5Delta32/Delta32 stem cell transplantation. Blood 2011;117(10):2791–9.

20. Hutter G, Nowak D, Mossner M, et al. Long-term control of HIV by CCR5 Delta32/Delta32 stem-cell transplantation. N Engl J Med 2009;360(7):692–8.

21. Holt N, Wang J, Kim K, et al. Human hematopoietic stem/progenitor cells modified by zinc-finger nucleases targeted to CCR5 control HIV-1 in vivo. Nat Biotechnol 2010;28(8):839–47.

22. Glass WG, McDermott DH, Lim JK, et al. CCR5 deficiency increases risk of symptomatic West Nile virus infection. J Exp Med 2006;203(1):35–40.

23. Wang GP, Levine BL, Binder GK, et al. Analysis of lentiviral vector integration in HIV+ study subjects receiving autologous infusions of gene modified CD4+ T cells. Mol Ther 2009;17(5):844–50.

24. Kleinstiver BP, Pattanayak V, Prew MS, et al. High-fidelity CRISPR-Cas9 nucleases with no detectable genome-wide off-target effects. Nature 2016;529(7587):490–5.

25. Schultz LB, Chehab NH, Malikzay A, et al. p53 binding protein 1 (53BP1) is an early participant in the cellular response to DNA double-strand breaks. J Cell Biol 2000;151(7):1381–90.

26. Rogakou EP, Boon C, Redon C, et al. Megabase chromatin domains involved in DNA double-strand breaks in vivo. J Cell Biol 1999;146(5):905–16.

27. Rappold I, Iwabuchi K, Date T, et al. Tumor suppressor p53 binding protein 1 (53BP1) is involved in DNA damage-signaling pathways. J Cell Biol 2001;153(3):613–20.

28. Burma S, Chen BP, Murphy M, et al. ATM phosphorylates histone H2AX in response to DNA double-strand breaks. J Biol Chem 2001;276(45):42462–7.

29. Ward IM, Minn K, Jorda KG, et al. Accumulation of checkpoint protein 53BP1 at DNA breaks involves its binding to phosphorylated histone H2AX. J Biol Chem 2003;278(22):19579–82.

30. Dimitrova N, Chen YC, Spector DL, et al. 53BP1 promotes non-homologous end joining of telomeres by increasing chromatin mobility. Nature 2008;456(7221): 524–8.

31. Vilenchik MM, Knudson AG. Endogenous DNA double-strand breaks: production, fidelity of repair, and induction of cancer. Proc Natl Acad Sci U S A 2003; 100(22):12871–6.

32. Anderson DE, Trujillo KM, Sung P, et al. Structure of the Rad50 x Mre11 DNA repair complex from Saccharomyces cerevisiae by electron microscopy. J Biol Chem 2001;276(40):37027–33.

33. Puck TT, Marcus PI, Cieciura SJ. Clonal growth of mammalian cells in vitro - growth characteristics of colonies from single HeLa cells with and without a "feeder" layer. J Exp Med 1956;103:273–83.

34. Shultz LD, Lyons BL, Burzenski LM, et al. Human lymphoid and myeloid cell development in NOD/LtSz-SCID IL2R gamma null mice engrafted with mobilized human hemopoietic stem cells. J Immunol 2005;174(10):6477–89.

35. Cao X, Shores EW, Hu-Li J, et al. Defective lymphoid development in mice lacking expression of the common cytokine receptor gamma chain. Immunity 1995;2(3): 223–38.

36. Risueno RM, Campbell CJ, Dingwall S, et al. Identification of T-lymphocytic leukemia-initiating stem cells residing in a small subset of patients with acute myeloid leukemic disease. Blood 2011;117(26):7112–20.

37. Agliano A, Martin-Padura I, Mancuso P, et al. Human acute leukemia cells injected in NOD/LtSz-SCID/IL-2R gamma null mice generate a faster and more efficient disease compared to other NOD/SCID-related strains. Int J Cancer 2008; 123(9):2222–7.

38. Quintana E, Shackleton M, Sabel MS, et al. Efficient tumour formation by single human melanoma cells. Nature 2008;456(7222):593–8.

Opening Marrow Niches in Patients Undergoing Autologous Hematopoietic Stem Cell Gene Therapy

Morton J. Cowan, MD[a],*, Christopher C. Dvorak, MD[a],
Janel Long-Boyle, PharmD, PhD[b]

KEYWORDS

- Marrow niches • Gene therapy • Pharmacokinetics • Conditioning
- Primary immune deficiency • Inborn errors of metabolism • Hemoglobinopathies

KEY POINTS

- Gene therapy for bone marrow disorders and inborn errors requires sufficient open marrow niches to allow gene-corrected autologous stem cells to engraft and correct all disease manifestations.
- In young children, the clearance of alkylating agents used for opening marrow niches can vary significantly, making it essential that pharmacokinetic studies be done to ensure optimal therapy.
- To minimize/eliminate late effects, nonchemotherapy approaches to opening marrow niches are being developed and may replace the need for chemotherapy as conditioning.

INTRODUCTION

The concept of opening marrow niches or "making space" for allogeneic hematopoietic stem cells (HSC) to engraft is well known. Hematopoietic cell transplants (HCT) for many patients with severe combined immunodeficiency (SCID) typically require no marrow ablative conditioning and result in at least T- and sometimes B-cell reconstitution, although rarely is multilineage engraftment seen.[1] A limited number of reports

Disclosure Statement: M.J. Cowan is on the Scientific Advisory Boards for Homology Medicine, Inc and Exogen, Inc and the Data and Safety Monitoring Board for bluebird bio, Inc; C.C. Dvorak and J. Long-Boyle have nothing to disclose.
Due to word limits, only essential references could be included.
[a] Pediatric Allergy Immunology and Blood and Marrow Transplant Division, UCSF Benioff Children's Hospital, 550 16th Street, Floor 4, San Francisco, CA 94143-0434, USA; [b] Department of Clinical Pharmacy, University of California San Francisco, 600 16th Street, Room N474F, San Francisco, CA 94158-0622, USA
* Corresponding author. Department of Pediatrics, 550 16th Street, Floor 4, San Francisco, CA 94143-0434.
E-mail address: mort.cowan@ucsf.edu

suggest that small numbers of donor HSC are engrafted; however, even this concept is controversial, because it is also thought that either some stem cells may engraft in the thymus or long-lived autonomous T- and B-lymphocytes may be able to reconstitute sufficient immunity in SCID patients to achieve long-term survival.[2] For malignant diseases, full donor chimerism is the goal, whereas for nonmalignant disorders, the degree of chimerism that is necessary, and whether multilineage engraftment is even required, depends on the specific disorder. With the exception of SCID, durable grafts generally require the achievement of some degree of multilineage engraftment involving donor T cells and the specific defective lineage or lineages. Donor T cells are needed to ensure tolerance of the graft by the recipient immune system.

For inborn errors of metabolism (in which marrow lineages are typically not involved) such as Hurlers mucopolysaccharidosis and adrenoleukodystrophy (ALD), the ultimate therapeutic goal is delivering the maximum amount of missing/defective enzyme to affected tissues. The rationale is that donor myeloid cells that are precursors of microglial cells can populate the brain and provide a source of enzyme.[3] Generally, this requires maximum engraftment of donor HSC. For the hemoglobinopathies, it is apparent that full allogeneic donor chimerism is not essential to correct the anemia and that even less than 50% donor chimerism will correct the disease manifestations in both thalassemia and sickle cell disease; whether this will be true for gene therapy remains to be determined and will be influenced by the transduction efficiency. For the primary immune deficiencies (PIDs) other than SCID, the degree of donor chimerism needed for disease correction varies. In Wiskott-Aldrich syndrome (WAS), it appears that mixed chimerism is adequate to correct the T-cell defect but that closer to full donor chimerism may be required to correct the thrombocytopenia and autoimmune manifestations, the latter likely mediated by abnormal B cells.[4] Studies in a mouse model of Chronic Granulomatous Disease (CGD) demonstrates as little as 20% donor chimerism is adequate to correct the disease with respect to infection and inflammation.[5] Even for some types of SCID-related disorders, in particular, Omenn syndrome, full donor chimerism may be needed in order to eliminate all disease manifestations.

The major chemotherapy agents that are used today for opening marrow niches for allogeneic HCT in patients with nonmalignant diseases are busulfan and melphalan. Treosulfan, an analogue of busulfan with both myeloablative and immunosuppressive activities, is also in use primarily in Europe. Finally, thiotepa has both myeloablative and immunosuppressive activities and has been used in combination with busulfan or melphalan. Because most of the diseases for which gene therapy is currently being used involve children, and drug clearance may change with age, it is critical that discussions regarding conditioning include what is known about the pharmacokinetics (PK) and pharmacodynamics (PD) of each agent.

Finally, at least for the nonmalignant disorders, the ideal approach to opening marrow niches would be to avoid or minimize the use of these drugs, all of which are alkylating agents associated with early and late side effects, especially in infants and young children. Significant progress has been made in understanding the biology of the marrow niche, in particular, the critical cells and their receptors. With this information, there has been a variety of approaches taken to use small molecules and monoclonal antibodies (mAbs) to either block homing receptors or specifically target HSC in order to open marrow niches without the need for alkylating therapy.

This article focuses on what is currently known about the need for opening marrow niches in recipients of gene-corrected autologous HSC, the PK of the currently available chemotherapy agents to minimize exposure, and the novel approaches that may be available in the future to eliminate the need for any chemotherapy-based conditioning before gene therapy.

CONDITIONING PATIENTS BEFORE AUTOLOGOUS GENE-CORRECTED HEMATOPOIETIC CELL TRANSPLANTATION

This section reviews the experience with autologous gene therapy for PIDs, inborn errors of metabolism, hemoglobinopathies, and marrow failure syndromes in order to better understand conditioning and the degree to which marrow niches need to be opened to correct disease manifestations. The first disease successfully treated by gene-corrective therapy was adenosine deaminase (ADA) -deficient SCID. Initial attempts at gene correction using a γ-retroviral vector with transduced autologous cord blood or bone marrow stem cells did not use any conditioning therapy.[6] In these early trials, only a tiny fraction of cells (<0.01%) could be detected long term, and there was no discernible improvement in T- or B-cell immunity off enzyme replacement therapy (ERT). The addition of low total doses of busulfan (4 mg/kg vs 16 mg/kg or 60–90 mg*h/L cumulative area under the curve [AUC] for myeloablation) as conditioning resulted in significant durable engraftment with reconstitution of T-cell and B-cell immunity.[7] Of a total of 18 patients treated, 15 durably engrafted and remained off ERT; of those 15, 12 came off immunoglobulin replacement therapy, and busulfan PK studies were not reported. In the first US trial of gene therapy for ADA-SCID using a γ-retroviral vector in 6 patients receiving low-dose busulfan (2.4–3.3 mg/kg), 3 remained off ERT. A more recent experience with low-dose busulfan using a lentiviral vector appears to result in improved multilineage engraftment and both T- and B-cell reconstitution. Although targeted busulfan was not used, PK measurements indicate an average cumulative AUC of ∼18 mg*h/L was achieved (D. Kohn, personal communication, 2017).

The second PID treated effectively with gene therapy using a γ-retroviral vector was X (γc)-SCID. Conditioning did not appear to be necessary, and initially, most patients seemed able to come off immunoglobulin supplementation, an indication of B-cell reconstitution, even though transduced B-cell chimerism was relatively low (<1%). However, over time, most of these patients required reinitiation of immunoglobulin replacement.[8] The need for conditioning was confirmed in a second trial using a modified γ-retroviral vector in a joint European/US trial. Recently, De Ravin and colleagues[9] reported on a small cohort of γc-SCID patients who had failed a prior allogeneic transplant and were treated with autologous gene correction using a lentiviral vector and a relatively low total dose (6 mg/kg) of busulfan. Busulfan was not targeted; however, PK studies were performed, and the average cumulative AUC in these 5 recipients was ∼30 mg*h/L (H. Malech, personal communication). This dose was a higher busulfan dose than that used for ADA-SCID. The optimal cumulative exposure of busulfan and the minimal threshold of stem cell engraftment for ADA or γc-SCID are unknown, but it does appear that targeted conditioning to open marrow niches and allow gene-corrected donor stem cells to engraft is essential for both diseases.

The need for conditioning to open marrow niches is likely to be true for other SCID genotypes, at least those in which there is an intrinsic B-cell defect, for example, RAG SCID and Artemis-deficient (ART) SCID.[10,11] In the latter, a mouse model of gene therapy demonstrates that some approach that opens marrow niches is necessary to achieve multilineage engraftment with both T- and B-cell reconstitution (M. Cowan, personal communication and Ref.[11]). In the mouse model of ART-SCID, the marrow is more susceptible to alkylating agents than wild-type marrow, so that lower doses of chemotherapy may suffice in humans (M. Cowan, personal communication). Regardless, in ART-SCID and other radiation-sensitive types of SCID, it will be critical to minimize or, if possible, eliminate the need for alkylating agents in order to avoid long-term side effects. Finally, for Omenn syndrome occurring in patients with hypomorphic SCID gene mutations (often RAG1/2), resulting in hyperinflammation with auto-reactive T cells, it is likely that a significant amount of marrow ablation resulting in a high degree of donor chimerism will be necessary to correct all of the disease manifestations,[10] just as it is for allogeneic HCT. For SCID secondary to IL7Rα or CD3 receptor defects, cytoreduction with busulfan may not be necessary, because B cells in these SCID disorders are intrinsically normal.

Based on the experience with allogeneic transplantation for CGD and WAS, it is likely that submyeloablative conditioning should be effective for the former, whereas ablative doses of busulfan will be required for the latter in order to correct all of the disease manifestations.[4,12] In the initial trial of gene therapy for WAS using a γ-retroviral vector, the total busulfan dose without PK studies was 8 mg/kg with 9/10 patients showing sustained engraftment and correction of WAS protein expression in lymphoid and myeloid cells and platelets between 60 and greater than 90%.[13] Unfortunately, 6 of the patients developed T-cell acute lymphoblastic leukemia, thought to be due to the vector configuration. Subsequently, a limited clinical trial in 3 patients using a lentiviral construct with similar subablative conditioning (busulfan 8 mg/kg) was reported with good correction in all 3 patients. These investigators added fludarabine to control autoimmunity and reduce the autologous T-cell burden. In a third trial using a lentiviral vector, 7 patients were conditioned with busulfan 12 mg/kg and fludarabine 120 mg/m^2.[14] One patient died of herpes viral infection. In the remaining 6 patients, all resolved their eczema and susceptibility to infections. There were also major improvements in vasculitis and bleeding episodes. However, at the time of the report, only 2 of the patients no longer needed immunoglobulin replacement therapy. The extent of gene marking in nonlymphoid cells was variable from 0.4 to 0.01 copies per cell. The expression of WAS protein was highest in T cells (34%–84%) and lower in NK and B cells (13%–85%). At last follow-up, only one patient had normal platelets, with 5 patients having platelet counts ranging from 6 to 87 × 10^9/L. Three patients had platelet counts less than 15 × 10^9/L, suggesting that busulfan total doses of 12 mg/kg may be insufficient to achieve adequate donor chimerism and full disease correction. Conversely, in a preliminary report of 4 patients treated with a lentiviral vector and conditioning consisting of 12 to 15 mg/kg total dose of busulfan and 120 mg/m^2 fludarabine, all patients had improvement in eczema and were platelet transfusion independent. The median follow-up of this small cohort was only 13.5 months, so that longer follow-up will be necessary to fully evaluate outcome. These early results suggest that ablative exposure busulfan will be necessary in future trials of gene therapy for WAS to fully correct disease manifestations. It is not clear whether the addition of fludarabine is of any benefit.

The experience to date with gene therapy for CGD is very limited, and it is impossible to know if mixed chimerism will be curative after autologous gene therapy, although in mouse models it appears that as little as 20% chimerism with gene-corrected cells is sufficient to protect against infection and inflammation.[15] However, in human trials of gene therapy for CGD, achievement of durable engraftment using nonmyeloablative regimens (busulfan 6.4–10 mg/kg or melphalan 140 mg/m^2) has been unsuccessful.[5] In a study of gene therapy in a mouse model of CGD, the pretreatment of recipient mice with granulocyte colony-stimulating factor (G-CSF), a cytokine that stimulates granulopoiesis, before nonmyeloablative (300 cGy) total body irradiation (TBI), significantly improved donor cell engraftment. The potential synergistic effect of G-CSF with busulfan, rather than TBI, in this mouse model was not reported.

For the inborn errors of metabolism, including ALD and metachromatic leukodystrophy (MLD), myeloablation will be necessary, with either reduced intensity or full myeloablative regimens.[16,17] Similar to allogeneic HCT for ALD, myeloablation with high-dose busulfan and immunosuppression with cyclophosphamide are being used for Gene Therapy trials. With this regimen, 9% to 14% of cells express the ALD protein. A larger study is ongoing with targeted myeloablative dosing. The rationale for the immunosuppression for this autologous HCT is unclear, although some of the central nervous system (CNS) damage is thought to be secondary to an immune response. In one reported trial for MLD in which myeloablative (11–16.8 mg/kg) dosing of busulfan was given to 9 patients, enzyme activity in myeloid cells was at or above the healthy donor range in all of them at a median of 36 months follow-up.[17] There was also no evidence of disease progression by brain MRI, although longer follow-up is needed.

There is great interest in gene therapy for thalassemia and sickle cell disease due to the prevalence of these hemoglobinopathies in certain populations and the selective advantage for corrected erythroid precursors.[18] The initial gene therapy trial in 2 patients with thalassemia in which myeloablative doses (12.8 mg/kg) of busulfan were administered resulted in transfusion independence in both patients.[19] International clinical trials for both thalassemia and sickle cell disease are ongoing using targeted myeloablative dosing of busulfan. Whether nonmyeloablative conditioning with less chimerism will also be effective, comparable to what has been seen with allogeneic HCT, remains to be determined.[20,21]

For Fanconi anemia, a marrow failure disorder associated with a DNA repair defect, either immunosuppression alone or immunosuppression with relatively low exposure to alkylating agents or ionizing radiation has been used before allogeneic HCT. For alternative donor sources (unrelated or haploidentical donors), low-dose radiation has been used,[22] although a more recent trial suggests it may be replaced with low-dose busulfan. Whether any myeloablative therapy will be needed for autologous gene therapy remains to be determined.[23]

Finally, any discussion regarding conditioning for autologous gene-corrective HCT must take into account the transduction efficiency in CD34$^+$ HSC. Even with lentiviral vectors, the percent of autologous donor cells that are transduced can vary from 10% to 60%. Also, the fraction of these cells that are truly repopulating stem cells is much less than 100%, so that the transduced stem cell dose is considerably less than optimal. The lower efficiency is reflected in the vector copy numbers (VCN) that are seen in hematopoietic cell lineages after infusion. In most cases, the average VCN is significantly less than 1 per cell. Until the efficiency is closer to 100% in HSC, higher marrow ablation may be required to achieve disease correction in some of these disorders compared with what will be necessary in the future as the efficiency improves.

CHEMOTHERAPEUTIC AGENTS USED AS PRETREATMENT IN HEMATOPOIETIC CELL GENE THERAPY

Intervention early in life is often considered critical to effectively treat several childhood diseases, including many immunodeficiencies and genetic metabolic disorders.[24–26] With newborn screening (NBS) for SCID nearly universal in the United States, and NBS for inborn errors of metabolism on the horizon, children are now being diagnosed within the first few weeks of life, allowing corrective interventions such as gene therapy to be offered at a young age when outcomes are superior. It is well recognized the PK and PD of drugs in infants can differ widely between children and adults.[27] Within the first year of life, age-related developmental changes in physiologic and metabolic processes can lead to significantly altered drug disposition.[28] This section summarizes what is currently understood about the PK and PD of alkylating agents used in the setting of autologous and allogeneic HCT, which then may be applied to autologous gene therapy.

Busulfan

Busulfan is a bifunctional alkylating agent widely used in conditioning regimens before both autologous and allogeneic HCT. The rationale for its use as pretreatment before gene therapy resides in its ability to target both slowly proliferating and nonproliferating cells. Through the formation of DNA and DNA-protein crosslinks, busulfan suppresses HSC function by inducing senescence, thus creating space in the bone marrow microenvironment to support stem cell engraftment. In the case of lysosomal disorders, busulfan may also facilitate the depletion of microglial cells in the brain parenchyma, allowing for engraftment of gene-modified monocytes in the CNS and the delivery of deficient proteins past the blood-brain barrier. Historically, the inclusion of busulfan in the conditioning regimens of infants has often been preferred to promote stem cell engraftment and avoid long-term consequences of total body irradiation, including growth and developmental delay, poor tooth development, endocrinopathies, and increased risk of malignancy later in life. Allewelt and colleagues[29] have recently described significant late effects of high-dose busulfan (primarily in combination with cyclophosphamide) in children undergoing cord blood HCT at a very young age. However, the results of this study must be interpreted with caution given a significant number of the patients had either inborn errors of metabolism with preexisting CNS abnormalities or leukemia and were therefore exposed to induction and consolidation chemotherapy before conditioning for allogeneic HCT.

The PK of busulfan has been studied extensively in the setting of pediatric allogeneic HCT. Busulfan clearance is a combined function of patient-specific and clinical covariates impacting drug metabolism and distribution. Population PK (PopPK) studies in infants and children have shown that in model-based algorithms for busulfan that incorporate body size and metabolic maturation provide improved targeted therapy when compared with stratified weight- or age-based regimens alone.[30–33] Busulfan undergoes extensive conversion in the liver through conjugation with glutathione by glutathione S-transferases (GST) enzymes, predominantly via GSTA1, and minor contributions from GSTM1 and GSTP1.[34] Based on popPK modeling, the clearance of busulfan increases approximately 1.7-fold between 6 weeks to 2 years of life, an effect largely attributed to changes in expression of GST enzymes.[33]

Moreover, because busulfan PK displays large interpatient variability and exposure-response relationships have been described, the therapeutic drug monitoring (TDM) of busulfan should be routinely performed in children undergoing HCT.[35–37] Strategies for the TDM of busulfan differ among treatment centers, such as concentration at steady state or cumulative AUC exposure over the entire course of therapy. Improved rates of engraftment and lower drug-related toxicity in the setting of allogeneic transplantation have been demonstrated with cumulative AUCs of 60 to 90 mg*h/L for a variety of both malignant and nonmalignant disorders.[36–38] However, the need for myeloablative versus low-exposure busulfan (cumulative AUC <45 mg*h/L) as a requirement to support long-term engraftment and immune reconstitution, particularly in the setting of PID, continues to be debated and warrants further study.

Advantages of low-exposure busulfan as pretreatment for gene therapy that can still support stem cell engraftment would be an expected reduction of acute drug-related toxicity and minimization of the risk for severe long-term complications, particularly in the very young. With recent advancements in Bayesian software, model-based dosing can be easily implemented into clinical protocols and used to individualize therapy irrespective of the therapeutic target or dose interval.[37] Model-based dosing signifies an important shift in the paradigm of busulfan dosing away from predefined dose intensity (eg, 1 mg/kg/dose or 16 mg/kg total over 4 days) to a more tailored approach to therapy. However, even with a model-based strategy, there will be a proportion of patients who fail to achieve the therapeutic target with the first dose of busulfan, therefore reinforcing the need for repeat evaluation of drug levels in some patients.

Melphalan

Similar to busulfan, melphalan is cell cycle independent and exerts its cytotoxic effect on HSCs through the formation of interstrand or intrastrand DNA and DNA-protein crosslinks.[39] It undergoes active transport into cells by the high-affinity L-amino-acid transport system, a process inhibited in HSCs in vitro in the presence of high concentrations of either glutamine or leucine.[39] There are varying data available describing the ability and extent of melphalan to penetrate the blood-brain barrier.

For children of all ages, the knowledge of the PK properties of melphalan is extremely limited. When dosed on a milligram per square meter basis, wide interpatient variability has been demonstrated, with estimates for clearance and exposure (AUC) highly variable up to 10-fold.[40] The plasma half-life of melphalan is relatively short (17–75 minutes) and biphasic. It is eliminated by both renal excretion and spontaneous chemical degradation to its monohydroxy and dihydroxy metabolites, with the latter pathway shown to be a relatively minor contributor (<5%). PopPK analyses have identified several potential clinical covariates, which may contribute significantly to drug clearance, including weight and renal function.[40] However, larger studies spanning a wide range of ages are needed to confirm these results. Exposure-response studies in the setting of pediatric allogeneic HCT are to date completely lacking, but an association with an increase in gastrointestinal toxicity, including severe mucositis, has been found with high melphalan AUC in children undergoing autologous peripheral HCT for neuroblastoma and medulloblastoma.[40,41]

Thiotepa

Thiotepa is a polyfunctional alkylating agent commonly added to high-dose combination chemotherapy before autologous and allogeneic HCT at doses ranging from 200 to 300 mg/m^2 (7–10 mg/kg). However, despite its widespread use in the setting of pediatric HCT, the PK of thiotepa remains largely unknown, especially in children under the age of 2. Administered as a prodrug, thiotepa requires conversion in the liver by the cytochrome P450 (CYP) enzymes, CYP2B6 and CYP3A4, to its primary active metabolite TEPA.[42] Although CYP3A4 is the most abundantly expressed hepatic CYP, accounting for approximately 30% to 40% of the total content in the adult liver, it is not the predominate isoform present early in life.[43] Instead, CYP3A7 activity is high during embryonic and fetal stages of life, decreasing rapidly within the first few weeks of life.[43] Conversely, CYP3A4 expression is low at birth, increasing thereafter and reaching 50% of typical adult levels between 6 and 12 months of life.[43] Substrate specificity for the fetal isoform has not been fully characterized, and understanding the ontogeny of hepatic isozymes as it relates to thiotepa would contribute significantly to its application in gene therapy.

The further detoxification of thiotepa and TEPA is mediated by glutathione conjugation.[42] Although inconsistent, dose-dependent kinetics of thiotepa and TEPA have been described over doses ranging from 180 to 900 mg/m^2, suggesting saturable clearance. Renal elimination of TEPA accounts for approximately 11% of an administered dose, with a single case report describing altered PK in the presence of moderate renal insufficiency.[42,44] In the setting of high-dose combination chemotherapy and HCT, thiotepa-containing regimens have been associated with veno-occlusive disease, pulmonary complications, severe mucositis, and neurotoxicity. Studies in mice evaluating neurologic effects of thiotepa demonstrate that long-term cognitive deficits may result.

Treosulfan

Treosulfan is an analogue of busulfan differing by the addition of 2 hydroxyl groups and improved solubility.[45] Administered intravenously as a prodrug, treosulfan undergoes nonenzymatic transformation upon administration to the active monoepoxide and diepoxide metabolites.[46] The mechanism of action of treosulfan has not yet been clearly established and may differ in target pathways from that of busulfan.[45]

Unlike busulfan, the monoepoxide and diepoxide metabolites are not thought to undergo further metabolism via the liver and are primarily excreted through the kidneys. Only recently has the PK of treosulfan given as part of conditioning before allogeneic HCT in a pediatric population been reported.[47] The small number of patients evaluated is not sufficient to draw formal conclusions about the PK properties of treosulfan in children but does demonstrate a high degree of variability in exposure among similar dose cohorts. Whether PK-guided dosing of treosulfan will lead to optimal clinical outcomes, as seen with busulfan, is not known. The acute toxicity profile of treosulfan is considered favorable, with the main toxicities including mucositis, diarrhea, skin and liver toxicity; however, no long-term effects of treosulfan have been reported.[46] It is commercially available in Europe with an official indication for use in ovarian cancer. Treosulfan remains under clinical development and has not yet received approval from the US Food and Drug Administration, although a trial is ongoing and several are planned.

NONCHEMOTHERAPY APPROACHES TO CONDITIONING BEFORE INFUSION OF GENE-MODIFIED HEMATOPOIETIC STEM CELLS

In an ideal world, the conditioning used to make space in the bone marrow niches before infusion of gene-modified HSC would not use alkylating chemotherapy because of its known risks for short- and long-term side effects. The identification of HSC-specific targets should potentially allow for non-chemotherapy-based targeted HSC suppression.

CD45

First attempts in this direction used mAbs directed at CD45. CD45, also known as the leukocyte common antigen, is expressed on all hemato-lymphoid cells. It was shown in rats that lytic anti-CD45 mAbs can produce marrow aplasia and death in the absence of HSC rescue. In mice, however, a lytic anti-CD45 mAb produced only transient myeloid and lymphoid depletion.[48] Treatment with anti-CD45 mAb alone was insufficient to permit engraftment of syngeneic HSC. However, in combination with a submyeloablative dose of total body irradiation (5.5 Gy), the anti-CD45 mAb activity appeared synergistic, allowing the engraftment of allogeneic HSC.

In 2003, a phase 1 clinical trial assessed the safety of 2 unconjugated rat antihuman CD45 mAbs, YT25.4 and YTH54.12, in patients who were being conditioned for allogeneic HCT for advanced malignancies.[49] The study was a dose escalation of this mAb pair, which was given before the administration of standard conditioning therapy. At mAb dose levels greater than 400 μg/kg, significant decreases in blood neutrophils and lymphocytes were noted. However, examination of the marrow to assess the effect of the antibodies on the myeloid precursors revealed that at the greater than 400 μg/kg dose levels, the precursor cells (promyelocytes, metamyelocytes, and myelocytes) were not reduced. Furthermore, colony assays from pretreatment and posttreatment marrow samples revealed no effect on the colony forming units, thereby suggesting no depletion of hematopoietic stem/progenitors.

The combination of YT25.4/YTH54.12 anti-CD45 mAbs was subsequently tested as part of a minimally intensive conditioning regimen for patients with primary immunodeficiencies.[50] The 2 anti-CD45 mAbs were administered in combination with antilymphocyte reagents anti-CD52 (alemtuzumab), fludarabine, and low-dose cyclophosphamide. The regimen was well tolerated, and 15 of 16 patients engrafted, with 11 achieving full or high-level mixed chimerism in both the lymphoid and the myeloid lineages. At a median of 40 months after transplant, 13/16 patients were alive and cured of their underlying disease. However, there were only 2 patients with typical SCID included, one of whom had no detectable myeloid engraftment and the other had 58% myeloid engraftment. Furthermore, the rates of acute and chronic graft-versus-host disease (GVHD) were 36% and 31%, respectively. Although the anti-CD45 mAbs were the only potentially myeloablative components of the conditioning treatment, the grafts infused in this study were replete with T cells (hence the high GVHD incidence), which may have conferred a graft-versus-marrow effect and been at least partly responsible for the clearance of niche space for donor cells. Thus, although these data are promising, the exact contribution of the anti-CD45 mAbs remains to be clarified.

Additional studies have been performed using anti-CD45 mAbs conjugated to radionuclides, including beta particle emitters (Iodine-131, Yttrium-90) and alpha emitters (Astatine-211). The principle behind the use of radioimmunoconjugates is to enable delivery of higher radiation exposures specifically to hematopoietic tissues, thus sparing exposure to other critical organs. This approach has been well characterized in mouse and dog models of HCT[51,52]; however, in humans, its use has been limited to patients with hematologic malignancies for which intensifying and localizing a toxic effect to the bone marrow is desired. Given the significant long-term safety concerns of administering radionuclides to infants and children, this may not be applicable for conditioning before infusion of gene-corrected HSCs. However, the very short linear pathway (only a few cell diameters) and half-life (7.2 hours) of alpha emitters suggests that this approach deserves further study to define efficacy and off-target side effects.

Anti-CD45 has also been conjugated to various agents in order to produce an immunotoxin. One example involves the ricin-family-member molecule saporin (SAP), a catalytic N-glycosidase ribosome-inactivating protein that halts protein synthesis. Unlike other ricin family members, SAP lacks a general cell entry domain and is therefore nontoxic unless conjugated to a targeting antibody or ligand capable of receptor-mediated internalization. A recent study in an immunocompetent mouse model of sickle-cell disease demonstrated high-level peripheral blood and bone marrow engraftment (75%–90%) of congenic and syngeneic cells at 4 months following administration of anti-CD45-SAP.[53] Equivalent levels of chimerism were observed for cells transplanted between 2 and 12 days after CD45-SAP administration, demonstrating a wide transplantation window. Peripheral chimerism was stable and reached greater than 90% at 15 months. Myeloid chimerism was established rapidly within 2 months, whereas the highest levels of T- and B-cell donor chimerism appeared after longer intervals, likely due to the longer lifespan of resident host lymphoid cells. Stem cell engraftment was further confirmed by serial transplantation into lethally irradiated secondary recipients. In comparison to mice treated with TBI, recipients of anti-CD45–SAP had superior bone marrow cellularity and vascular integrity, suggesting a lower toxicity profile. However, to the authors' knowledge, an SAP-conjugated immunotoxin has not yet been trialed in humans.

CD117

A competing approach to anti-CD45 in the field of using mAbs to create space in the bone marrow niche is mAbs directed against CD117. CD117, also known as c-kit, is a cytokine receptor expressed on HSC, erythroid and lymphoid progenitors, mast cells, and other nonhematologic progenitor cells, including melanocytes, and neural and cardiomyocyte precursors. The ligand for CD117 is a stem cell factor, a cytokine that promotes survival, self-renewal, differentiation, and proliferation of HSC and other cell types. A study in immunodeficient mice demonstrated that administration of an mAb against murine CD117 (termed ACK2) resulted in transient removal of greater than 90% of endogenous HSCs, with subsequent recovery by around 2 weeks after ACK2. When these animals were transplanted with congenic HSCs 9 days after ACK2 administration, donor myeloid engraftment of approximately 15% was seen and persisted for at least 9 months.[54] ACK2 can also be given to fetal wild-type mice and results in similar levels of donor myeloid chimerism.[55] In 2 mouse models of Fanconi anemia, administration of ACK2 before HCT resulted in 22% to 24% donor multilineage chimerism by 4 months. Finally, in a mouse model of gene therapy for ART-SCID, ACK2 pretreatment resulted in durable multilineage engraftment of gene-transduced cells with both T- and B-cell reconstitution.[11] This effect has been more difficult to replicate in mature immunocompetent mice. However, when ACK2 was combined with low doses of nonmyeloablative TBI (3 Gy), there was a synergistic effect in wild-type mice and in a mouse model of CGD.[56] In this setting, donor myeloid chimerism of approximately 80% was seen; unfortunately, busulfan does not appear to have the same synergy with ACK2 that is seen with TBI (M. Cowan and M. Dinauer, personal communication). Besides anticipated drops in blood counts, the major off-target side effects of ACK2 noted in mice have been coat discoloration, presumably due to targeting of CD117-positive melanocytes, reduction in spermatogenesis, and histamine release.[54,55]

A human analogue of ACK2, termed AMG191, has been generated and shown to target human HSCs engrafted in mice (J. Shizuru, personal communication). This antibody has been tested in more than 70 healthy adult volunteers, and no serious adverse effects were noted beyond one transient hypotensive anaphylactic reaction. A clinical trial of AMG191-based conditioning in previously transplanted SCID patients with either poor T- or B-cell function has been initiated at Stanford University and the University of California–San Francisco (NCT02963064). If AMG191 proves to be safe and effective, the use of AMG191 will then be moved into the front-line conditioning for patients with newly diagnosed SCID for both allogeneic HCT and autologous gene therapy.

The 15% average donor chimerism seen in SCID mice treated with ACK2, if replicated in human trials of patients with SCID, should be sufficient to correct the immune deficiency. However, for non-SCID disorders, additional approaches will likely be required given the poor efficacy of this single agent in immune-competent mice. To this end, a recent report demonstrated a synergistic effect of blocking CD47 plus targeting c-kit.[57] CD47, a transmembrane protein expressed on HSCs and many other cell types, is a "don't eat me" signal that is an innate immune checkpoint and acts as a critical "marker of self" to attenuate antibody-dependent cell-mediated cytotoxicity/phagocytosis via its interaction with neutrophils and macrophages. Mobilized or naturally circulating HSCs in peripheral blood upregulate expression of surface CD47 to avoid destruction by macrophages in the perisinusoidal spaces in bone marrow, spleen, and liver. In this study, blockade of CD47 markedly enhanced the attenuate antibody-dependent cell-mediated phagocytosis activity of ACK2 in wild-type mice undergoing congenic HCT, resulting in donor myeloid chimerism of 45% to 60%.[57] Anti-CD47 is currently undergoing clinical trials in patients with cancer, and if proven to be safe, the next generation of human clinical trials might test this combination approach for the opening of bone marrow niches before infusion of gene-modified cells.

SUMMARY

It is clear that for the successful application of autologous gene therapy for marrow disorders and inborn errors of metabolism, sufficient marrow niches need to be open for engraftment of gene-corrected HSC. The degree of transduced cell engraftment will depend on the particular disease with some disorders requiring full chimerism and others only limited chimerism to correct all of the disease manifestations. Unlike allogeneic HCT in which all donor-derived cells are normal, with gene therapy, the efficiency of gene transduction is a critical factor that influences the degree of chimerism needed. Alkylating chemotherapy is the standard approach to opening marrow niches. Because the clearance of these drugs varies considerably with age and weight in children less than 12 years old, knowledge of the PK and PD of these agents is essential. Targeting specific dose exposures to safely achieve the desired transduced cell chimerism should be a critical component of any hematopoietic gene therapy trial. To avoid the potential side effects of alkylating agents, newer approaches are being developed and evaluated in animal models and human clinical trials. The most effective ones appear to utilize mAb and/or immunotoxins that target HSC. These and other approaches will likely replace the need for most if not all chemotherapy at least for the nonmalignant hematopoietic disorders. A non-chemotherapy-based approach to conditioning before infusion of gene-modified cells that sustains high-level chimerism would be a major advance in the safe and effective treatment of both children and adults with these life-threatening diseases.

REFERENCES

1. Pai SY, Logan BR, Griffith LM, et al. Transplantation outcomes for severe combined immunodeficiency, 2000-2009. N Engl J Med 2014;371(5):434–46.
2. Stiehm ER, Roberts RL, Hanley-Lopez J, et al. Bone marrow transplantation in severe combined immunodeficiency from a sibling who had received a paternal bone marrow transplant. N Engl J Med 1996;335(24):1811–4.
3. Aubourg P. Gene therapy for rare central nervous system diseases comes to age. Endocr Dev 2016;30:141–6.
4. Moratto D, Giliani S, Bonfim C, et al. Long-term outcome and lineage-specific chimerism in 194 patients with Wiskott-Aldrich syndrome treated by hematopoietic cell transplantation in the period 1980-2009: an international collaborative study. Blood 2011;118(6):1675–84.
5. Grez M, Reichenbach J, Schwable J, et al. Gene therapy of chronic granulomatous disease: the engraftment dilemma. Mol Ther 2011;19(1):28–35.
6. Kohn DB, Weinberg KI, Nolta JA, et al. Engraftment of gene-modified umbilical cord blood cells in neonates with adenosine deaminase deficiency. Nat Med 1995;1(10):1017–23.
7. Aiuti A, Slavin S, Aker M, et al. Correction of ADA-SCID by stem cell gene therapy combined with nonmyeloablative conditioning. Science 2002;296(5577):2410–3.
8. Cavazzana M, Six E, Lagresle-Peyrou C, et al. Gene therapy for X-linked severe combined immunodeficiency: where do we stand? Hum Gene Ther 2016;27(2):108–16.

9. De Ravin SS, Wu X, Moir S, et al. Lentiviral hematopoietic stem cell gene therapy for X-linked severe combined immunodeficiency. Sci Transl Med 2016;8(335): 335ra357.

10. van Til NP, Sarwari R, Visser TP, et al. Recombination-activating gene 1 (Rag1)-deficient mice with severe combined immunodeficiency treated with lentiviral gene therapy demonstrate autoimmune Omenn-like syndrome. J Allergy Clin Immunol 2014;133(4):1116–23.

11. Punwani D, Kawahara M, Yu J, et al. Lentivirus mediated correction of Artemis-deficient severe combined immunodeficiency. Hum Gene Ther 2016;28(1): 112–24.

12. Gungor T, Teira P, Slatter M, et al. Reduced-intensity conditioning and HLA-matched haemopoietic stem-cell transplantation in patients with chronic granulomatous disease: a prospective multicentre study. Lancet 2014;383(9915): 436–48.

13. Braun CJ, Boztug K, Paruzynski A, et al. Gene therapy for Wiskott-Aldrich syndrome–long-term efficacy and genotoxicity. Sci Transl Med 2014;6(227): 227ra233.

14. Hacein-Bey Abina S, Gaspar HB, Blondeau J, et al. Outcomes following gene therapy in patients with severe Wiskott-Aldrich syndrome. JAMA 2015;313(15): 1550–63.

15. Farinelli G, Jofra Hernandez R, Rossi A, et al. Lentiviral vector gene therapy protects XCGD mice from acute staphylococcus aureus pneumonia and inflammatory response. Mol Ther 2016;24(10):1873–80.

16. Cartier N, Hacein-Bey-Abina S, Bartholomae CC, et al. Hematopoietic stem cell gene therapy with a lentiviral vector in X-linked adrenoleukodystrophy. Science 2009;326(5954):818–23.

17. Sessa M, Lorioli L, Fumagalli F, et al. Lentiviral haemopoietic stem-cell gene therapy in early-onset metachromatic leukodystrophy: an ad-hoc analysis of a non-randomised, open-label, phase 1/2 trial. Lancet 2016;388(10043):476–87.

18. Goodman MA, Malik P. The potential of gene therapy approaches for the treatment of hemoglobinopathies: achievements and challenges. Ther Adv Hematol 2016;7(5):302–15.

19. Cavazzana-Calvo M, Payen E, Negre O, et al. Transfusion independence and HMGA2 activation after gene therapy of human beta-thalassaemia. Nature 2010;467(7313):318–22.

20. Saraf SL, Oh AL, Patel PR, et al. Nonmyeloablative stem cell transplantation with alemtuzumab/low-dose irradiation to cure and improve the quality of life of adults with sickle cell disease. Biol Blood Marrow Transplant 2016;22(3):441–8.

21. Andreani M, Testi M, Lucarelli G. Mixed chimerism in haemoglobinopathies: from risk of graft rejection to immune tolerance. Tissue Antigens 2014;83(3):137–46.

22. MacMillan ML, DeFor TE, Young JA, et al. Alternative donor hematopoietic cell transplantation for Fanconi anemia. Blood 2015;125(24):3798–804.

23. Tolar J, Becker PS, Clapp DW, et al. Gene therapy for Fanconi anemia: one step closer to the clinic. Hum Gene Ther 2012;23(2):141–4.

24. Lipstein EA, Vorono S, Browning MF, et al. Systematic evidence review of newborn screening and treatment of severe combined immunodeficiency. Pediatrics 2010;125(5):e1226–1235.

25. Myers LA, Patel DD, Puck JM, et al. Hematopoietic stem cell transplantation for severe combined immunodeficiency in the neonatal period leads to superior thymic output and improved survival. Blood 2002;99(3):872–8.

26. Boelens JJ, Aldenhoven M, Purtill D, et al. Outcomes of transplantation using various hematopoietic cell sources in children with Hurler syndrome after myeloablative conditioning. Blood 2013;121(19):3981–7.

27. van den Anker JN, Schwab M, Kearns GL. Developmental pharmacokinetics. Handb Exp Pharmacol 2011;205:51–75.

28. Hines RN. The ontogeny of drug metabolism enzymes and implications for adverse drug events. Pharmacol Ther 2008;118(2):250–67.

29. Allewelt H, El-Khorazaty J, Mendizabal A, et al. Late effects after umbilical cord blood transplantation in very young children after busulfan-based, myeloablative conditioning. Biol Blood Marrow Transplant 2016;22(9):1627–35.

30. Bartelink IH, van Kesteren C, Boelens JJ, et al. Predictive performance of a busulfan pharmacokinetic model in children and young adults. Ther Drug Monit 2012;34(5):574–83.

31. Paci A, Vassal G, Moshous D, et al. Pharmacokinetic behavior and appraisal of intravenous busulfan dosing in infants and older children: the results of a population pharmacokinetic study from a large pediatric cohort undergoing hematopoietic stem-cell transplantation. Ther Drug Monit 2012;34(2):198–208.

32. Long-Boyle JR, Savic R, Yan S, et al. Population pharmacokinetics of busulfan in pediatric and young adult patients undergoing hematopoietic cell transplant: a model-based dosing algorithm for personalized therapy and implementation into routine clinical use. Ther Drug Monit 2015;37(2):236–45.

33. Savic RM, Cowan MJ, Dvorak CC, et al. Effect of weight and maturation on busulfan clearance in infants and small children undergoing hematopoietic cell transplantation. Biol Blood Marrow Transplant 2013;19(11):1608–14.

34. Gibbs JP, Liacouras CA, Baldassano RN, et al. Up-regulation of glutathione S-transferase activity in enterocytes of young children. Drug Metab Dispos 1999;27(12):1466–9.

35. McCune JS, Gooley T, Gibbs JP, et al. Busulfan concentration and graft rejection in pediatric patients undergoing hematopoietic stem cell transplantation. Bone Marrow Transplant 2002;30(3):167–73.

36. Bolinger AM, Zangwill AB, Slattery JT, et al. Target dose adjustment of busulfan in pediatric patients undergoing bone marrow transplantation. Bone Marrow Transplant 2001;28(11):1013–8.

37. Bartelink IH, Lalmohamed A, van Reij EM, et al. Association of busulfan exposure with survival and toxicity after haemopoietic cell transplantation in children and young adults: a multicentre, retrospective cohort analysis. Lancet Haematol 2016;3(11):e526–36.

38. Vassal G, Michel G, Esperou H, et al. Prospective validation of a novel IV busulfan fixed dosing for paediatric patients to improve therapeutic AUC targeting without drug monitoring. Cancer Chemother Pharmacol 2008;61(1):113–23.

39. Samuels BL, Bitran JD. High-dose intravenous melphalan: a review. J Clin Oncol 1995;13(7):1786–99.

40. Nath CE, Shaw PJ, Montgomery K, et al. Population pharmacokinetics of melphalan in paediatric blood or marrow transplant recipients. Br J Clin Pharmacol 2007;64(2):151–64.

41. Nath CE, Shaw PJ, Montgomery K, et al. Melphalan pharmacokinetics in children with malignant disease: influence of body weight, renal function, carboplatin therapy and total body irradiation. Br J Clin Pharmacol 2005;59(3):314–24.

42. Maanen MJ, Smeets CJ, Beijnen JH. Chemistry, pharmacology and pharmacokinetics of N,N',N"-triethylenethiophosphoramide (ThioTEPA). Cancer Treat Rev 2000;26(4):257–68.

43. de Wildt SN, Kearns GL, Leeder JS, et al. Cytochrome P450 3A: ontogeny and drug disposition. Clin Pharmacokinet 1999;37(6):485–505.
44. Ekhart C, Kerst JM, Rodenhuis S, et al. Altered cyclophosphamide and thiotepa pharmacokinetics in a patient with moderate renal insufficiency. Cancer Chemother Pharmacol 2009;63(2):375–9.
45. Galaup A, Paci A. Pharmacology of dimethanesulfonate alkylating agents: busulfan and treosulfan. Expert Opin Drug Metab Toxicol 2013;9(3):333–47.
46. ten Brink MH, Zwaveling J, Swen JJ, et al. Personalized busulfan and treosulfan conditioning for pediatric stem cell transplantation: the role of pharmacogenetics and pharmacokinetics. Drug Discov Today 2014;19(10):1572–86.
47. Ten Brink MH, Ackaert O, Zwaveling J, et al. Pharmacokinetics of treosulfan in pediatric patients undergoing hematopoietic stem cell transplantation. Ther Drug Monit 2014;36(4):465–72.
48. Wulf GG, Luo K-L, Goodell MA, et al. Anti-CD45–mediated cytoreduction to facilitate allogeneic stem cell transplantation. Blood 2003;101(6):2434–9.
49. Krance RA, Kuehnle I, Rill DR, et al. Hematopoietic and immunomodulatory effects of lytic CD45 monoclonal antibodies in patients with hematologic malignancy. Biol Blood Marrow Transplant 2003;9(4):273–81.
50. Straathof K, Rao K, Eyrich M, et al. Haemopoietic stem-cell transplantation with antibody-based minimal-intensity conditioning: a phase 1/2 study. Lancet 2009;374(9693):912–20.
51. Orozco JJ, Kenoyer A, Balkin ER, et al. Anti-CD45 radioimmunotherapy without TBI before transplantation facilitates persistent haploidentical donor engraftment. Blood 2016;127(3):352–9.
52. Chen Y, Kornblit B, Hamlin DK, et al. Durable donor engraftment after radioimmunotherapy using α-emitter astatine-211-labeled anti-CD45 antibody for conditioning in allogeneic hematopoietic cell transplantation. Blood 2012;119(5):1130–8.
53. Palchaudhuri R, Saez B, Hoggatt J, et al. Non-genotoxic conditioning for hematopoietic stem cell transplantation using a hematopoietic-cell-specific internalizing immunotoxin. Nat Biotechnol 2016;34(7):738–45.
54. Czechowicz A, Kraft D, Weissman I, et al. Efficient transplantation via antibody-based clearance of hematopoietic stem cell niches. Science 2007;318(5854):1296–9.
55. Derderian SC, Togarrati PP, King C, et al. In utero depletion of fetal hematopoietic stem cells improves engraftment after neonatal transplantation in mice. Blood 2014;124(6):973–80.
56. Xue X, Pech NK, Shelley WC, et al. Antibody targeting KIT as pretransplantation conditioning in immunocompetent mice. Blood 2010;116(24):5419–22.
57. Chhabra A, Ring AM, Weiskopf K, et al. Hematopoietic stem cell transplantation in immunocompetent hosts without radiation or chemotherapy. Sci Transl Med 2016;8(351):351ra105.

Gene Therapy Approaches to Immunodeficiency

Sujal Ghosh, MD[a,b], H. Bobby Gaspar, MBBS, PhD[a],*

KEYWORDS

- Gene therapy • Primary immunodeficiency • Adenosine deaminase deficiency
- X-linked severe combined immunodeficiency • Chronic granulomatous disease
- Wiskott-Aldrich syndrome

KEY POINTS

- Ex vivo gene transfer can be used in different primary immune disorders.
- Initial results were tempered by genotoxicity associated with the gammaretroviral design.
- New "safer" vector designs combined with nonmyeloablative or fully myeloablative conditioning regimens allow enhanced engraftment and efficient transgene expression, while maintaining a robust safety profile.

INTRODUCTION

More than 300 gene defects have been associated with primary immunodeficiency syndromes (PID).[1] Treatment strategies encompass anti-infective prophylaxis and immunoglobulin substitution. However, hematopoietic stem cell transplantation has been the only option for definitive correction and functional reconstitution. Transplant-related mortality due to toxicity and infections is a major concern even in a fully matched setting. Despite emerging reduced-intensity conditioning regimens, a mismatched donor may lead to a fatal outcome in some patients.[2] Ex vivo gene transfer of autologous hematopoietic stem cells has been progressively developed in the past decades. Initial studies using gammaretroviral vectors showed success but also major safety issues because of insertional mutagenesis, which ultimately led to a range of newly developed safer vectors and promising current phase 1/phase 2 trials. In at least in one of the diseases, namely adenosine deaminase (ADA) deficiency, it seems gene therapy is an equal or even slightly superior treatment to current

Disclosure of Conflicts of Interest: H.B. Gaspar is a founder and advisory board member of Orchard Therapeutics and has financial interests in the company.
^a Infection, Immunity, Inflammation, Molecular and Cellular Immunology Section, University College London, UCL Great Ormond Street Institute of Child Health, 30 Guilford Street, London WC1N 1EH, UK; ^b Department of Pediatric Oncology, Hematology and Clinical Immunology, Center of Child and Adolescent Health, Heinrich-Heine-University, Moorenstraße 5, 40225 Düsseldorf, Germany
* Corresponding author.
E-mail address: h.gaspar@ucl.ac.uk

Hematol Oncol Clin N Am 31 (2017) 823–834
http://dx.doi.org/10.1016/j.hoc.2017.05.003
hemonc.theclinics.com
0889-8588/17/© 2017 Elsevier Inc. All rights reserved.

standards of treatment with fully matched unrelated donors. Besides safety concerns, one major challenge of the future will certainly be the accessibility of gene therapy in other centers than the current few ones in high-resource countries.

ADENOSINE DEAMINASE DEFICIENCY

ADA is essential in the purine salvage pathway and catalyses the deamination of metabolites into deoxyinosine and inosine. Because it is ubiquitously expressed, mutations in *ADA* lead to accumulation of toxic deoxyadenosine triphosphate and adenosine triphosphate and subsequently to immunologic, pulmonary, gastrointestinal, skeletal, and neurologic abnormalities.[3] Affected infants present usually with a T-B-NK- severe combined immunodeficiency (SCID) phenotype in the first months of life with failure to thrive and severe infections. Weekly enzyme replacement therapy with pegylated bovine ADA allows partial numeric and functional T-cell reconstitution; however, long-term results show limited sustained efficacy. Hematopoietic stem cell transplant (HSCT) has been considered the only curative treatment for a long time, and success rates reach 90% in patients with a matched-sibling or matched-family donor without the need of any conditioning. However, the transplantation of matched unrelated donor (MUD) or haploidentical grafts is associated with inferior results (1-year survival: matched family donor [MFD] 90%, MUD 67%, haplo 43%).[4]

Gene correction of peripheral blood lymphocytes and later of hematopoietic progenitor cells has been attempted from the early 1990s. Initial studies at National Institutes of Health (NIH) Bethesda and San Raffaele in Milan with gammaretroviral vectors and concomitant enzyme replacement therapy (ERT) showed low toxicity, but lack of substantial immunologic and clinical benefit due to low levels of marked cells in the peripheral circulation.[5–8] The next generation of trials in Milan and London incorporated the idea of conferring a greater competitive advantage to transduced cells and so polyethylene glycol (PEG)-ADA was stopped before gene therapy; furthermore, a nonmyeloablative reduced intensity conditioning regimen with Busulfan or Melphalan was given to enhance engraftment. The trial at Children's Hospital Los Angeles and NIH amended its protocol after treating the first patients without conditioning.[4,9,10] Implementation of conditioning led to a more favorable outcome in all patients compared with the initial studies. Murine studies confirmed the findings of the positive effect of prior cytoreduction; however, it seems that cessation of ERT is of less importance, and ERT continuation showed significantly increased levels of gene-modified cells in the thymus in mice.[11] Based on that, current trials allow the continuation of ERT until day 30. Together the 3 gammaretroviral studies treated more than 40 patients with gammaretroviral vectors, and all patients are alive. Approximately 75% of patients are off ERT, and transduced cells engrafted permanently with partial reconstitution in all lineages 4 (Gaspar), 9 (Aiuti), 10 (Candotti). Notably, none of the patients have developed insertional mutagenesis, although in all studies, patients harbor integration events near protooncogenes, including LMO2 as a consequence of being treated with a gammaretroviral vector. The positive outcome and the excellent survival in ADA deficiency led to the market authorization of the Milan gammaretroviral vector by the European Medicines Agency (Strimvelis).[12]

Given the adverse events using gammaretroviral vectors in other gene therapy studies, the authors' group in London and the group at University of California, Los Angeles decided to proceed to further trials using a lentiviral vector. A codon-optimized human complementary DNA (cDNA) ADA gene under the control of the short form elongation factor-1 alpha promoter (EF1α) was shown to have efficacy in the murine model.[13] Furthermore, safety issues assessed through in vitro immortalization indicated a reduced transformation potential compared with gammar-etroviral vectors. Interim data from these 2 studies using the lentiviral vector again show 100% survival and impressive immune and metabolic correction.[14]

X-LINKED SEVERE COMBINED IMMUNODEFICIENCY

Mutations in the *IL2RG* gene encoding the common gamma chain on the X-chromo-some led to one of the most common forms of SCID. The gamma chain is a key sub-unit shared by different cytokine receptor complexes for interleukin-2 (IL-2), IL-4, IL-7, IL-9, IL-15, and IL-21. Hence, SCID-X1 patients with defective gamma chain function have profound cellular (due to decreased T-cell number and function) and humoral (due to decreased B-cell function) defects with typically a T-B+NK- phenotype.[15]

There are rare cases of patients with spontaneous reversion of the mutation in a frac-tion of cells leading to the correction of immunodeficiency in these individuals.[16] This phenomenon supported the concept of selective advantage of "gene-corrected" cells over mutated lymphocytes and thus the principle of gene therapy. The first generation of gammaretroviral vectors was applied to hematopoietic stem cells in a total of 20 pa-tients, lacking an HLA-identical donor, in studies in Hôpital Necker, Paris and Great Ormond Street Hospital, London.[17–19] In both studies, a gammaretroviral vector derived from a defective Moloney murine leukemia virus (Mo-MLV) was used, in which *IL2RG* expression was driven by the viral long terminal repeat (LTR). Ex vivo transduced autologous CD34+ cells were given to patients without any conditioning, and in most patients, a rapid and sustained functional and numeric reconstitution of T cells (with high levels of gene marking) was seen. NK cells engrafted transiently, to a lesser extent, and humoral reconstitution allowed the discontinuation of immunoglobulin replace-ment therapy in less than 50% of treated patients. It is likely that this level of reconsti-tution results from the engraftment of more committed progenitor cells rather than true hematopoietic stem cells as has been observed in other unconditioned allogeneic HSCT procedures. A similar approach was initiated in 5 older patients with hypomor-phic *IL2RG* mutations (including 3 treated at the NIH), but despite good marking in all lineages, functional reconstitution was not achieved. A lack of thymopoietic capacity due to age-related decreased function may be related to the insufficient outcome.[20]

The promising outcome in X-linked severe combined immunodeficiency (XSCID) patients was shadowed by the occurrence of genotoxicity from approximately 2 years after treatment.[18,21,22] A total of 5 clinically well patients in both centers developed acute lymphoblastic T-cell leukemia, 4 of whom entered remission with standard chemotherapy and then showed recovery of gene corrected cells and restored im-munity. One patient died because of incurable refractory leukemia despite allogeneic HSCT. Extensive investigations performed at this time revealed the pathophysiology of insertional mutagenesis in all cases of malignancies, which could be linked to fea-tures of the gammaretroviral vector used. The tendency for preferential gammaretro-viral integration near transcription start sites together with enhancing activity of the viral LTR most likely led to aberrant transcription and expression of neighboring on-cogenes (*LMO2*) or cell cycle regulators (*BMI1* and *CCND2*). Furthermore, accumu-lation of other abnormalities in genes such as *NOTCH1* and *CDKN2A* were detected in the blast population and most likely led finally to leukemic transformation. The se-vere outcome seen in these and other PID trials (see later discussion) led to a global redesign of most ongoing clinical gene therapy trials, notably in the configuration of the vectors. Self-inactivating (SIN) gammaretroviral and lentiviral vectors incorporate safety features such as the deletion of the viral LTR with transcription of the trans-gene under the control of an internal mammalian promoter. Various in vivo and in vitro models showed that the risk of insertional mutagenesis was significantly reduced with the use of SIN vector designs. Based on these concerns, 2 SIN vectors have been developed. One SIN gammaretroviral vector under the control of an internal EF1α promoter and deletion of the original Mo-MLV U3 LTR enhancer[23] has been used in a multicenter approach to XSCID in Boston, Cincinnati, London, Los Angeles, and Paris, and 10 patients have been treated so far.[24] Conditioning was initially not given to most patients (only in those with maternal engraftment or maternal graft-versus-host disease), and 9/10 boys survived. One patient died because of preexisting adenoviremia, and one patient had to undergo another stem cell procedure with a mismatched cord blood graft because of absent gene marking. All other patients show a similar T-cell reconstitution to that seen in the previous gammaretroviral studies, with significant reduction of infections, but with the majority still retaining dependence on immunoglobulin replacement. With regards to genotoxicity, clustering of viral integrations around oncogenes was significantly decreased in comparison to gammaretroviral studies. Moreover, clonal expansion, persistence, or dominance was not seen in any of the patients treated, with the longest follow-up greater than 5 years in the first patient treated. Another trial in older patients (7–23 years old), conducted at NIH, included the application of an SIN lentivirus using an EF1α promoter to drive a codon-optimized gamma chain cDNA flanked by 400-bp chicken insulators.[25,26] The same vector will be applied to infants with XSCID in the future as well. The older patients treated so far received a mild conditioning regime. These patients had all previously failed haploidentical HSCT attempts. After treatment with autologous corrected CD34 cells, patients had gene marking in all lineages, functional T cell, NK, and humoral reconstitution. Interestingly, they were able to clear persistent norovirus (whereas prior immunoglobulin G replacement failed), warts, and molloscum (associated with NK cell reconstitution). Unfortunately, one patient, with prior severely compromised pulmonary function and irreversible airway damage, died because of fatal pulmonary hemorrhage 27 months after gene therapy. Vector integration site analysis showed dynamic fluctuation in clonal integration sites near known oncogenes, but without any enrichment. Although follow-up in these patients is still too short to rule out any possible genotoxic adverse effects, both studies applying an SIN concept show promising results.

CHRONIC GRANULOMATOUS DISEASE

Chronic granulomatous disease (CGD) is caused by mutations in one of the subunits of the NADPH oxidase complex leading to disturbance in the phagocytic activity of neutrophils. The fully assembled complex consists of cytosolic phox proteins (p47^{phox}, p67^{phox}, and p40^{phox}) translocated to the membrane-bound flavocytochrome (gp91^{phox} and p22^{phox}), and upon assembly, reactive oxygen species (ROS) are produced to kill invading microbes. Mutations in the CYBB gene (encoding gp91phox) account for most CGD patients, are inherited in an X-linked manner, and have been the target for gene therapy trials. Patients are susceptible to recurrent bacterial and fungal infections, and furthermore, sterile inflammation involves the respiratory, gastrointestinal, and genitourinary tract. HSCT is successful in the early course; however, the outcome declines with existing comorbidities and lack of a suitable donor.[27–29] Unlike in SCID, patients with defects in CGD have a fully replete marrow because the defect is due to a lack of peripheral neutrophil function and not of impaired development. For this reason, myeloablative conditioning is required to allow stem cell engraftment and achieve long-term correction because restoration of gp91 protein does not confer selective advantage over noncorrected cells.

Furthermore, CGD patients have an inflammatory bone marrow milieu that might negatively influence hematopoietic stem cell (HSC) gene transfer and engraftment of gene-modified cells.[30,31] The first trials in the late 1990s used a Mo-MLV-based gammaretrovirus on granulocyte colony stimulating factor–mobilized CD34+ HSCs. Five patients were treated without any preconditioning, and as a result of this, only a transient production of neutrophils producing ROS could be detected; these studies failed to show any long-term clinical benefit.[32,33] Other clinical trials around the world used LTR-based gammaretroviral vectors and included the administration of a nonmyeloablative conditioning regimen before gene transfer. A total of 13 patients were treated, and 10 patients experienced a transient clinical benefit with initial correction of NADPH activity. Up to 50% of neutrophils showed gene marking, but over time, functional neutrophils did not persist.[34–39] In 2 adults and one child, the increase of gene-marked neutrophils reflected clonal expansion, and the viral spleen focus-forming virus LTR drove transactivation of the *MDS/EVI1* and *PRDM16* oncogenes leading to myelodysplasia (MDS) with monosomy 7. Both adult patients died because of complications in the context of MDS.[34,37,40] The other child displayed clonal expansion without monosomy 7, and currently, both the younger patients are alive after HSCT.[35,38] Current clinical trials now use SIN lentiviral vectors and include a fully myeloablative conditioning regime. Notably, one multicenter trial uses a lentiviral vector, in which gp91^{phox} is driven by a synthetic chimeric promoter, created by the fusion of Cathepsin G and c-Fes minimal 5′-flanking regions. This vector allows preferential expression in myeloid cells and differentiated granulocytes and has a reduced potential regarding insertional mutagenesis.[41]

WISKOTT-ALDRICH SYNDROME

Wiskott-Aldrich syndrome (WAS) is an X-linked inherited disorder arising by mutations in the *WAS* gene, encoding WASp, a main actin cytoskeleton regulator protein. Patients usually manifest with microthrombocytopenia, eczema, infections, and autoimmunity.[42–44] HSCT in a matched-donor setting can cure most patients; however, as in other genetic disorders, a mismatched setting is associated with a higher rate of morbidity and mortality. Early murine studies have suggested a selective survival advantage of wild-type over diseased cells.[45] The first clinical gene therapy trial was conducted in Hannover in the 2000s and included 10 patients lacking a matched family donor. An LTR intact gammaretroviral vector restored gene expression in the myeloid and lymphoid compartment in 9 of 10 patients with increased platelet numbers and normalized T-, B-, and NK-cell function and clear initial clinical benefit[46]; however, 7 of 9 reconstituted patients developed acute leukemia revealing dominant clones with integration in *LMO2*, *MDS1/EVI1*, and *MN1* oncogenes.[47]

Several SIN-LV vectors for the treatment of WAS have been developed by various groups[48–51] to comply with safety requirements and have shown efficient transduction. A lentiviral vector consisting of the endogenous 1.6-kb human WAS promoter was chosen for clinical trials in Boston, London, Milan, and Paris with preliminary results published recently.[52–55] All studies used a conditioning regime consisting of busulfan and fludarabine, and a total of 21 patients have been treated so far. In most patients, a stable engraftment of gene-marked cells could be seen associated with clear clinical benefits, in terms of bleeding episodes, infections, autoimmunity, and eczema. However, platelet recovery has been variable in all studies, indicating that WASp expression in this lineage might be suboptimal. There has been no evidence of any genotoxicity so far.

PRECLINICAL APPROACHES IN OTHER PRIMARY IMMUNE DISORDERS

In light of promising results in the 4 above-mentioned disorders and other inherited diseases of the bone marrow, preclinical approaches to target other monogenic PIDs are currently being developed. V(D)J recombination defects account for one-third of patients with SCID and lead to an inability to generate T- and B-cell receptor. Patients suffering from recombinase activating gene (*RAG1/2*), Artemis (*DCLRE1C*), and Ligase IV (*LIG4*) deficiency usually present with a T-B-NK+ phenotype.[56,57] The latter, both being DNA repair disorders, are additionally associated with radiosensitivity, which is relevant for both HSCT and gene therapy. Several studies have highlighted lentivirus-mediated correction of murine and human HSCs in Artemis deficiency. Two early in vivo studies showed sustained correction of T- and B-cell dysfunction in the mouse model. A lentiviral vector, in which Artemis expression was driven from an internal phosphoglycerate kinase (PGK) promoter, was used with Artemis knock-out HSCs, which were transplanted to either nonmyeolablative Busulfan conditioned or irradiated Artemis knock-out mice.[58,59] Furthermore, bone marrow–derived CD34+ cells from Artemis patients were successfully transduced, and repopulation studies in NSG mice showed the capability for further B- and T-cell differentiation of these cells.[60] Two groups in the United States have recently published their experience with an SIN lentiviral vector containing human Artemis cDNA under transcriptional regulation of the endogenous Artemis promoter.[61,62] Because the moderate-strength PGK gives insufficient immune reconstitution and human EF1α-driven Artemis overexpression can be toxic, the use of the most "endogenous" promoter may have potential to be superior. Fibroblasts from patients transduced with that lentivirus showed correction of radiosensitivity. Furthermore, the group demonstrated that transduced peripheral blood CD34+ cells from a patient as well as HSCs from Artemis-deficient mice are able to differentiate to T and B cells. Vector copy number and tight regulation of protein expression are also of major concern in preclinical models of both recombinase-activating genes. Early attempts corrected the murine model of RAG1 and 2 with MLV-derived gammaretroviral vector, allowing high vector copy numbers in all organs.[63,64] However, to avoid risk of insertional mutagenesis, new lentiviral vectors delivering a codon-optimized transgene have been developed.[65,66] In RAG-1 reconstitution studies in the murine model, low vector copy number (VCN) leads to autoreactive T cells and an Omenn-like syndrome with a reduced thymic cellularity, emphasizing the need for appropriate RAG-1 regulation to fully correct the disease phenotype. RAG-2 correction appears to be more readily achieved using an LV with a ubiquitous promoter and suggests that for RAG-2, there is a less stringent need for regulated gene expression.[65,67]

Inherited diseases associated with a reduced NK and CD8 cytotoxicity, such as hemophagocytic lymphohistiocytosis (HLH), are also amenable to corrective strategies using gene therapy. Proof-of-concept studies have been performed in murine models of perforin deficiency, Munc 13-4 deficiency, and X-linked lymphoproliferative disease.[68–70] Autologous T-cell gene therapy is an equally attractive strategy in these disorders, as is known from early ADA trials (see earlier discussion), that transplanted gene-transduced peripheral lymphocytes remain in the circulation for decades.[71] The safety profile and long-term effects of these products have been investigated in numerous adoptive cell trials in cancer and infectious disease, so that the authors and other groups have performed murine T-cell gene therapy studies in defects of the cytolytic pathway. Further genetic correction is currently investigated in preclinical models of IPEX syndrome, CD40L deficiency, p47 autosomal recessive CGD, Bruton agammaglobulinemia, and leukocyte adhesion deficiency type I.[72–76]

Table 1
Gene therapy clinical trials for primary immunodeficiencies

Disease	Center	Status	Patients	NCT	Viral Vector	Conditioning
ADA	Los Angeles, Bethesda	R	8	NCT01852071; NCT02022696	LV	Busulfan/ERT till d+30
	London	R	12	NCT01380990	LV	Busulfan/ERT till d+30
	Milan, Jerusalem	C	18	NCT00599781; NCT00598481	γ-RV	None/Busulfan
	Bethesda	C	16	NCT00018018	γ-RV	Melphalan/Busulfan
	London	C	8	NCT01279720	γ-RV	
SCID-X1	Boston, Cincinnati London, Los Angeles, Paris	R	11	NCT01410019; NCT01175239; NCT01129544	SIN-γ-RV	None
	Memphis, Seattle	R	0	NCT01512888	LV	None
	Bethesda, Memphis	R	5	NCT01306019	LV	Busulfan
	Bethesda	C	3	NCT00028236	γ-RV	None
	London	C	11	—	γ-RV	None
	Paris	C	11	—	γ-RV	None
CGD	Frankfurt	R	0	NCT01906541	SIN-γ-RV	Busulfan
	Frankfurt, London, Paris, Zürich	R	1	NCT01855685	LV	Busulfan
	Bethesda, Boston, Los Angeles	R	1	NCT02234934	LV	Busulfan
	London	C	4	—	γ-RV	Melphalan
	Frankfurt	C	2	NCT00564759	γ-RV	Busulfan
	Zürich	C	2	NCT00927134	γ-RV	Busulfan
	Seoul	C	2	NCT00778882	γ-RV	Busulfan/Fludarabine
	Bethesda	C	3	NCT00394316	γ-RV	Busulfan
	Bethesda	C	10	NCT00001476	γ-RV	None
WAS	Boston, London, Paris	R	13	NCT01347242; NCT01347346; NCT01410825	LV	Busulfan/Fludarabine
	Milan	R	10	NCT01515462	LV	—
	Hannover	C	10	—	γ-RV	Busulfan

Abbreviations: C, completed/terminated/not recruiting any longer; R, recruiting or not yet recruiting; LV, lentivirus; RV, retrovirus.

SUMMARY

The new generation of gene therapy trials (**Table 1**) used safer vectors and the use of myeloablative and nonmyeloablative conditioning regimens. The occurrence of insertional mutagenesis and subsequent malignancies was strongly linked to the use of gammaretroviral vectors. An SIN configuration, lacking the enhancers of the LTR in U3 to avoid enhancer-mediated activation, and using well-designed different internal promoters to drive transgene expression, are the main changes in vector design. Short-term results are encouraging in terms of both safety and efficacy. Furthermore, gene editing, especially for diseases where there is a need for more physiologic gene regulation (which is discussed in Andy Scharenberg and Christopher Lux'article, "Therapeutic Gene Editing Safety and Specificity," and Dale Ando and Kathleen Meyer'article, "Gene Editing: Regulatory and Translation to Clinic," in this issue), will certainly lead to new opportunities in the treatment of these patients.

REFERENCES

1. Picard C, Al-Herz W, Bousfiha A, et al. Primary immunodeficiency diseases: an update on the classification from the International Union of Immunological Societies Expert Committee for Primary Immunodeficiency 2015. J Clin Immunol 2015;35(8):696–726.
2. Booth C, Silva J, Veys P. Stem cell transplantation for the treatment of immunodeficiency in children: current status and hopes for the future. Expert Rev Clin Immunol 2016;12(7):713–23.
3. Whitmore KV, Gaspar HB. Adenosine deaminase deficiency - more than just an immunodeficiency. Front Immunol 2016;7:314.
4. Gaspar HB, Cooray S, Gilmour KC, et al. Hematopoietic stem cell gene therapy for adenosine deaminase-deficient severe combined immunodeficiency leads to long-term immunological recovery and metabolic correction. Sci Transl Med 2011;3(97):97ra80.
5. Blaese RM, Culver KW, Miller AD, et al. T lymphocyte-directed gene therapy for ADA-SCID: initial trial results after 4 years. Science 1995;270(5235):475–80.
6. Bordignon C, Notarangelo LD, Nobili N, et al. Gene therapy in peripheral blood lymphocytes and bone marrow for ADA- immunodeficient patients. Science 1995;270(5235):470–5.
7. Onodera M, Ariga T, Kawamura N, et al. Successful peripheral T-lymphocyte-directed gene transfer for a patient with severe combined immune deficiency caused by adenosine deaminase deficiency. Blood 1998;91(1):30–6.
8. Aiuti A, Vai S, Mortellaro A, et al. Immune reconstitution in ADA-SCID after PBL gene therapy and discontinuation of enzyme replacement. Nat Med 2002;8(5):423–5.
9. Aiuti A, Cattaneo F, Galimberti S, et al. Gene therapy for immunodeficiency due to adenosine deaminase deficiency. N Engl J Med 2009;360(5):447–58.
10. Candotti F, Shaw KL, Muul L, et al. Gene therapy for adenosine deaminase-deficient severe combined immune deficiency: clinical comparison of retroviral vectors and treatment plans. Blood 2012;120(18):3635–46.
11. Carbonaro DA, Jin X, Wang X, et al. Gene therapy/bone marrow transplantation in ADA-deficient mice: roles of enzyme-replacement therapy and cytoreduction. Blood 2012;120(18):3677–87.
12. Schimmer J, Breazzano S. Investor outlook: rising from the ashes; GSK's European Approval of Strimvelis for ADA-SCID. Hum Gene Ther Clin Dev 2016;27(2):57–61.

13. Carbonaro DA, Zhang L, Jin X, et al. Preclinical demonstration of lentiviral vector-mediated correction of immunological and metabolic abnormalities in models of adenosine deaminase deficiency. Mol Ther 2014;22(3):607–22.
14. Gaspar HB, Buckland K, Carbonaro DA, et al. Immunological and metabolic correction after lentiviral vector gene therapy for ADA deficiency. Paper presented at: 18th Annual Meeting of the American Society of Gene and Cell Therapy (ASGCT). New Orleans, LA, May 13–16, 2015.
15. Fischer A, Notarangelo LD, Neven B, et al. Severe combined immunodeficiencies and related disorders. Nat Rev Dis Primers 2015;1:15061.
16. Stephan V, Wahn V, Le Deist F, et al. Atypical X-linked severe combined immunodeficiency due to possible spontaneous reversion of the genetic defect in T cells. N Engl J Med 1996;335(21):1563–7.
17. Hacein-Bey-Abina S, Le Deist F, Carlier F, et al. Sustained correction of X-linked severe combined immunodeficiency by ex vivo gene therapy. N Engl J Med 2002;346(16):1185–93.
18. Hacein-Bey-Abina S, Garrigue A, Wang GP, et al. Insertional oncogenesis in 4 patients after retrovirus-mediated gene therapy of SCID-X1. J Clin Invest 2008;118(9):3132–42.
19. Gaspar HB, Cooray S, Gilmour KC, et al. Long-term persistence of a polyclonal T cell repertoire after gene therapy for X-linked severe combined immunodeficiency. Sci Transl Med 2011;3(97):97ra79.
20. Chinen J, Davis J, De Ravin SS, et al. Gene therapy improves immune function in preadolescents with X-linked severe combined immunodeficiency. Blood 2007;110(1):67–73.
21. Deichmann A, Hacein-Bey-Abina S, Schmidt M, et al. Vector integration is nonrandom and clustered and influences the fate of lymphopoiesis in SCID-X1 gene therapy. J Clin Invest 2007;117(8):2225–32.
22. Howe SJ, Mansour MR, Schwarzwaelder K, et al. Insertional mutagenesis combined with acquired somatic mutations causes leukemogenesis following gene therapy of SCID-X1 patients. J Clin Invest 2008;118(9):3143–50.
23. Thornhill SI, Schambach A, Howe SJ, et al. Self-inactivating gammaretroviral vectors for gene therapy of X-linked severe combined immunodeficiency. Mol Ther 2008;16(3):590–8.
24. Hacein-Bey-Abina S, Pai SY, Gaspar HB, et al. A modified gamma-retrovirus vector for X-linked severe combined immunodeficiency. N Engl J Med 2014;371(15):1407–17.
25. Zhou S, Mody D, DeRavin SS, et al. A self-inactivating lentiviral vector for SCID-X1 gene therapy that does not activate LMO2 expression in human T cells. Blood 2010;116(6):900–8.
26. De Ravin SS, Wu X, Moir S, et al. Lentiviral hematopoietic stem cell gene therapy for X-linked severe combined immunodeficiency. Sci Transl Med 2016;8(335):335ra357.
27. Cole T, Pearce MS, Cant AJ, et al. Clinical outcome in children with chronic granulomatous disease managed conservatively or with hematopoietic stem cell transplantation. J Allergy Clin Immunol 2013;132(5):1150–5.
28. Holland SM. Chronic granulomatous disease. Hematol Oncol Clin North Am 2013;27(1):89–99, viii.
29. Seger RA. Advances in the diagnosis and treatment of chronic granulomatous disease. Curr Opin Hematol 2011;18(1):36–41.
30. Grez M, Reichenbach J, Schwable J, et al. Gene therapy of chronic granulomatous disease: the engraftment dilemma. Mol Ther 2011;19(1):28–35.

31. Weisser M, Demel UM, Stein S, et al. Hyperinflammation in patients with chronic granulomatous disease leads to impairment of hematopoietic stem cell functions. J Allergy Clin Immunol 2016;138(1):219–28.e9.

32. Malech HL, Maples PB, Whiting-Theobald N, et al. Prolonged production of NADPH oxidase-corrected granulocytes after gene therapy of chronic granulomatous disease. Proc Natl Acad Sci U S A 1997;94(22):12133–8.

33. Goebel WS, Dinauer MC. Gene therapy for chronic granulomatous disease. Acta Haematol 2003;110(2–3):86–92.

34. Ott MG, Schmidt M, Schwarzwaelder K, et al. Correction of X-linked chronic granulomatous disease by gene therapy, augmented by insertional activation of MDS1-EVI1, PRDM16 or SETBP1. Nat Med 2006;12(4):401–9.

35. Bianchi M, Hakkim A, Brinkmann V, et al. Restoration of NET formation by gene therapy in CGD controls aspergillosis. Blood 2009;114(13):2619–22.

36. Kang EM, Choi U, Theobald N, et al. Retrovirus gene therapy for X-linked chronic granulomatous disease can achieve stable long-term correction of oxidase activity in peripheral blood neutrophils. Blood 2010;115(4):783–91.

37. Stein S, Ott MG, Schultze-Strasser S, et al. Genomic instability and myelodysplasia with monosomy 7 consequent to EVI1 activation after gene therapy for chronic granulomatous disease. Nat Med 2010;16(2):198–204.

38. Bianchi M, Niemiec MJ, Siler U, et al. Restoration of anti-Aspergillus defense by neutrophil extracellular traps in human chronic granulomatous disease after gene therapy is calprotectin-dependent. J Allergy Clin Immunol 2011;127(5): 1243–52.e7.

39. Kang HJ, Bartholomae CC, Paruzynski A, et al. Retroviral gene therapy for X-linked chronic granulomatous disease: results from phase I/II trial. Mol Ther 2011;19(11):2092–101.

40. Aiuti A, Bacchetta R, Seger R, et al. Gene therapy for primary immunodeficiencies: part 2. Curr Opin Immunol 2012;24(5):585–91.

41. Santilli G, Almarza E, Brendel C, et al. Biochemical correction of X-CGD by a novel chimeric promoter regulating high levels of transgene expression in myeloid cells. Mol Ther 2011;19(1):122–32.

42. Thrasher AJ. New insights into the biology of Wiskott-Aldrich syndrome (WAS). Hematology Am Soc Hematol Educ Program 2009;132–8.

43. Massaad MJ, Ramesh N, Geha RS. Wiskott-Aldrich syndrome: a comprehensive review. Ann N Y Acad Sci 2013;1285:26–43.

44. Blundell MP, Worth A, Bouma G, et al. The Wiskott-Aldrich syndrome: the actin cytoskeleton and immune cell function. Dis Markers 2010;29(3–4):157–75.

45. Moratto D, Giliani S, Bonfim C, et al. Long-term outcome and lineage-specific chimerism in 194 patients with Wiskott-Aldrich syndrome treated by hematopoietic cell transplantation in the period 1980-2009: an international collaborative study. Blood 2011;118(6):1675–84.

46. Boztug K, Schmidt M, Schwarzer A, et al. Stem-cell gene therapy for the Wiskott-Aldrich syndrome. N Engl J Med 2010;363(20):1918–27.

47. Braun CJ, Boztug K, Paruzynski A, et al. Gene therapy for Wiskott-Aldrich syndrome–long-term efficacy and genotoxicity. Sci Transl Med 2014;6(227): 227ra233.

48. Avedillo Diez I, Zychlinski D, Coci EG, et al. Development of novel efficient SIN vectors with improved safety features for Wiskott-Aldrich syndrome stem cell based gene therapy. Mol Pharm 2011;8(5):1525–37.

49. Dupre L, Marangoni F, Scaramuzza S, et al. Efficacy of gene therapy for Wiskott-Aldrich syndrome using a WAS promoter/cDNA-containing lentiviral vector and nonlethal irradiation. Hum Gene Ther 2006;17(3):303–13.

50. Marangoni F, Bosticardo M, Charrier S, et al. Evidence for long-term efficacy and safety of gene therapy for Wiskott-Aldrich syndrome in preclinical models. Mol Ther 2009;17(6):1073–82.

51. Bosticardo M, Draghici E, Schena F, et al. Lentiviral-mediated gene therapy leads to improvement of B-cell functionality in a murine model of Wiskott-Aldrich syndrome. J Allergy Clin Immunol 2011;127(6):1376–84.e5.

52. Aiuti A, Biasco L, Scaramuzza S, et al. Lentiviral hematopoietic stem cell gene therapy in patients with Wiskott-Aldrich syndrome. Science 2013;341(6148): 1233151.

53. Bosticardo M, Ferrua F, Cavazzana M, et al. Gene therapy for Wiskott-Aldrich syndrome. Curr Gene Ther 2014;14(6):413–21.

54. Castiello MC, Scaramuzza S, Pala F, et al. B-cell reconstitution after lentiviral vector-mediated gene therapy in patients with Wiskott-Aldrich syndrome. J Allergy Clin Immunol 2015;136(3):692–702.e2.

55. Hacein-Bey Abina S, Gaspar HB, Blondeau J, et al. Outcomes following gene therapy in patients with severe Wiskott-Aldrich syndrome. JAMA 2015;313(15): 1550–63.

56. Moshous D, Callebaut I, de Chasseval R, et al. Artemis, a novel DNA double-strand break repair/V(D)J recombination protein, is mutated in human severe combined immune deficiency. Cell 2001;105(2):177–86.

57. Schwarz K, Gauss GH, Ludwig L, et al. RAG mutations in human B cell-negative SCID. Science 1996;274(5284):97–9.

58. Benjelloun F, Garrigue A, Demerens-de Chappedelaine C, et al. Stable and functional lymphoid reconstitution in Artemis-deficient mice following lentiviral artemis gene transfer into hematopoietic stem cells. Mol Ther 2008;16(8):1490–9.

59. Mostoslavsky G, Fabian AJ, Rooney S, et al. Complete correction of murine Artemis immunodeficiency by lentiviral vector-mediated gene transfer. Proc Natl Acad Sci U S A 2006;103(44):16406–11.

60. Lagresle-Peyrou C, Benjelloun F, Hue C, et al. Restoration of human B-cell differentiation into NOD-SCID mice engrafted with gene-corrected CD34+ cells isolated from Artemis or RAG1-deficient patients. Mol Ther 2008;16(2):396–403.

61. Multhaup MM, Podetz-Pedersen KM, Karlen AD, et al. Role of transgene regulation in ex vivo lentiviral correction of artemis deficiency. Hum Gene Ther 2015; 26(4):232–43.

62. Punwani D, Kawahara M, Yu J, et al. Lentivirus mediated correction of artemis-deficient severe combined immunodeficiency. Hum Gene Ther 2017;28(1): 112–24.

63. Lagresle-Peyrou C, Yates F, Malassis-Seris M, et al. Long-term immune reconstitution in RAG-1-deficient mice treated by retroviral gene therapy: a balance between efficiency and toxicity. Blood 2006;107(1):63–72.

64. Yates F, Malassis-Seris M, Stockholm D, et al. Gene therapy of RAG-2-/- mice: sustained correction of the immunodeficiency. Blood 2002;100(12):3942–9.

65. Pike-Overzet K, Rodijk M, Ng YY, et al. Correction of murine Rag1 deficiency by self-inactivating lentiviral vector-mediated gene transfer. Leukemia 2011;25(9): 1471–83.

66. van Til NP, de Boer H, Mashamba N, et al. Correction of murine Rag2 severe combined immunodeficiency by lentiviral gene therapy using a codon-optimized RAG2 therapeutic transgene. Mol Ther 2012;20(10):1968–80.

67. van Til NP, Sarwari R, Visser TP, et al. Recombination-activating gene 1 (Rag1)-deficient mice with severe combined immunodeficiency treated with lentiviral gene therapy demonstrate autoimmune Omenn-like syndrome. J Allergy Clin Immunol 2014;133(4):1116–23.

68. Rivat C, Booth C, Alonso-Ferrero M, et al. SAP gene transfer restores cellular and humoral immune function in a murine model of X-linked lymphoproliferative disease. Blood 2013;121(7):1073–6.

69. Carmo M, Risma KA, Arumugam P, et al. Perforin gene transfer into hematopoietic stem cells improves immune dysregulation in murine models of perforin deficiency. Mol Ther 2015;23(4):737–45.

70. Tiwari S, Hontz A, Terrell CE, et al. High level of perforin expression is required for effective correction of hemophagocytic lymphohistiocytosis. Hum Gene Ther 2016;27(10):847–59.

71. Oliveira G, Ruggiero E, Stanghellini MT, et al. Tracking genetically engineered lymphocytes long-term reveals the dynamics of T cell immunological memory. Sci Transl Med 2015;7(317):317ra198.

72. Leon-Rico D, Aldea M, Sanchez-Baltasar R, et al. Lentiviral vector-mediated correction of a mouse model of leukocyte adhesion deficiency type I. Hum Gene Ther 2016;27(9):668–78.

73. Passerini L, Rossi Mel E, Sartirana C, et al. CD4(+) T cells from IPEX patients convert into functional and stable regulatory T cells by FOXP3 gene transfer. Sci Transl Med 2013;5(215):215ra174.

74. Brown MP, Topham DJ, Sangster MY, et al. Thymic lymphoproliferative disease after successful correction of CD40 ligand deficiency by gene transfer in mice. Nat Med 1998;4(11):1253–60.

75. Schejtman A, Cutrim Arago Filho W, Zinicola M, et al. Establishing the platform for clinical gene therapy of p47phox chronic granulomatous disease (CGD). Paper presented at: Changing the face of modern medicine: stem cells and gene therapy - 24th Annual Congress of European Society of Gene & Cell Therapy. Florence, Italy, October 18 – 21, 2016.

76. Zinicola M, Schejtman A, Calero-Garcia M, et al. Targeted gene therapy for the treatment of X-linked agammaglobulinemia (XLA). Paper presented at: Changing the face of modern medicine: stem cells and gene therapy - 24th Annual Congress of European Society of Gene & Cell Therapy. Florence, Italy, October 18 – 21, 2016.

Gene Therapy Approaches to Hemoglobinopathies

Giuliana Ferrari, PhD[a,b], Marina Cavazzana, MD[c,d], Fulvio Mavilio, PhD[e,*]

KEYWORDS

- Thalassemia • Sickle cell disease • Gene transfer • Retroviral vectors
- Lentiviral vectors • Globin gene regulation • Stem cell transplantation
- Hematopoiesis

KEY POINTS

- Gene therapy for hemoglobinopathies requires the transfer to hematopoietic stem cells of large globin gene expression cassettes driven by complex regulatory elements.
- Preclinical and early clinical studies proved safety and efficacy of stem cell–based gene therapy while showing hurdles and limitations of the existing technology, particularly for sickle cell disease.
- Stem cell procurement, cell dose, transduction efficiency, gene expression level, conditioning regimen, and patient's age at the time of intervention are key factors affecting the therapeutic range and clinical efficacy of gene therapy.
- The bone marrow microenvironment is a crucial yet poorly understood factor for both stem cell mobilization and engraftment.

INTRODUCTION

Hemoglobinopathies are a family of inherited blood disorders characterized by the defective synthesis of 1 of the 2 polypeptide chains of hemoglobin (α- or β-thalassemia [β-thal]) or by the synthesis of an abnormal hemoglobin variant, such as the hemoglobin S (HbS) mutation (β^{A-E6V}) that causes sickle cell diseases (SCD). Hemoglobinopathies are found all over the world, although the carriers' relative resistance to malaria established a high frequency of thalassemia in the Mediterranean areas, India, and the Far East, and of SCD in sub-Saharan Africa.[1] Migration

Disclosure Statement: No interest to disclose.
Disclaimer: Due to word limits, only essential references are included.
[a] San Raffaele-Telethon Institute for Gene Therapy (SR-TIGET), Istituto Scientifico Ospedale San Raffaele, Via Olgettina 58, Milan 20132, Italy; [b] Vita-Salute San Raffaele University, Milan, Italy; [c] Biotherapy Department, Necker Children's Hospital, Imagine Institute, 149 rue de Sèvres, Paris 75015, France; [d] Paris Descartes University, INSERM UMR 1163, Paris, France; [e] Department of Life Sciences, University of Modena and Reggio Emilia, Via Campi 287, 41125 Modena, Italy
* Corresponding author.
E-mail address: fulvio.mavilio@unimore.it

Hematol Oncol Clin N Am 31 (2017) 835–852
http://dx.doi.org/10.1016/j.hoc.2017.06.010
0889-8588/17/© 2017 Elsevier Inc. All rights reserved.

phenomena caused their spreading to other regions of the world, notably the United States and Europe. Overall, hemoglobinopathies are the most frequent monogenic diseases worldwide, with approximately 5% of the world population carrying a hemoglobin disorder trait.[2]

The only curative treatment of thalassemias and SCD is allogeneic transplantation of hematopoietic stem cells (HSCs) from HLA-matched sibling donors, which is associated with greater than 90% disease-free survival but is available to only less than 20% of patients.[3] Transplants with matched unrelated or mismatched donors carry a progressively higher risk of morbidity and mortality, unacceptable given the current high standards of care for both diseases. Gene therapy, or the autologous transplantation of genetically corrected HSCs, would be a potential alternative available to all patients and carries low transplant–related risks.

Over the past 2 decades, gene therapy has been successfully applied to primary immunodeficiencies, such as adenosine deaminase–deficient severe combined immunodeficiency (ADA-SCID), X-linked SCID (SCID-X1), Wiskott-Aldrich syndrome, and X-linked chronic granulomatous disease (X-CGD) (reviewed in Booth and colleagues, 2016[4]). The first clinical trials were based on vectors derived from the Moloney murine leukemia retrovirus (MLV), carrying a therapeutic gene under the control of the promoter/enhancer elements contained in the MLV long terminal repeats (LTRs). Although gene therapy has been beneficial for most patients, all trials except those for ADA-SCID were characterized by the occurrence of leukemia or myelodysplasia in most patients.[4] The molecular bases of these events are still ill defined, although it is likely that insertional deregulation of proto-oncogenes led to clonal expansion and eventually malignant progression.[5,6] The recognition of the MLV LTR as a major component of proto-oncogene activation led to the design of self-inactivating (SIN) vectors devoid of LTR regulatory sequences and incorporating cellular, short-range promoters to drive the expression of the therapeutic gene. This vector design proved safe and efficacious in a clinical trial of gene therapy for SCID-X1.[7]

To reduce the risk of insertional oncogenesis, SIN lentiviral vectors (LVs) derived from the human immunodeficiency virus–replaced MLV-derived vectors in all clinical trials involving genetically modified HSCs. Although MLV preferentially targets transcriptional regulatory elements,[5,8,9] LVs integrate throughout transcribed genes[5,6] in proximity of the nuclear membrane,[10] an inherently safer integration pattern as indicated by in vitro as well as in vivo studies (reviewed in Naldini, 2015[11]). LVs are currently used in early- or advanced-phase clinical trials of gene therapy for Wiskott-Aldrich syndrome, ADA-SCID, X-CGD, and nonimmune disorders such as adrenoleukodystrophy or metachromatic leukodystrophy. These trials are providing strong evidence of clinical efficacy in the absence of treatment-related adverse events or clonal abnormalities in the genetically modified HSC repertoire.[11]

Gene therapy for hemoglobinopathies presents additional challenges. Globin genes are subjected to a sophisticated regulation relying on the molecular interaction of globin promoters with a locus-control region (LCR), which regulates high-level, lineage-restricted gene expression as well as the choice of embryonic, fetal, or adult genes in different phases of development.[12,13] The combination of a full LCR and an adult β-globin gene, which requires its introns and 3′ untranslated region for proper function, is too large to be accommodated by an LV. Size reduction has been achieved, although globin-expressing LVs remain large and complex and have a lower transduction efficiency compared with simpler vectors. LVs have been developed and successfully tested in preclinical models of hemoglobinopathies, whereas recent clinical trials are showing remarkable safety and promising clinical efficacy.

DEVELOPING GENE TRANSFER VECTORS FOR HEMOGLOBINOPATHIES

The first pioneering studies on gene therapy for β-thal were based on MLV-derived retroviral vectors expressing a human β-globin gene. They achieved successful gene transfer in mouse repopulating stem/progenitor cells but showed low, nontherapeutic levels of β-globin expression, variegation of gene expression due to promoter silencing, and proviral rearrangements. Introduction of essential elements of the β-globin LCR and elimination of portions of an intron and multiple cryptic polyadenylation and splicing signals improved the vector characteristics, although transduction efficiency in HSCs remained insufficient and globin gene expression was subtherapeutic (reviewed in Rivella and Sadelain, 1998[14]).

A major breakthrough occurred with the development of the first LVs, which featured an optimized β-globin gene under the control of the β-globin promoter, 3′ enhancer, and the DNase I hypersensitive sites 2, 3, and 4 (HS2, HS3, and HS4) of the β-globin LCR.[15,16] This new generation of vectors, belonging to the TNS9 and HPV569 families, expressed β-globin at much higher levels and proved their therapeutic efficacy in correcting 2 murine models of β-thal[15,17,18] and SCD.[16] Major advantages of globin LVs were higher transduction of HSCs and persistent gene expression even after serial transplantation in mice. LV vectors combine reduced genotoxic properties to the strict lineage specificity of the β-globin promoter, enhancer, and LCR, which have only minimal, if any, capacity to activate neighboring genes in stem and progenitor cells.[19] Different combinations of LCR elements have been tested in an attempt to improve vector titer and infectivity, a persistent problem due to the size and the complex nature of the β-globin regulatory sequences. The GLOBE vector contains an extended HS2 and an HS3 element, but lacks the HS4 and the 3′ β-globin enhancer. This vector showed higher infectivity compared with larger vectors while achieving comparable efficacy in correcting murine β-thal[20] and reducing globin chain imbalance in human β-thalassemic cells.[21]

To further improve safety, several investigators inserted chromatin "insulators" in the LV LTRs, to shield the vector from the repressive effect of neighboring chromatin and/or the promoter of neighboring genes from any vector influence. Examples of such elements are the chicken β-globin HS4[22,23] or a synthetic element (FB) that combines sequences from the chicken HS4 and the T-cell receptor BEAD-1 insulator.[24] Unfortunately, the presence of these elements led in most cases to loss of vector titer, decreased transduction efficiency, and genetic instability, whereas enhancer-blocking activity proved to be modest and integration site dependent, leading to the removal of these elements from LVs used in clinical applications (reviewed in Negre and colleagues, 2016[25]).

GENE THERAPY FOR β-THALASSEMIA: RATIONALE AND REQUIREMENTS

β-Thal is caused by greater than 200 mutations in the *HBB* gene that reduce the synthesis of β-globin chains.[26] The excess, uncoupled α-chains cause ineffective erythropoiesis, intramedullary hemolysis, and hemolytic anemia. Clinical classification is based on the severity of the anemia, which is in turn related to the genetic defect that either abolishes (β^0) or reduces (β^+) β-chain synthesis. An estimated 1.5% of the global population carries a β-thal mutation, and 60,000 β-thal symptomatic individuals are born each year.[2] Most patients with β-thal live in Mediterranean countries, the Middle East, South-East Asia, and China, although, because of increasing migratory flows, more β-thal carriers are entering Europe, Australia, and North America.[27] Clinical presentation depends on the association of different mutations, the concomitant presence of α-thalassemia, or compensatory mechanisms, such as persistence of fetal hemoglobin (HbF).[28,29] Patients with severe β-thal are affected by anemia, chronic hemolysis, iron overload, hepatosplenomegaly, skeletal abnormalities related to bone marrow (BM) expansion, and extramedullary hematopoiesis. Complications include heart, liver, and endocrine dysfunction, with onset depending on the severity of the disease and the adequacy of the supportive treatment.[30] Approximately 8% of β-thal children worldwide die within the first 5 years of life because of lack of adequate treatment.[31] In developed countries, an optimal clinical management based on regular blood transfusions and iron chelation has greatly improved the survival and quality of life of patients with β-thal, who may expect to live well into adulthood. Nevertheless, complications caused by iron accumulation still affect quality of life and represent a major cause of death.[32]

The only curative approach for β-thal is allogeneic HSC transplantation with high-dose chemotherapy and long-term immunosuppression.[33] Donor options include an HLA-identical sibling, a matched unrelated donor (MUD), or a mismatched family donor. In the pediatric population, transplant from a matched sibling donor results in 80% to 89% disease-free survival with 3% to 10% mortality on an up to 20-year follow-up.[3,34–36] Transplant from MUDs results in 66% to 82% disease-free survival at 2 to 4 years and up to 21% mortality.[37,38] Alternative donor sources such as umbilical cord blood lead to higher mortality and lower disease-free survival,[39] whereas haploidentical transplantation is not routinely proposed because of unacceptable transplant-related risks. The most common side effects of HSC transplantation are chronic graft-versus-host disease, infections, and chemotherapy-related toxicity, affecting both survival and quality of life. According to the European Society for Blood and Marrow Transplantation registry, the probability of finding a matched sibling or unrelated donor is 25% to 30% and 58%, respectively,[40] leaving half of the patients' population without a well-matched donor. Gene therapy would be available to all patients and likely associated with reduced toxicity and treatment-related morbidity.

Gene therapy for β-thal needs to address several fundamental issues, among which include the following:

- The source of hematopoietic stem/progenitor cells (HSPCs), which should contain an adequate dose of stem cells with long-term engraftment capacity;
- The choice of the BM conditioning regimen, which should aim at creating space for the transduced cells while reducing toxicity and erythroid expansion before transplant;
- The dose of transduced HSPCs and the therapeutic level of transgene expression in erythroid progenitors, which depends on the vector output and the average vector copy number (VCN);
- The presence of a favorable BM microenvironment enabling regeneration of a complete hematopoiesis starting from the corrected HSCs.

Conventional sources of transplantable HSCs are either the BM, harvested from the iliac crests, or peripheral blood mobilized CD34$^+$ cells. The latter have essentially replaced BM as a source of stem cells because of higher yield of HSPCs, less invasive procedure (apheresis), faster engraftment, enhanced immune reconstitution, and shorter hospitalization. Adequate doses and clonal diversity of transduced cells are required to reduce the risk of skewed or stressed hematopoiesis engraftment. The issue of HSC procurement is critical in particular for adult patients, because the minimal target dose of CD34$^+$ (usually >5 × 10^6 cells per kilogram) poses a challenge for a steady-state BM. The gold standard mobilization agent for gene therapy is granulocyte colony-stimulating factor (G-CSF), which yields acceptable doses of CD34$^+$ HSPCs in most conditions but must be used with caution in patients with β-thal with splenomegaly, thrombophilia, or a chronic hypercoagulable state.[41,42] An alternative mobilization agent is Plerixafor (AMD3100; Mozobil), a bicyclam molecule that mobilizes HSPCs by selectively and reversibly antagonizing the binding of stromal cell derived factor-1 to the chemokine CXC receptor-4.[43] The use of Plerixafor + G-CSF is currently approved by US Food and Drug Administration and European Medicines Agency in conditions resulting in poor mobilization with G-CSF alone.[44] Clinical trials demonstrated that Plerixafor, alone or in combination with G-CSF, safely and rapidly mobilizes HSCs also in patients with β-thal.[45–47] Comparative in vitro and in vivo analysis of HSPCs collected from BM or mobilized by G-CSF and/or Plerixafor highlighted the superior biological characteristics, homing capacity, and repopulation potential of Plerixafor-mobilized HSPCs.[48] The reduced overall yield of CD34+ cells by Plerixafor-only mobilization is counterbalanced by the superior stem cell characteristics of the harvest, which may support the elimination of G-CSF provided that an adequate cell dose is achieved in its absence.

The clinical history of gene therapy for SCIDs has indicated that in vivo selective advantage improves the efficacy of the treatment and allows the use of non-myeloablative, minimally toxic conditioning regimens.[4] In the absence of selective advantage, high doses of transduced HSPCs and fully myeloablative conditioning are mandatory to achieve engraftment of therapeutic levels of genetically corrected HSCs, as clearly demonstrated in recent gene therapy trials for metachromatic leukodystrophy[49] and CGD (D. Williams and H. Malech, unpublished data, 2017). In the case of β-thal, partial myeloablation resulted in insufficient engraftment of corrected HSCs.[50] The toxicity of myeloablative conditioning is reduced in gene therapy protocols compared with allogeneic HSC transplantation, because immune suppression is not required in an autologous setting. Nevertheless, for nonlethal disorders such as β-thal, there remains a strong rationale for developing minimally toxic conditioning regimens. Recent examples are the use of anti-cKit or anti-CD45-SAP antibodies that empty the marrow niche in the absence of chemical myeloablation (reviewed in Aiuti and Naldini, 2016[51]).

Engraftment of HSCs requires the support of the nonhematopoietic component of the BM microenvironment. Anemia, extramedullary hematopoiesis, iron accumulation, and bone deformities due to marrow expansion alter the microenvironment in patients with β-thal by inducing stress signals such as oxidation, inflammation, and hypoxia. Preliminary data from a mouse β-thal model point to the impact of an altered microenvironment on HSC behavior and function.[52] Further investigation in a human context is necessary to understand the basis for reconstituting hematopoiesis and effective erythropoiesis in a chronic stressed environment.

GENE THERAPY FOR β-THALASSEMIA: PRECLINICAL STUDIES

Preclinical testing of globin vectors is usually carried out in β-thal mice, carrying mutations in the murine β-globin locus. They are characterized by anemia, abnormal hematological parameters, ineffective erythropoiesis, splenomegaly, and iron overload and are considered clinically relevant and predictive models of the human disease. Long-term correction of murine thalassemia intermedia by transplantation of HSCs transduced with a globin LV (TNS9, **Fig. 1**) was reported in 2000.[15] Since then, several laboratories have shown that LVs carrying the human β- or γ-globin gene under the control of β-globin promoter and LCR elements are able to rescue murine models of β-thal intermedia and major.[17,18,20,53–55] One of these studies showed that genetically corrected erythroblasts have a survival advantage and undergo in vivo selection in mice,[20] predicting that suboptimal HSC transduction may provide sufficient clinical

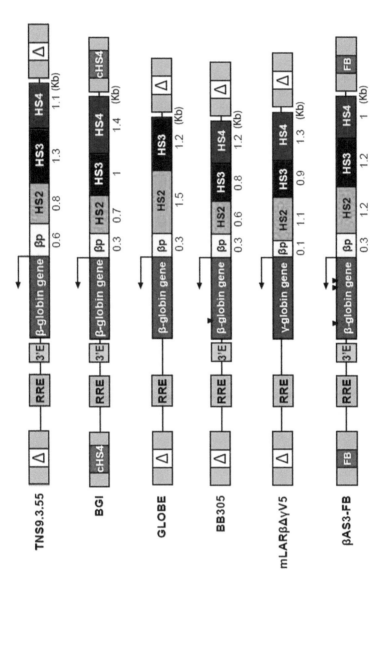

Fig. 1. Structure of the proviral form of LVs used in preclinical and clinical studies of gene therapy for hemoglobinopathies: TNS9.3.55,[50] BGI,[59] GLOBE,[20] BB305,[25] mLARβΔγV5,[71] and βAS3-FB.[24] Δ, U3-deleted LTR; βp, β-globin promoter; 3′E, 3′ β-globin enhancer; cHS4, chicken β-globin HS4 insulator; FB, hybrid chicken HS4/T-cell receptor BEAD-1 insulator; HS2, HS3, HS4, DNase I hypersensitive sites of the β-globin locus LCR; size (in kb) is indicated under each element; RRE, Rev-responsive element.

benefit in patients. Several investigators attempted to improve the expression characteristics of globin LVs by introducing larger portions of the β-LCR, or incorporating insulator or GATA-1 elements to reduce chromatin position effect on β-globin expression[23,56–58] (see **Fig. 1**). Most of these changes provided at best modest improvements at the expense of vector titer and infectivity, which remain the 2 most critical parameters for clinical translation.

Several studies addressed the correction of globin chain imbalance in human β^0- or β^+-thal by transducing patient-derived $CD34^+$ HSPCs and analyzing globin synthesis after differentiation in vitro or ex vivo after xenotransplantation in immunodeficient mice. These studies showed potentially therapeutic levels of correction, predicting clinical efficacy.[21,59] The potential genotoxicity caused by LV integration was also analyzed in these models.[19,50,60] Interference with stem cell endogenous gene regulation is expected to be limited for globin LVs, because of the erythroid-restricted activity of the regulatory elements driving the β-globin gene. However, constitutive and cryptic splice and polyadenylation signals contained in a globin vector may interfere with endogenous gene splicing with potentially deleterious effects.[61] Potential genotoxicity was rigorously tested for the 2 vectors currently used in clinical trials (BB305 and GLOBE) with results that fully supported clinical application (G. Ferrari, unpublished results, 2017).[19]

CLINICAL GENE THERAPY FOR β-THALASSEMIA

In June 2007, a patient affected by transfusion-dependent hemoglobin E (HbE)/β-thal was treated for the first time by gene therapy with an SIN LV expressing the β^{T87Q} globin.[62] In the HbE/β-thal conditions, the HbE variant is produced at low level, mimicking a mild β^+ allele and reducing the overall requirement for therapeutic β-globin synthesis. The patient received myeloablative conditioning followed by infusion of 3.9×10^6 transduced $CD34^+$ cells per kilogram. After engraftment, he had a gradual increase in gene-marked cells up to 10% to 20% and became transfusion independent 1 year after gene therapy with stable hemoglobin levels of 8.5 to 9 g/dL, contributed in almost equal proportions by the vector, elevated HbF synthesis, and the HbE allele. Integration site analysis showed that the vector-derived globin synthesis was sustained in large part by expansion of a single clone in which the provirus was inserted in the *HMGA2* (high-mobility-group AT-hook 2) proto-oncogene. The gene was activated posttranscriptionally by a vector-induced abnormal splicing and premature transcript termination caused by the presence of a cryptic splice site in the cHS4 insulator. The benign clonal dominance persisted for almost 9 years, after which it started to decline and currently contributes to less than 10% of the circulating nucleated cells (M. Cavazzana, unpublished observations, 2017). The patient maintains stable although low levels of therapeutic hemoglobin and requires occasional transfusion. This case proved that gene therapy may provide significant clinical benefit and identified gene transfer efficiency and polyclonality within the transduced HSC repertoire as crucial factors in maintaining long-term therapeutic efficacy. The need for full myeloablation was demonstrated by a trial carried out with the TNS9.3.55 vector (**Table 1**), where partially myeloablative conditioning achieved insufficient gene marking and showed minimal clinical benefit.[50]

Clinical trials currently running in the United States and Europe are based on mobilized peripheral blood HSPCs, improved cell transduction, and full BM conditioning. The currently used procedure is summarized in **Fig. 2**. The multicenter Northstar HGB204 study and the single-center HGB205 study are based on the BB305 vector (see **Fig. 1**) and are ongoing in the United States, Australia, Thailand, and France (see **Table 1**). As of December 2016, all patients with genotypes different from β^0/β^0 and a follow-up of ≥ 12 months have discontinued transfusions. Patients with β^0/β^0 genotypes (n = 5) still

Table 1
Ongoing gene therapy clinical trials for hemoglobinopathies

Indication	Country	Sponsor	Gene	Vector	Conditioning (TD)	Enrollment	Identifier	Status
β-thal	USA	MSKCC	β-globin	TNS9.3.55	Busulfan: 8 mg/kg	Adults, up to 10 patients (pts)	NCT01639690	Active: 4 pts treated
β-thal	France	Bluebird bio	β^{A-T87Q} globin	BB305	Busulfan: 12.8 mg/kg, pk-adjusted	Ages 5–37 y, up to 7 pts	NCT02151526	Active: 4 pts treated
β-thal	USA, Thailand, Australia	Bluebird bio	β^{A-T87Q} globin	BB305	Busulfan: 12.8 mg/kg	Adults, up to 8 pts	NCT02906202	Active: 18 pts treated
β-thal	Italy	Telethon Foundation	β-globin	GLOBE	Treosulfan 42 g/m^2 + thiotepa 8 mg/kg	Age 3–64 y, up to 10 pts	NCT02453477	Active: 7 pts treated
SCD	France	Bluebird bio	β^{A-T87Q} globin	BB305	Busulfan: 12.8 mg/kg, pk-adjusted	Ages 5–37 y, up to 7 pts	NCT02151526	Active: 1 pt treated
SCD	USA	Bluebird bio	β^{A-T87Q} globin	BB305	Busulfan: 12.8 mg/kg	Adults, up to 8 pts	NCT02140554	Active: 7 pts treated
SCD	USA	UCLA	βAS3 globin	βAS3-FB	Busulfan: 12.8 mg/kg, pk-adjusted	Adults, up to 6 pts	NCT02247843	Active: 1 pt treated
SCD	USA	Cincinnati Children's Hosp	γ-globin	mLARβΔγV5	Melphalan: 140 mg/m^2	Adults to 35 y, up to 10 pts	NCT02186418	Recruiting

Abbreviations: TD, total dose; pk-adjusted pharmacokinetics-adjusted.

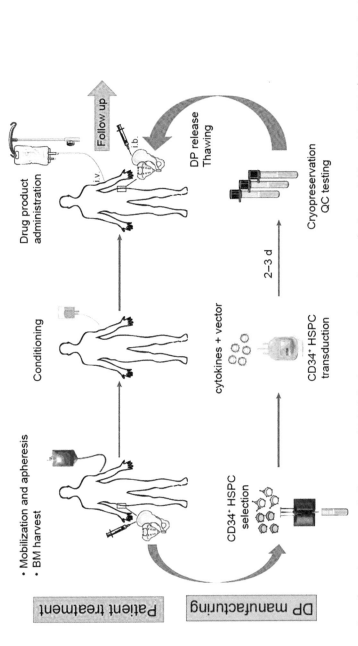

Fig. 2. Transplantation of autologous genetically corrected HSPCs in the context of gene therapy for hemoglobinopathies. CD34⁺ HSPCs are obtained by BM harvest or peripheral blood mobilization, purified by immunoselection on GMP-compliant equipment, transduced in bags or flasks with the therapeutic vector in appropriate cytokine-containing media, and cryopreserved. After BM conditioning, the "drug product" (DP) is thawed and re-infused by either intravenous (i.v.) or intrabone (i.b.) injection. GMP, good manufacturing practices; QC, quality control.

require transfusions, although with requirements decreased to 60% with respect to base-line. In both studies, gene therapy was well tolerated, with no gene transfer–related severe adverse event. When performed, integration site analysis showed polyclonal reconstitution and no apparent clonal dominance[63] (M. Cavazzana, unpublished results, 2016).

Plerixafor + G-CSF mobilization of HSPCs was introduced in a phase 1/2 clinical trial addressing transfusion-dependent β-thal, based on the GLOBE vector[64] (see **Table 1**). The study includes 3 cohorts of adult ($\geq$18 years, n = 3), adolescent (8–17 years, n = 3), and pediatric (3–7 years, n = 4) subjects, with Data and Safety Monitoring Board–monitored safety assessment after each cohort. The rationale to treat pediatric patients is based on their better HSC quality, less damaged microenvironment, and less compromised organ function, all factors potentially improving the long-term efficacy of the treatment and the overall risk-benefit ratio. A myeloablative, reduced toxicity conditioning regimen based on treosulfan and thiotepa is used to favor engraftment while ablating extramedullary hematopoiesis.[37] The transduced cell product is administered by intraosseous injection in both posterior-superior iliac crests to boost homing and engraftment of genetically modified HSCs particularly in patients with constitutive hepatosplenomegaly, which enhances filtering of intravenously delivered cells and delays/reduces engraftment. As of June 2017, seven patients (3 adults, 3 adolescents, and 1 child) with different genotypes (β^0/β^0, β^+/β^+, and β^0/β^+) have been treated with GLOBE-transduced CD34$^+$ cells at a dose ranging from 16.3 to 19.5 $\times$ 10^6 cells per kilogram and a VCN of 0.7 to 1.5. The procedure was well tolerated, with no product-related adverse events. Multilineage engraftment of gene-marked cells was observed in all tested patients, whereas polyclonal vector integration profiles have been detected in the first 3 patients with no evidence of clonal skewing. The clinical outcome indicates so far significant reduction in transfusion requirement and improved quality of life in adult patients and greater clinical benefit in younger patients (G. Ferrari, unpublished results, 2017).

GENE THERAPY FOR SICKLE CELL DISEASE: CHALLENGES AND INITIAL STUDIES

SCD is caused by a mutation (E6V) in the sixth amino acid of the Hb β-chain that induces polymerization of Hb tetramers upon deoxygenation. As a consequence, red blood cells (RBCs) lose flexibility and adopt the characteristic sickle shape in the capillary circulation, causing ischemia, stroke, multiorgan damage, severe pain, hemolytic anemia, and shortened lifespan.[1,65] Current treatments include chronic blood transfusions and hydroxyurea, an inducer of HbF synthesis.[65,66] SCD is endemic in Africa, where an estimated 300,000 children are born annually with the disease, and the majority do not survive to adulthood.[67] SCD is frequent also in the Western world: approximately 100,000 Americans and 10,000 French people of African descent are affected by the disease, with an incidence of 1:5000 and 1:2500, respectively. Despite improvements in supportive care in these countries, disease morbidities remain severe and life expectancy remains significantly shortened.[65,66] The only definitive therapy for SCD is allogeneic HSC transplantation from matched sibling donors, with a reported greater than 90% disease-free survival over 6 years.[3] Allogeneic HSC transplantation is not frequently performed in SCD patients given the variable clinical severity, the toxicity associated with the procedure, and the often limited donor availability. As for β-thal, gene therapy could be a less toxic therapeutic option available to all patients, which however faces comparable issues in terms of HSC source, BM conditioning, transgene expression levels, and quality of the BM microenvironment.

The current source of HSPCs in SCD patients is BM harvest, a risky procedure that often fails to provide an optimal cell dose due in part to an altered BM microenvironment. Vaso-occlusion caused by sickling leads to ischemia and inflammation, with production of reactive oxygen species from activated lymphocytes. Cycles of ischemia and reperfusion cause additional oxidative stress that worsens inflammation in the BM stroma.[68] The altered microenvironment influences the quality of the HSC harvest as well as homing and engraftment of incoming cells upon transplantation. In addition, HbS polymerization changes the density characteristics of RBCs and causes the formation of aggregates that further affect the recovery of CD34$^+$ cells from BM harvests. Attempts to mobilize HSPCs by low-dose G-CSF treatment caused severe adverse events and one fatality and is no longer used.[69] Recently, Plerixafor has been proposed as a potentially safe mobilizer of high-quality HSCs also in SCD patients: clinical trials are ongoing in France (NCT02212535) and the United States (NCT02193191, NCT02140554, NCT02989701) to prove the treatment's safety and provide an estimate of the overall recovery of CD34$^+$ HSPCs after apheresis in adult and juvenile patients.

Preclinical studies showed the potential of LV-based gene therapy in correcting the SCD phenotype. The vectors used in these studies carry expression cassettes based on the same β-globin promoter/LCR combinations used for β-thal, but express globins with the potential to interfere with Hb polymerization. The design of antisickling globins is based on genetic considerations: SCD patients experience less severe symptoms when HbF is elevated due to conditions known as hereditary persistence of fetal hemoglobin (HPFH). The protective activity of HbF is due to the incorporation of γ-globin chains into mixed hemoglobin tetramers that do not participate in polymer formation and inhibit sickling. The severity of SCD correlates with HbF levels: patients who produce HbF at levels of greater than 20% experience less severe disease and improved survival, whereas asymptomatic disease has been reported in patients with greater than 30% HbF expression.[36,70] Based on these observations, investigators developed LVs expressing γ-globin under the control of β-globin promoter (mLARβΔγV5 in **Fig. 1**), which efficiently corrected a murine model of SCD.[71,72] Other investigators developed mutant β-globin chains that interfere with axial and lateral contacts in the HbS polymer, with potent antisickling properties.[73] An LV expressing one such mutant, the β^{A-T87Q}, effectively corrected a murine model of SCD[16] and is currently used in clinical trials for both β-thal and SCD[25] (BB305 in **Fig. 1**). A second mutant, the AS3 globin, carries the T87Q mutation and 2 additional ones, G16D and E22A, which contribute to the antisickling activity and also increase affinity for the α-chain.[74] The AS3 globin, expressed in the βAS3-FB vector (see **Fig. 1**), corrects a murine model of SCD[75] and reduces HbS and RBC sickling at potentially therapeutic levels when transferred in human CD34$^+$ progenitors from SCD patients.[24,76]

As for β-thal, allogeneic stem cell transplantation provides important predictions about the minimal level of corrected HSCs necessary to achieve clinical benefit in SCD patients. Stable mixed chimerism with donor HSC levels as low as 10% to 30% provides significant hematologic and clinical improvement because of the selective survival advantage of normal, donor-derived RBCs against sickling RBCs in the peripheral circulation.[77–79] These data, combined with the evidence coming from SCD + HPFH subjects, predict that engraftment of ∼20% of autologous HSC producing a progeny of RBCs with greater than 30% antisickling Hb levels could provide therapeutic levels of phenotypic correction in SCD patients.

CLINICAL GENE THERAPY FOR SICKLE CELL DISEASE

The results obtained in patients with severe β-thal encouraged attempts to extend gene therapy also to SCD patients. A first subject was treated in France with the BB305 LV vector expressing the β^{A-T87Q} globin. He received full myeloablative chemotherapy and was transplanted with 5×10^6 CD34$^+$ cells per kilogram coming from 2 BM harvests transduced at an average VCN of 1. Reconstitution of all hematopoietic lineages was rapid and sustained, and no treatment-related adverse event was observed at 2-year follow-up. The patient achieved a level of therapeutic β^{A-T87Q} globin around 50% and transfusion independence, with a clinical picture comparable to that of an HbS carrier.[80] Integration site analysis showed polyclonal hematopoietic reconstitution and no clonal abnormality (M. Cavazzana, unpublished observations, 2017).

The results obtained in the first patient encouraged the treatment of additional severe SCD patients in the context of 2 clinical trials ongoing in France and the United States (see **Table 1**). The interim report of the first 7 adult patients treated in the multi-center US trial failed, however, to achieve a level of correction comparable to that observed in the first patient. Patients received a median dose of 2×10^6 CD34$^+$ HSPCs coming from at least 2 BM harvests, with a median VCN of 0.6. A follow-up of 8 to 17 months showed a VCN in peripheral blood of less than 0.12, hemoglobin A (HbA)^{T87Q} levels of less than 2 g/dL and an average HbA^{T87Q}/HbS ratio of less than 15%.[81] These results pointed to the difficulty in obtaining adequate doses and robust engraftment of transduced HSCs in SCD patients, particularly adult ones. Stem cell procurement, transduction efficiency, and patient conditioning appear the most critical factors that need improving in order to achieve the minimal stem cell chimerism and antisickling Hb production levels predicted to provide a sustained clinical benefit. Two more trials have recently opened in the United States based on the use of LV vectors expressing the βAS3 or the γ-globin (see **Table 1**).

GENE THERAPY FOR HEMOGLOBINOPATHIES: FUTURE DIRECTIONS

New strategies have recently emerged for gene therapy for β-hemoglobinopathies, aimed at correcting the β^S mutation or activating endogenous HbF synthesis rather than providing a therapeutic β–like gene by vector-mediated transfer. Direct correction of the β^S mutation has been attempted by several groups by using zinc-finger nucleases or CRISPR/Cas9 to specifically cleave the β^S locus, and viral genomes or single-stranded oligonucleotides as donor templates to correct the mutation by homology-directed DNA repair (HDR).[82–85] In all cases, correction of the β^S mutation was achieved in HSPCs, although with subtherapeutic efficiency, and the HbA/HbS ratio was favorably altered in the erythroid progeny of edited HSPCs in vitro or after xenotransplantation in immunodeficient mice.

A different approach, aimed at activating HbF synthesis by reversing the fetal-to-adult Hb switch, is based on the knowledge that the transcription factor BCL11A plays a major role in silencing γ-globin expression in adult erythroblasts (reviewed in Bauer and Orkin[86] and Smith and Orkin[13]). Downregulating BCL11A by restricted expression of a short-hairpin RNA in the erythroid compartment is a potentially effective strategy,[87] although fine modulation is necessary because it is an essential factor in HSCs, lymphoid cell development,[88] and RBC enucleation.[89] Alternatively, BCL11A down-modulation can be obtained by deleting the enhancer elements controlling its expression in an erythroid-restricted fashion by CRISPR/Cas9-mediated genome editing.[90,91]

Re-creating genomic deletions in the β-globin locus or mutations in the γ-globin promoters associated with HPFH is an alternative strategy to increase HbF, validated by clinical genetics data.[1,70] Re-creating HPFH mutations in adult HSPCs by CRISPR/Cas9-mediated deletion does lead to increased γ-globin expression in their erythroid progeny,[92,93] although the efficiency of gene editing is still subtherapeutic compared with LV-mediated gene replacement. Generating deletions in the BCL11A or the β-globin locus is less complex compared with direct editing of the $β^S$ mutation, because it does not require the concomitant delivery of a DNA template and relies on nonhomologous end joining, which appears to be the dominant DNA repair pathway in HSPCs with respect to HDR.[82,94] An alternative approach to manipulating the Hb switch is based on the use of zinc-finger proteins with an effector domain forcing the formation of a loop between the LCR and the γ-globin promoters, which reactivates γ-globin expression and concomitantly reduces $β^S$-globin expression.[95] This approach does not require DNA cleavage as in the case of gene editing.

Gene and genome editing hold great promise as a second-generation approach to gene therapy for hemoglobinopathies. Provided that off-target effects are appropriately controlled, they would offer advantages in terms of biosafety and, at least in the case of nonviral delivery of the editing machinery, of complexity and overall cost of treatment. Nevertheless, gene editing is at the moment much less efficient than LV-mediated gene replacement, and its safety profile is still untested in vivo.

SUMMARY

Gene therapy for hemoglobinopathies is showing its safety and potential efficacy in both preclinical and early clinical studies. However, source, quality, and dose of repopulating stem cells, suboptimal transduction efficiency and gene expression levels, and toxicity and efficacy of current conditioning regimens and an altered BM microenvironment remain significant hurdles limiting generalized application. In addition, the complexity and costs associated with vector and cell manufacturing are limiting the applicability and commercial future of this therapeutic approach, particularly in less developed countries. Despite the encouraging results and the current enthusiasm by both investigators and industrial sponsors, these limiting factors need to be systematically addressed for gene therapy for hemoglobinopathies to become a clinical reality. The emerging gene editing technology may overcome at least some of these limitations and provide additional therapeutic alternatives, although its safety and efficacy are yet to be tested in the clinical reality.

REFERENCES

1. Stamatoyannopoulos G, editor. The molecular basis of blood diseases. 3rd edition. Philadelphia: W.B. Saunders Co; 2001.
2. Modell B. Global epidemiology of hemoglobin disorders and derived service indicators. London: World Health Organization; 2008. p. 417–96.
3. Locatelli F, Kabbara N, Ruggeri A, et al. Outcome of patients with hemoglobinopathies given either cord blood or bone marrow transplantation from an HLA-identical sibling. Blood 2013;122(6):1072–8.
4. Booth C, Gaspar HB, Thrasher AJ. Treating Immunodeficiency through HSC gene therapy. Trends Mol Med 2016;22(4):317–27.
5. Cavazza A, Moiani A, Mavilio F. Mechanisms of retroviral integration and mutagenesis. Hum Gene Ther 2013;24(2):119–31.
6. Biasco L, Baricordi C, Aiuti A. Retroviral integrations in gene therapy trials. Mol Ther 2012;20(4):709–16.
7. Hacein-Bey-Abina S, Pai SY, Gaspar HB, et al. A modified gamma-retrovirus vector for X-linked severe combined immunodeficiency. N Engl J Med 2014;371(15): 1407–17.
8. Cattoglio C, Pellin D, Rizzi E, et al. High-definition mapping of retroviral integration sites identifies active regulatory elements in human multipotent hematopoietic progenitors. Blood 2010;116(25):5507–17.

9. De Ravin SS, Su L, Theobald N, et al. Enhancers are major targets for murine leukemia virus vector integration. J Virol 2014;88(8):4504–13.

10. Marini B, Kertesz-Farkas A, Ali H, et al. Nuclear architecture dictates HIV-1 integration site selection. Nature 2015;521(7551):227–31.

11. Naldini L. Gene therapy returns to centre stage. Nature 2015;526(7573):351–60.

12. Wilber A, Nienhuis AW, Persons DA. Transcriptional regulation of fetal to adult hemoglobin switching: new therapeutic opportunities. Blood 2011;117(15):3945–53.

13. Smith EC, Orkin SH. Hemoglobin genetics: recent contributions of GWAS and gene editing. Hum Mol Genet 2016;25(R2):R99–105.

14. Rivella S, Sadelain M. Genetic treatment of severe hemoglobinopathies: the combat against transgene variegation and transgene silencing. Semin Hematol 1998;35(2):112–25.

15. May C, Rivella S, Callegari J, et al. Therapeutic haemoglobin synthesis in beta-thalassaemic mice expressing lentivirus-encoded human beta-globin. Nature 2000;406(6791):82–6.

16. Pawliuk R, Westerman KA, Fabry ME, et al. Correction of sickle cell disease in transgenic mouse models by gene therapy. Science 2001;294(5550):2368–71.

17. May C, Rivella S, Chadburn A, et al. Successful treatment of murine beta-thalassemia intermedia by transfer of the human beta-globin gene. Blood 2002;99(6):1902–8.

18. Rivella S, May C, Chadburn A, et al. A novel murine model of Cooley anemia and its rescue by lentiviral-mediated human beta-globin gene transfer. Blood 2003;101(8):2932–9.

19. Negre O, Bartholomae C, Beuzard Y, et al. Preclinical evaluation of efficacy and safety of an improved lentiviral vector for the treatment of beta-thalassemia and sickle cell disease. Curr Gene Ther 2015;15(1):64–81.

20. Miccio A, Cesari R, Lotti F, et al. In vivo selection of genetically modified erythroblastic progenitors leads to long-term correction of beta-thalassemia. Proc Natl Acad Sci U S A 2008;105(30):10547–52.

21. Roselli EA, Mezzadra R, Frittoli MC, et al. Correction of beta-thalassemia major by gene transfer in haematopoietic progenitors of pediatric patients. EMBO Mol Med 2010;2(8):315–28.

22. Emery DW, Yannaki E, Tubb J, et al. A chromatin insulator protects retrovirus vectors from chromosomal position effects. Proc Natl Acad Sci U S A 2000;97(16):9150–5.

23. Arumugam PI, Scholes J, Perelman N, et al. Improved human beta-globin expression from self-inactivating lentiviral vectors carrying the chicken hypersensitive site-4 (cHS4) insulator element. Mol Ther 2007;15(10):1863–71.

24. Romero Z, Urbinati F, Geiger S, et al. beta-globin gene transfer to human bone marrow for sickle cell disease. J Clin Invest 2013;123(8):3317–30.

25. Negre O, Eggimann AV, Beuzard Y, et al. Gene therapy of the beta-hemoglobinopathies by lentiviral transfer of the beta(A(T87Q))-globin gene. Hum Gene Ther 2016;27(2):148–65.

26. Higgs DR, Engel JD, Stamatoyannopoulos G. Thalassaemia. Lancet 2012;379(9813):373–83.

27. Weatherall DJ. The definition and epidemiology of non-transfusion-dependent thalassaemia. Blood Rev 2012;26(Suppl 1):S3–6.

28. Chang YP, Littera R, Garau R, et al. The role of heterocellular hereditary persistence of fetal haemoglobin in beta(0)-thalassaemia intermedia. Br J Haematol 2001;114(4):899–906.

29. Panigrahi I, Agarwal S. Genetic determinants of phenotype in beta-thalassemia. Hematology 2008;13(4):247–52.
30. Rund D, Rachmilewitz E. Beta-thalassemia. N Engl J Med 2005;353(11):1135–46.
31. Vento S, Cainelli F, Cesario F. Infections and thalassaemia. Lancet Infect Dis 2006;6(4):226–33.
32. Borgna-Pignatti C. The life of patients with thalassemia major. Haematologica 2010;95(3):345–8.
33. Angelucci E. Hematopoietic stem cell transplantation in thalassemia. Hematol Am Soc Hematol Educ Program 2010;2010:456–62.
34. Chiesa R, Cappelli B, Crocchiolo R, et al. Unpredictability of intravenous busulfan pharmacokinetics in children undergoing hematopoietic stem cell transplantation for advanced beta thalassemia: limited toxicity with a dose-adjustment policy. Biol Blood Marrow Transplant 2010;16(5):622–8.
35. Lucarelli G, Gaziev J. Advances in the allogeneic transplantation for thalassemia. Blood Rev 2008;22(2):53–63.
36. Akinsheye I, Alsultan A, Solovieff N, et al. Fetal hemoglobin in sickle cell anemia. Blood 2011;118(1):19–27.
37. Bernardo M, Piras E, Vacca A, et al. Allogeneic hematopoietic stem cell transplantation in thalassemia major: results of a reduced-toxicity conditioning regimen based on the use of treosulfan. Blood 2012;120(122):473–6.
38. La Nasa G, Caocci G, Argiolu F, et al. Unrelated donor stem cell transplantation in adult patients with thalassemia. Bone Marrow Transplant 2005;36(11):971–5.
39. Ruggeri A, Eapen M, Scaravadou A, et al. Umbilical cord blood transplantation for children with thalassemia and sickle cell disease. Biol Blood Marrow Transplant 2011;17(9):1375–82.
40. Angelucci E, Matthes-Martin S, Baronciani D, et al. Hematopoietic stem cell transplantation in thalassemia major and sickle cell disease: indications and management recommendations from an international expert panel. Haematologica 2014;99(5):811–20.
41. Eldor A, Rachmilewitz EA. The hypercoagulable state in thalassemia. Blood 2002;99(1):36–43.
42. Taher AT, Otrock ZK, Uthman I, et al. Thalassemia and hypercoagulability. Blood Rev 2008;22(5):283–92.
43. De Clercq E. The bicyclam AMD3100 story. Nat Rev Drug Discov 2003;2(7):581–7.
44. DiPersio JF, Stadtmauer EA, Nademanee A, et al. Plerixafor and G-CSF versus placebo and G-CSF to mobilize hematopoietic stem cells for autologous stem cell transplantation in patients with multiple myeloma. Blood 2009;113(23):5720–6.
45. Yannaki E, Karponi G, Zervou F, et al. Hematopoietic stem cell mobilization for gene therapy: superior mobilization by the combination of granulocyte-colony stimulating factor plus plerixafor in patients with beta-thalassemia major. Hum Gene Ther 2013;24(10):852–60.
46. Yannaki E, Papayannopoulou T, Jonlin E, et al. Hematopoietic stem cell mobilization for gene therapy of adult patients with severe beta-thalassemia: results of clinical trials using G-CSF or plerixafor in splenectomized and nonsplenectomized subjects. Mol Ther 2012;20(1):230–8.
47. Karponi G, Psatha N, Lederer CW, et al. Plerixafor+G-CSF-mobilized CD34+ cells represent an optimal graft source for thalassemia gene therapy. Blood 2015;126(5):616–9.

48. Lidonnici MR, Aprile A, Frittoli MC, et al. Plerixafor and G-CSF combination mobilizes hematopoietic stem and progenitors cells with a distinct transcriptional profile and a reduced in vivo homing capacity compared to Plerixafor alone. Haematologica 2017;102(4):e120–4.

49. Sessa M, Lorioli L, Fumagalli F, et al. Lentiviral haemopoietic stem-cell gene therapy in early-onset metachromatic leukodystrophy: an ad-hoc analysis of a non-randomised, open-label, phase 1/2 trial. Lancet 2016;388(10043): 476–87.

50. Mansilla-Soto J, Riviere I, Boulad F, et al. Cell and gene therapy for the beta-thalassemias: advances and prospects. Hum Gene Ther 2016;27(4):295–304.

51. Aiuti A, Naldini L. Safer conditioning for blood stem cell transplants. Nat Biotechnol 2016;34(7):721–3.

52. Aprile ALM, Gulino A, Tripodo C, et al. Alteration of HSC functions in thalassemia. Blood 2015;126:4752.

53. Imren S, Payen E, Westerman KA, et al. Permanent and panerythroid correction of murine beta thalassemia by multiple lentiviral integration in hematopoietic stem cells. Proc Natl Acad Sci U S A 2002;99(22):14380–5.

54. Hanawa H, Hargrove PW, Kepes S, et al. Extended beta-globin locus control region elements promote consistent therapeutic expression of a gamma-globin lentiviral vector in murine beta-thalassemia. Blood 2004;104(8):2281–90.

55. Persons DA, Allay ER, Sawai N, et al. Successful treatment of murine {beta}-thalassemia using in vivo selection of genetically-modified, drug-resistant hematopoietic stem cells. Blood 2003;102(2):506–16.

56. Lisowski L, Sadelain M. Locus control region elements HS1 and HS4 enhance the therapeutic efficacy of globin gene transfer in beta-thalassemic mice. Blood 2007;110(13):4175–8.

57. Miccio A, Poletti V, Tiboni F, et al. The GATA1-HS2 enhancer allows persistent and position-independent expression of a beta-globin transgene. PLoS One 2011; 6(12):e27955.

58. Breda L, Casu C, Gardenghi S, et al. Therapeutic hemoglobin levels after gene transfer in beta-thalassemia mice and in hematopoietic cells of beta-thalassemia and sickle cells disease patients. PLoS One 2012;7(3):e32345.

59. Puthenveetil G, Scholes J, Carbonell D, et al. Successful correction of the human beta-thalassemia major phenotype using a lentiviral vector. Blood 2004;104(12): 3445–53.

60. Lidonnici M, Salvatori F, Tiboni F, et al. High dose of transduced HPSCs provides safe long term correction of beta-thalassemia. Hum Gene Ther 2013; 24(12):A109.

61. Moiani A, Paleari Y, Sartori D, et al. Lentiviral vector integration in the human genome induces alternative splicing and generates aberrant transcripts. J Clin Invest 2012;122(5):1653–66.

62. Cavazzana-Calvo M, Payen E, Negre O, et al. Transfusion independence and HMGA2 activation after gene therapy of human beta-thalassaemia. Nature 2010;467(7313):318–22.

63. Thompson AA, Kwiatkowski J, Rasko J, et al. Lentiglobin gene therapy for transfusion-dependent β-thalassemia: update from the Northstar Hgb-204 phase 1/2 clinical study. Blood 2016;128:1165.

64. Marktel SGF, Cicalese MP, Casiraghi M, et al. A phase I/II study of autologous hematopoietic stem cells genetically modified with globe lentiviral vector for the treatment of transfusion dependent beta-thalassemia. Haematologica 2016; 101(s1):168.

65. Madigan C, Malik P. Pathophysiology and therapy for haemoglobinopathies. Part I: sickle cell disease. Expert Rev Mol Med 2006;8(9):1–23.
66. Platt OS. Hydroxyurea for the treatment of sickle cell anemia. N Engl J Med 2008; 358(13):1362–9.
67. Piel FB, Patil AP, Howes RE, et al. Global epidemiology of sickle haemoglobin in neonates: a contemporary geostatistical model-based map and population estimates. Lancet 2013;381(9861):142–51.
68. Zhang D, Xu C, Manwani D, et al. Neutrophils, platelets, and inflammatory pathways at the nexus of sickle cell disease pathophysiology. Blood 2016;127(7): 801–9.
69. Fitzhugh CD, Hsieh MM, Bolan CD, et al. Granulocyte colony-stimulating factor (G-CSF) administration in individuals with sickle cell disease: time for a moratorium? Cytotherapy 2009;11(4):464–71.
70. Steinberg MH, Chui DH, Dover GJ, et al. Fetal hemoglobin in sickle cell anemia: a glass half full? Blood 2014;123(4):481–5.
71. Pestina TI, Hargrove PW, Jay D, et al. Correction of murine sickle cell disease using gamma-globin lentiviral vectors to mediate high-level expression of fetal hemoglobin. Mol Ther 2009;17(2):245–52.
72. Perumbeti A, Higashimoto T, Urbinati F, et al. A novel human gamma-globin gene vector for genetic correction of sickle cell anemia in a humanized sickle mouse model: critical determinants for successful correction. Blood 2009;114(6): 1174–85.
73. McCune SL, Reilly MP, Chomo MJ, et al. Recombinant human hemoglobins designed for gene therapy of sickle cell disease. Proc Natl Acad Sci U S A 1994; 91(21):9852–6.
74. Levasseur DN, Ryan TM, Reilly MP, et al. A recombinant human hemoglobin with anti-sickling properties greater than fetal hemoglobin. J Biol Chem 2004;279(26): 27518–24.
75. Levasseur DN, Ryan TM, Pawlik KM, et al. Correction of a mouse model of sickle cell disease: lentiviral/antisickling beta-globin gene transduction of unmobilized, purified hematopoietic stem cells. Blood 2003;102(13):4312–9.
76. Urbinati F, Hargrove PW, Geiger S, et al. Potentially therapeutic levels of anti-sickling globin gene expression following lentivirus-mediated gene transfer in sickle cell disease bone marrow CD34+ cells. Exp Hematol 2015;43(5):346–51.
77. Andreani M, Testi M, Gaziev J, et al. Quantitatively different red cell/nucleated cell chimerism in patients with long-term, persistent hematopoietic mixed chimerism after bone marrow transplantation for thalassemia major or sickle cell disease. Haematologica 2011;96(1):128–33.
78. Walters MC, Patience M, Leisenring W, et al. Stable mixed hematopoietic chimerism after bone marrow transplantation for sickle cell anemia. Biol Blood Marrow Transplant 2001;7(12):665–73.
79. Wu CJ, Gladwin M, Tisdale J, et al. Mixed haematopoietic chimerism for sickle cell disease prevents intravascular haemolysis. Br J Haematol 2007;139(3): 504–7.
80. Ribeil JA, Hacein-Bey-Abina S, Payen E, et al. Gene therapy in a patient with sickle cell disease. N Engl J Med 2017;376(9):848–55.
81. Kanter J, Walters MC, Hsieh MM, et al. Interim results from a phase 1/2 clinical study of lentiglobin gene therapy for severe sickle cell disease. Blood 2016; 128(1176).

82. Hoban MD, Cost GJ, Mendel MC, et al. Correction of the sickle cell disease mutation in human hematopoietic stem/progenitor cells. Blood 2015;125(17):2597–604.

83. Hoban MD, Lumaquin D, Kuo CY, et al. CRISPR/Cas9-mediated correction of the sickle mutation in human CD34+ cells. Mol Ther 2016;24(9):1561–9.

84. DeWitt MA, Magis W, Bray NL, et al. Selection-free genome editing of the sickle mutation in human adult hematopoietic stem/progenitor cells. Sci Transl Med 2016;8(360):360ra134.

85. Dever DP, Bak RO, Reinisch A, et al. CRISPR/Cas9 beta-globin gene targeting in human haematopoietic stem cells. Nature 2016;539(7629):384–9.

86. Bauer DE, Orkin SH. Hemoglobin switching's surprise: the versatile transcription factor BCL11A is a master repressor of fetal hemoglobin. Curr Opin Genet Dev 2015;33:62–70.

87. Brendel C, Guda S, Renella R, et al. Lineage-specific BCL11A knockdown circumvents toxicities and reverses sickle phenotype. J Clin Invest 2016;126(10):3868–78.

88. Tsang JC, Yu Y, Burke S, et al. Single-cell transcriptomic reconstruction reveals cell cycle and multi-lineage differentiation defects in Bcl11a-deficient hematopoietic stem cells. Genome Biol 2015;16:178.

89. Chang K-H, Smith SE, Sullivan T, et al. Long-term engraftment and fetal globin induction upon BCL11A gene editing in bone-marrow-derived CD34+ hematopoietic stem and progenitor cells. Mol Ther Methods Clin Dev 2017;4:137–48.

90. Canver MC, Smith EC, Sher F, et al. BCL11A enhancer dissection by Cas9-mediated in situ saturating mutagenesis. Nature 2015;527(7577):192–7.

91. Vierstra J, Reik A, Chang K-H, et al. Functional footprinting of regulatory DNA. Nat Meth 2015;12(10):927–30.

92. Traxler EA, Yao Y, Wang Y-D, et al. A genome-editing strategy to treat [beta]-hemoglobinopathies that recapitulates a mutation associated with a benign genetic condition. Nat Med 2016;22(9):987–90.

93. Ye L, Wang J, Tan Y, et al. Genome editing using CRISPR-Cas9 to create the HPFH genotype in HSPCs: an approach for treating sickle cell disease and beta-thalassemia. Proc Natl Acad Sci U S A 2016;113(38):10661–5.

94. Genovese P, Schiroli G, Escobar G, et al. Targeted genome editing in human repopulating haematopoietic stem cells. Nature 2014;510(7504):235–40.

95. Breda L, Motta I, Lourenco S, et al. Forced chromatin looping raises fetal hemoglobin in adult sickle cells to higher levels than pharmacologic inducers. Blood 2016;128(8):1139–43.

Gene Therapy for Hemophilia

Amit C. Nathwani, MBChB, FRCP, FRCPath, PhD[a,b,*], Andrew M. Davidoff, MD[c],
Edward G.D. Tuddenham, MD[a]

KEYWORDS

- Gene therapy • Hemophilia • Clinical trials • Adeno-associated virus (AAV) vectors

KEY POINTS

- The best currently available treatments for hemophilia A and B (factor VIII or factor IX deficiency, respectively) require frequent intravenous infusion of highly expensive proteins that have short half-lives.
- Most hemophiliacs worldwide do not have access to even this level of care. In stark contrast, gene therapy holds out the hope of a cure by inducing continuous endogenous expression of factor VIII or factor IX following transfer of a functional gene to replace the hemophilic patient's own defective gene.
- Hemophilia may be considered a "low hanging fruit" for gene therapy because a small increment in blood factor levels (>2% of normal) significantly improves the bleeding tendency from severe to moderate, eliminating most spontaneous bleeds.
- In this review, the authors discuss the data from their own study – the first successful clinical gene transfer in hemophilia B, and results that are now emerging from many similar studies in both hemophilia A and B.

INTRODUCTION

The commonest severe inherited bleeding disorder in all ethnic groups worldwide is hemophilia A, followed by hemophilia B. These are X-linked recessive disorders that result from mutations in the genes for blood clotting factor VIII (FVIII) in hemophilia A or factor IX (FIX) in hemophilia B. The incidence of hemophilia A in live male births is approximately 1 in 5000, and of hemophilia B, 1 in 25,000. Bleeding tendency varies but correlates best with the residual circulating factor level, which in turn depends on

Due to word limits, only essential references are included.
[a] Department of Academic Haematology, UCL Cancer Institute, Katharine Dormandy Haemophilia and Thrombosis Centre, Rowland Hill Street, London NW3 2PF, United Kingdom;
[b] National Health Service Blood and Transplant, Oak House, Reeds Crescent, Watford, Hertfordshire, WD24 4QN, United Kingdom; [c] Department of Surgery, St. Jude Children's Research Hospital, 262 Danny Thomas Place Memphis, TN 38105-3678, USA
* Corresponding author. Department of Academic Haematology, UCL Cancer Institute, Katharine Dormandy Haemophilia and Thrombosis Centre, Rowland Hill Street, London NW3 2PF, United Kingdom.
E-mail addresses: amit.nathwani@ucl.ac.uk; a.nathwani@ucl.ac.uk

Hematol Oncol Clin N Am 31 (2017) 853–868
http://dx.doi.org/10.1016/j.hoc.2017.06.011
0889-8588/17/© 2017 Elsevier Inc. All rights reserved.

the genotype of the mutation that prevents synthesis and/or interferes with function of the affected factor. If the residual factor level is 5% of normal or greater, subjects can be assigned to the mild hemophilia category, in which spontaneous bleeding is absent and only occurs after significant trauma. Wherein residual factor level is less than 5% but greater than 1%, patients are considered to have moderate hemophilia with a variable bleeding tendency; some in this group seldom have any bleeding, whereas others experience frequent bleeding after minor trauma. About half of patients with hemophilia A or B have factor levels less than 1% of normal.[1] These individuals have a severe bleeding tendency with frequent spontaneous musculoskeletal and soft tissue bleeding. A recent careful study of the hemophilic patient population at a large Dutch clinic[2] confirmed these correlations and the basic division into severe, moderate, and mild, but added the insight that those mildly affected patients whose residual factor level is 13% or greater never experienced joint bleeding. Thus, factor levels of greater than 13% could be considered as a target for gene therapy to attain. Among those patients who do bleed into their joints, the ankles are most commonly affected starting in early childhood, with knees and elbows affected later. Repeated episodes of intra-articular bleeding cause severe, progressive, destructive arthropathy with deformity leading to complete loss of joint function and attendant disability.

In the absence of replacement therapy, the life expectancy of a boy with severe hemophilia is only about 10 years. This severe shortening of life still applies in many less-developed countries. Even in developed countries until the 1960s, treatment of hemophilia was limited to infusion of fresh frozen plasma. In 1968, the first widely available concentrate for hemophilia A, cryoprecipitate, was introduced.[3] During the 1970s and 1980s, many multidonor factor concentrates were developed to improve the purity, potency, stability, and convenience of administration of factor replacement therapy. However, these developments, depending as they did on large donor pools of often commercially sourced plasma, permitted transmission of human immunodeficiency virus (HIV) and hepatitis C virus. Almost a whole generation of hemophiliacs who were given the new products became HIV positive and died of AIDS before highly effective antiretroviral therapies were developed. During the period 1970 to 1986, every treated patient was also exposed to hepatitis C, and up to 25 years later, some are still succumbing to chronic liver failure resulting from continued infection. From 1986 onward, heat treatment and then the solvent detergent method inactivated both HIV and hepatitis C virus. Since then, there have been no new cases of transmission of those lipid enveloped viruses. Transmission by blood products of other pathogens resistant to inactivation, such as parvovirus,[3] hepatitis A,[4] and prions (variant Creutzfeldt-Jakob disease[5]), remain a major concern. Recombinant factor concentrates are of course free from blood-borne infections, but their availability has been limited to the most developed countries by very high cost and production constraints. With the expiry of patents on recombinant FVIII and FIX, biosimilars and other variants with enhanced pharmacokinetic or other properties are entering the market, with potential for wider availability than hitherto.

In developed countries, standard hemophilia care for severely affected patients now consists of home-administered prophylaxis with safe concentrates intended to maintain factor level greater than 1% of normal. This is a compromise based on cost and practical considerations, which reduces but does not eliminate bleeding. If started in early childhood after the first joint bleed, arthropathy can be largely prevented.[6] When continued throughout life, prophylaxis leads to near normalization of life expectancy.[7] However, the relatively short half-life of FVIII and FIX in the circulation necessitates frequent intravenous administration of factor concentrates (at least 2–3 times a week), which is demanding and extremely expensive; annualized costs of prophylaxis for an adult equal or exceed £120,000 for patients with hemophilia B. Even with prophylaxis, significant limitations remain because normal plasma clotting factor levels are not consistently restored; the short half-life of existing clotting factors results in peaks and troughs of circulating clotting factor associated with breakthrough bleeding. The saw-tooth pattern of factor level, high immediately after infusion, falling rapidly to near baseline, mandates careful planning of physical activities such as sports, which people living without hemophilia can hardly imagine. New modified synthetic formulations of FVIII and FIX that are pegylated or fused to proteins with long half-life such as albumin or Fcγ have greatly improved the activity profile for FIX but have been less impressive for FVIII because of the dominant role of von Willebrand factor in determining its half-life. In any case, these products do not remove the problems of lifelong intravenous administration, breakthrough bleeding, and ever-mounting cost. The cumulative effects of lifelong administration of pegylated proteins are unknown, as is the potential of fusion proteins to induce an immune response.[6] Two other entirely novel approaches to normalizing thrombin generation in hemophilia are undergoing extensive trials at the time of this writing (January 2017). The first is a synthetic FVIII mimic consisting of linked antibodies, one of which binds factor IXa and the other factor X (Emicizumab).[7] Although restoring thrombin generation to a degree comparable to FVIII level of about 15% in patients with or without inhibitory antibody, there is a major difference from wild-type FVIII. The mimic is under no control of its activity, being permanently active throughout the circulation, whereas native FVIII has very strictly controlled activity in both time and site of action. It circulates as a procofactor tightly bound to a carrier; it is activated only at sites of clot propagation, and it has a very short half-life after activation. The consequences of these differences have recently emerged in thrombotic events occurring in patients treated with Emicizumab and bypass clotting agents. The second alternative approach is to lower the natural antithrombin level with antisense RNA technology.[8] Both approaches have shown efficacy in reducing the rate of bleeding, but their use may be limited by risk of thrombogenicity, and both still require lifelong injections without restoring normal hemostasis.

Even set against this scenario of widening therapeutic choice, gene therapy offers a strikingly attractive potential for cure by means of the endogenous production of FVIII or FIX following transfer of a normal copy of the respective gene. The hemophilias were recognized in the 1980s as good candidates for gene therapy because all their clinical manifestations are due to lack of a single protein that circulates in minute amounts in the bloodstream. Years of clinical experience and the natural experiment of moderate hemophilia prove that a small increase to 1% to 2% in circulating levels of the deficient clotting factor significantly modifies the bleeding diathesis; even a modest response to gene therapy can be effective. Tight regulation of transgene expression is unnecessary because a wide range of FIX or FVIII levels is without toxicity and effective at reducing bleeding. Animal models such as FVIII- and FIX-knockout mice,[9–11] and dogs with hemophilia A or B,[12,13] have facilitated extensive preclinical evaluation of gene therapy strategies. The efficiency of therapy can be assessed easily just by measuring plasma levels of FVIII or FIX. The complementary DNA (cDNA) for the gene encoding FIX is small and adaptable to gene transfer in many viral systems. In addition, its expression pathway is significantly less complex than that of FVIII, and it is natively expressed at higher levels. Consequently, more gene transfer studies have focused on hemophilia B than hemophilia A, but this is rapidly changing as the technology evolves.

FIRST CLINICAL STUDIES OF GENE THERAPY IN HEMOPHILIA

The most efficient way to introduce therapeutic genes into target somatic cells, a process referred to as transduction, is to use adapted naturally occurring viruses as vectors, because they are highly evolved to transfer their own DNA in the central process of their life cycles. Targeted cells can be either in culture for ex vivo gene transfer or within organs for in vivo delivery of vector. Several gene transfer vehicles have been developed based on viral vectors (**Tables 1–4**). Early studies with nonviral, onco-retroviral, and adenoviral vectors appeared safe but did not result in sustained transgene expression at therapeutic levels.[14–17] Recombinant adeno-associated viral vectors (AAV) currently show the most promise for gene therapy for hemophilia. These vectors have the best safety profile among gene transfer vectors of viral origin, because wild-type AAV has never been associated with human disease. Safety is further enhanced by the dependence of AAV on coinfection with helper virus (usually adenovirus or herpesvirus) for productive infection. In addition, recombinant vectors based on AAV are entirely devoid of wild-type viral coding sequences, thus reducing the potential for invoking cell-mediated immune response to foreign viral proteins. Two clinical gene therapy trials for hemophilia B have been performed with AAV vectors based on serotype 2, the first serotype to be isolated and fully characterized (see **Table 4**).[18,19] The first study was a dose escalation phase 1/2 study entailing multiple intramuscular injections of AAV vector encoding the FIX gene. Vector administration was not associated with serious adverse events. However, sustained increase in plasma FIX levels of greater than 1% was not observed in any of the 7 subjects recruited to this study despite immunohistochemical evidence of FIX expression at the site of injection for more than 10 years.[18]

In the second study, AAV2 vector containing a liver-specific expression cassette was infused into the hepatic artery over 3 different doses ranging from 0.08 to 2 × 10^{12} vg/kg. In all patients, vector genomes were transiently detected in the semen, although there was no evidence of germ-line transmission because purified spermatozoa were negative by a polymerase chain reaction assay. The low and intermediate vector doses were safe but did not result in a detectable increase in plasma FIX levels. The results in the 2 subjects treated at the high-dose level (2 × 10^{12} vg/kg) were mixed. One had higher levels of neutralizing anti-AAV-2 antibodies before gene transfer which appeared to partly block successful transduction resulting in transgenic FIX expression peaking at 4% 4 weeks after vector infusion then declining to baseline. In contrast, FIX levels increased to around 10% of normal levels in the other subject for 4 weeks after vector administration and then unexpectedly declined to baseline values. This decline in transgenic protein coincided with a transient 10-fold increase in liver transaminases, which spontaneously returned to baseline values over the subsequent weeks, consistent with a self-limiting process. Further studies have led to the hypothesis that the decline in FIX expression and the liver toxicity were likely due to a capsid-specific cytotoxic T cells directed against the transduced hepatocytes following presentation of AAV2 capsid peptide in the context of major histocompatibility complex I molecules.[19]

Thus, both humoral and cell-mediated immune responses have the potential to limit persistent expression of FIX following administration of AAV vectors in humans.

CURRENT AND ON-GOING TRIALS OF GENE THERAPY FOR HEMOPHILIA A AND B

In what follows, on-going clinical trials of gene therapy for hemophilia using AAV-based vectors are presented and discussed. The pace of advance is now so rapid that data on recently opened trials are only available as meeting presentations and/or company news releases, not yet as peer-reviewed publications. Therefore, the authors are using those sources of information to bring readers of this review the most current available information, with the caveat that the data are not derived from peer-reviewed journals.

Table 1
Hemophilia gene therapy with a nonviral vector

A. Properties

Packaging Capacity	Ease of Production	Integration into Host Genome	Duration of Expression	Transduction of Postmitotic Cells	Preexisting Host Immunity	Safety Concerns	Germ-Line Transmission
Unlimited	+++	Rarely	Usually transient	++	None	—	—

B. Summary of Phase 1-2 Studies

Sponsor	Transgene	Promoter	Inclusion Criteria	Method of Vector Delivery	Safety	Peak Transgene Expression	Current Status
Transkaryotic therapies, Cambridge, MA	hFVIIIΔB	Fibronectin	Adults with severe hemophilia A	Electroporation of autologous fibroblast ex vivo followed by implantation into omentum	No significant side effects	Transient increase in FVIII activity to a maximum of 4%	Closed

Table 2
Hemophilia gene therapy with retroviral vectors

A. Properties

Packaging Capacity	Ease of Production	Integration into Host Genome	Duration of Expression	Transduction of Postmitotic Cells	Preexisting Host Immunity	Safety Concerns	Germ-Line Transmission
~8.0 kb	No reliable producer cell lines for lentiviral vectors	Yes	Long term	Lentiviral vectors ++ onco-retroviral vectors —	None	Insertional mutagenesis	–/+

B. Summary of Phase 1-2 Studies

Sponsor	Transgene	Vector	Inclusion Criteria	Method of Vector Delivery	Safety	Peak Transgene Expression	Current Status
Chiron Corp, Emeryville, CA	hFVIIIΔB	Onco-retroviral	Adults with severe hemophilia A, negative for hepatitis C virus	IV	Erroneous detection of vector genome in semen	Isolated increase in FVIII activity at low levels	Closed
Fudan University, China	hFIX	Onco-retroviral	Adults with moderate hemophilia B (baseline FIX of 2%)	3 monthly injections of ex vivo modified autologous fibroblasts	No significant side effects	Transient (<16 mo) increase in FIX activity to 4%	Closed
Bioverativ	Codon optimized FIX containing the Padua mutation	Lentivirus	Phase 1/2 trial expected to start in 2018				

Table 3

Hemophilia gene therapy with adenoviral vectors

A. Properties

Packaging Capacity	Ease of Production	Integration into Host Genome	Duration of Expression	Transduction of Postmitotic Cells	Preexisting Host Immunity	Safety Concerns	Germ-Line Transmission
~30.0 kb	+/−	No	Transient	Very efficient	+++	Inflammatory response	—

B. Summary of Phase 1-2 Studies

Sponsor	Transgene	Vector	Inclusion Criteria	Method of Vector Delivery	Safety	Peak Transgene Expression	Current Status
GenStar Therapeutics, Alameda, CA	Full-length FVIII	Gutless adenoviral vector containing the albumin promoter	Adults with severe hemophilia A with low titers of antiadenovirus antibodies	Peripheral venous infusion	Elevation of liver enzymes and thrombocytopenia observed in the first patient	Transient increase in FVIII activity to 3%	Closed

Table 4
Hemophilia gene therapy with adeno-associated viral vectors

A. Properties

Packaging Capacity	Ease of Production	Integration into Host Genome	Duration of Expression	Transduction of Postmitotic Cells	Preexisting Host Immunity	Safety Concerns
4.6 kb	Cumbersome	Infrequent	Long-term in postmitotic cells	Efficient	++	—

B. Summary of Gene Therapy Trials for Hemophilia B

Sponsor	Transgene	Vector	Method of Vector Delivery	Expression (% of Normal) Toxicity	Current Status
Avigen/CHOP	Wild-type FIX	AAV2	Intramuscularly	Transient <1.6% No significant side effects	Closed
Avigen/CHOP	Wild-type FIX	AAV2	Bolus infusion into hepatic artery	Transient FIX at 12% in 1 patient and 4% in 2nd patient at 2×10^{12} vg/kg Transient transaminitis at 3 wk after gene transfer in 2 out of 7 patients	Closed
St Jude/UCL	Codon optimized FIX	AAV8	Bolus peripheral vein infusion	Persistent (>6 y) dose-dependent expression of FIX at between 1% and 6% of normal level in all subjects recruited Transient transaminitis at 6–10 wk after gene transfer in 4 out of 10 patients	Open
Shire (Baxalta; BAX 335)	Codon optimized FIX containing the Padua mutation	AAV8	Bolus peripheral vein infusion	Persistent (>2 y) expression of FIX at 25% in 1 out of 7 patients recruited Transient transaminitis at 6–10 wk after gene transfer in 2 out of 7 patients	Closed
Spark Therapeutics (SPK-9001)	Codon optimized FIX containing the Padua mutation	AAV- SPK-100	Bolus peripheral vein infusion	Persistent (~1 y) expression of FIX at 12%–68% in 9 out of 9 patients recruited Transient transaminitis at 4–8 wk after gene transfer in 2 out of 9 patients	Open

Sponsor	Transgene	Vector	Method of Vector Delivery	Expression / Toxicity	Current Status
UniQure (AMT-060)	Codon optimized FIX	AAV5	Bolus peripheral vein infusion	Persistent (>1 y) expression of FIX at 3%–7% in 9 out of 10 patients recruited; Transient transaminitis at 6–10 wk after gene transfer in 3 out of 10 patients	Open
Dimension Therapeutics (DTX101)	Codon optimized FIX	AAVrh10	Bolus peripheral vein infusion	Persistent (~1 y) expression of FIX at 3%–8% in 6 out of 6 patients recruited; Transient transaminitis at 6–10 wk after gene transfer in 5 out of 6 patients	Open
Sangamo Bioscience (SB-FIX)	Codon optimized FIX	AAV6/Zinc-finger–mediated targeted integration into the albumin locus in hepatocytes	Study has US Food and Drug Administration approval		

C. Summary of Gene Therapy Trials for Hemophilia A

Sponsor	Transgene	Vector	Method of Vector Delivery	Expression (% of Normal) / Toxicity	Current Status
BioMarin (BMN 270)	Codon optimized BDD-FVIII	AAV5	Bolus peripheral vein infusion	Persistent (>1 y) expression of FVIII 2%–250% in 8 out of 9 patients recruited; Transient transaminitis at 6–20 wk after gene transfer in 8 out of 9 patients	Open
UCL/St Jude	Codon optimized FVIII; B domain replaced with V3 peptide	AAV8	Bolus peripheral vein infusion	Regulatory approvals granted in the UK	Open
Spark Therapeutics (SPK-8011)	BDD-FVIII	Hybrid capsid	Trial open; 3 patients enrolled		
Dimension Therapeutics/Bayer (DTX-201)	BDD-FVIII	? AAVRh10			
Shire (BAX-888)	BDD-FVIII	AAV8			
Sangamo Bioscience (SB-525)	BDD-FVIII	AAV6			

THE FIRST LONG-TERM SUCCESS IN A CLINICAL TRIAL OF GENE TRANSFER IN HEMOPHILIA

Building on earlier studies discussed above, an approach for gene therapy for hemophilia B was developed using a codon-optimized version of the human *FIX* (*hFIXco*) gene, which was cloned downstream of a compact synthetic liver-specific promoter (*LP1*) to enable packaging into self-complementary AAV vectors (scAAV), which have a packaging capacity of approximately 2.3 kb.[20] By this, it is meant that one-half of the AAV proviral palindromic sequence can be up to 2.3 kb, so that the whole self-complementary sequence does not exceed 4.6 kb, which is the packaging capacity of AAV. Preclinical studies in mice and nonhuman primates showed that scAAV vectors were more potent than comparable single-stranded AAV vectors, raising the possibility of achieving therapeutic levels of FIX using lower and potentially safer doses of vector.[20,21]

Another important aspect of this study was to use a vector pseudotyped with AAV serotype 8 capsid. This had the advantage over AAV2 vectors of the remarkable tropism of AAV8 for efficient transduction of the liver following administration of the vector in the peripheral circulation.[21,22] Hence, a simple noninvasive route of vector administration was used that is safer for patients with a bleeding diathesis. In addition, the lower seroprevalence of AAV8 in humans ($\sim$25% compared with >70% for AAV2[23]) enabled exclusion of fewer subjects with preexisting humoral immunity to AAV8.

Six subjects with severe hemophilia B were enrolled to the initial phase of this study with 2 subjects recruited sequentially at 1 of 3 vector doses (low [2×10^{11} vg/kg], intermediate [6×10^{11} vg/kg], or high dose [2×10^{12} vg/kg]) of scAAV2/8-LP1-hFIXco. FIX expression at 1% to 6% of normal was established in all 6 subjects with an initial follow-up of between 6 and 14 months following gene transfer. Asymptomatic, transient elevation of serum liver enzymes, perhaps a result of a cellular immune response to the AAV8 capsid, was observed in both subjects recruited to the high-dose level between 7 and 10 weeks after gene transfer. Treatment of each with a short course of prednisolone led to rapid normalization of liver enzymes and maintenance of FIX levels in the 2% to 4% range. Four of the 6 subjects have been able to discontinue routine prophylaxis without suffering spontaneous hemorrhage, even when they undertook activities that previously had provoked bleeds. The other 2 have increased the interval between FIX prophylaxes. This is consistent with the natural bleeding history in mild hemophilia patients (FIX levels of between 5% and 40%), where bleeding episodes generally only occur after trauma or surgery with very few or no spontaneous bleeds.[24]

Longer follow-up of these individuals shows that AAV-mediated FIX expression remained relatively stable over a period of at least 6 years.[25] One of the 4 subjects who discontinued prophylaxis has subsequently been started on a once-a-week prophylaxis regimen to avert trauma-related bleeding incurred in the course of his work as a geologist. The others remain off prophylaxis and free of spontaneous hemorrhage. The overall reduction in FIX usage in these 6 subjects over the duration of the study is several million units so far, and the resulting financial savings exceeds £5M. Subsequently, a further 4 subjects were recruited for treatment at the higher dose. Two of these subjects had no evidence of immune-mediated liver inflammation and achieved a level of stable FIX expression between 5% and 8%. Both have stopped prophylaxis and report no bleeding. One subject had a mild episode of immune hepatitis that responded promptly to steroids. His FIX level has been maintained at 5%, and he has no need for prophylaxis and does not experience spontaneous bleeding since gene transfer. The remaining subject experienced a more marked elevation of transaminase, which despite responding to a course of oral steroid was accompanied by a decrease in steady state FIX to 2%. He has less bleeding than before gene transfer, is not using prophylaxis, but has occasional trauma-related bleeding episodes requiring substitution therapy. In an on-going extension of the trial, the vector preparation has been further purified to remove empty capsids, and the optimum dose is being explored in dose escalation to determine if the immune hepatitis can be abrogated while attaining a therapeutically favorable FIX level.

RECENT TRIALS OF GENE TRANSFER IN HEMOPHILIA B

Five studies of similar vectors for transferring either wild-type FIX or the gain of function mutation known as Padua (R338L) have been initiated since the first reports of successful long-term expression noted above were published. The results of these trials as presented in meetings and/or released in communications from commercial sponsors are summarized in **Table 4**. Of note, the 2 studies using the Padua mutant are consistent with expression of a similar amount of protein as in the earlier St Jude/UCL trials but with 5- to 8-fold enhanced activity. Thus, FIX levels greater than 12% have been recorded in 9 subjects. Of further note, 2 out of 9 subjects so treated in the study carried out by Spark Therapeutics have had immune-mediated elevation of liver enzymes and were treated with a course of oral steroids.

ADENO-ASSOCIATED VIRAL VECTORS AND GENE THERAPY FOR HEMOPHILIA A

The limited packaging capacity of AAV vectors (4680 kb) and the poor expression profile of FVIII have hindered the use of these vectors for gene therapy for hemophilia A. Compared with other proteins of similar size, expression of FVIII is highly inefficient.[26] Bioengineering of the FVIII molecule has resulted in improvement of FVIII expression. For instance, deletion of the FVIII B domain, which is not required for cofactor activity, resulted in a 17-fold increase in mRNA levels over full-length wild-type FVIII and a 30% increase in secreted protein.[27,28] This has led to the development of BDD-FVIII protein concentrate, which is now widely used clinically (Refacto; Pfizer). Pipe and colleagues[29] have shown that the inclusion of the proximal 226 amino-acid portion of the B domain (FVIII-N6) that is rich in asparagine-linked oligosaccharides significantly increases expression over that achieved with BDD-FVIII. This may be due to improved secretion of FVIII facilitated by the interaction of 6 N-linked glycosylation triplets within this region with the mannose-binding lectin, LMAN1, or a reduced tendency to evoke an unfolded protein response.[30] These 6 N-linked glycosylation consensus sequences (Asn-X-Thr/Ser) are highly conserved in B domains from different species, suggesting that they play an important biological role.[31]

Another obstacle to AAV-mediated gene transfer for hemophilia A gene therapy is the size of the FVIII coding sequence, which at 7.0 kb far exceeds the normal packaging capacity of AAV vectors. AAV vectors encoding the canine BDD-FVIII variant that is around 4.4 kb have yielded promising results. Others have evaluated the coadministration of 2 AAV vectors separately encoding the FVIII heavy and light chains whose intracellular association in vivo leads to the formation of a functional molecule.[32] Another 2 AAV vector approach exploits the tendency of these vectors to form head-to-tail concatemers by splitting the FVIII expression cassette such that one AAV vector contains a promoter and part of the coding sequence, as well as a splice donor site, whereas the second AAV vector contains the splice acceptor site and the remaining coding sequence. Following in vivo head-to-tail concatemerization, a functional transcript is created that is capable of expressing full-length FVIII protein.[33–37] These 2 AAV vector approaches are however inefficient, cumbersome, and expensive and not easily transferred to the clinic.

The authors have developed an AAV-based gene transfer approach that addresses both the size constraints and inefficient FVIII expression. Expression of human FVIII was improved 10-fold by reorganization of the wild-type cDNA of human FVIII according to the codon usage of highly expressed human genes.[20,38–40] Expression from B domain deleted codon optimized FVIII molecule was further enhanced by the inclusion of a 17 amino-acid peptide that contains the 6 N-linked glycosylation signals from the B domain required for efficient cellular processing. These changes have resulted in a novel 5.2-kb AAV expression cassette (AAV-HLP-codop-hFVIII-V3) that is efficiently packaged into recombinant AAV vectors and is capable of mediating supraphysiologic levels of FVIII expression in animal models over the same dose range of AAV8 that proved to be efficacious in subjects with hemophilia B.

Juxtaposition of novel amino acid sequences as has been done in the authors' AAV-HLP-codop-hFVIII-V3 could lead to neoantigenicity, thereby increasing the risk of provoking a neutralizing antibody response to the transgenic protein. This was also a concern when recombinant BDD-FVIII (ReFacto) was first introduced for use in man. ReFacto contains the "SQ" link of 14 amino acids (SFSQNPPVLKRHQR) between the A2 and A3 domains, generated by fusion of Ser743 in the N-terminus with Gln1638 in the C-terminus of the B domain, creating a neoantigenic site. However, despite extensive clinical use of ReFacto, an increase in frequency of neutralizing human Factor VIII antibodies in patients treated with this product has not been observed.[41–43] In addition, antibodies to epitopes in the B domain that are occasionally seen in patients with severe hemophilia A treated with hFVIII protein concentrates are devoid of inhibitory activity because they bind to nonfunctional FVIII epitopes.[44]

Using an AAV5 containing the SQ linker codon optimized FVIII expression cassette described above, in a study sponsored by Biomarin, 9 subjects with severe hemophilia A have been treated at doses ranging from 6×10^{12} to 6×10^{13} vg/kg. Of 7 treated at the highest dose, 6 subjects now have FVIII level greater than 50% (see **Table 4**). Highly encouraged by this result, a new cohort of patients has been recruited to be treated at an intermediate lower dose level of 4×10^{13} vg/kg in order to find a dose to take forward in a phase 3 trial.

OBSTACLES TO WIDER USE OF ADENO-ASSOCIATED VIRAL VECTOR TECHNOLOGY
Safety Considerations

Thus far, the risk of liver toxicity accompanied by loss or reduction of transgene expression appears to be the most worrying toxicity associated with liver-targeted delivery of AAV. However, this phenomenon can be controlled with a short course of prednisolone and appears to be self-limiting with no evidence of persistent hepatocellular damage. The precise pathophysiologic basis for the hepatocellular toxicity remains unclear, in part because it has not been possible to recapitulate this toxicity in animal models. Longer follow-up of some of the high-dose subjects in the authors' study shows that cessation of prednisolone is not followed by a late increase in liver enzymes or reduction in transgene expression, presumably because capsid antigen has been degraded and cleared from the remaining transduced hepatocytes by this point.

As expected, all subjects exposed to AAV vectors develop long-lasting AAV capsid-specific humoral immunity. Although the increase in anti-AAV immunoglobulin G does not have direct clinical consequences, its persistence at high titers precludes subsequent successful gene transfer with vector of the same serotype, in the event that transgene expression should decrease to less than therapeutic levels. However, it has been established that it is possible to achieve successful transduction in animals including nonhuman primates with preexisting anti-AAV8 antibodies following administration of AAV vector pseudotyped with an alternate serotype.[21] On the basis of follow-up data in subjects with hemophilia B, it is likely that re-treatment may not be required for periods that extend beyond 6 years.

Another potential problem of systemic administration of AAV is spread of vector particles to nonhepatic tissues including the gonads. Vector genomes were transiently detectable in the semen of all subjects recruited to the AAV2 and AAV8 hemophilia B clinical trials.[24,45,46] The lack of persistence of the vector genome in semen of hemophilia B patients is consistent with animal data that suggested that AAV can transduce adventitial cells present in semen but not germ cells.

The risk of insertional mutagenesis following AAV-mediated gene transfer has been judged to be low because proviral DNA is maintained predominantly in an episomal form. This is consistent with the fact that wild-type AAV infection in humans, although common, is not associated with oncogenesis. However, deep sequencing studies show that integration of the AAV genome can occur in the liver.[47,48] Indeed, a recent publication has found wild-type AAV2 genome fragments integrated in the proximity of known proto-oncogenes in a small percentage of human hepatocellular carcinoma specimens.[49] However, the pathogenic role of AAV2 in these studies remains unclear.

Scale-Up of Vector Production

Continued progression toward flexible, scalable production and purification methodologies is required to support the commercialization of AAV biotherapeutics. The most widely used method for the generation of AAV entails the transient transfection of adherent HEK 293 cells with plasmids encoding the necessary vector, helper, and packaging genes. This method is cumbersome when scaled up and hence not suited for production of large quantities of clinical-grade vector required for phase 3/market authorization trials. Attention has recently shifted to transfection of suspension culture-adapted 293 cells because they are more amenable to scale-up than using adherent cells.[50] Another scalable method for production of AAV is based on baculovirus grown in SF9 insect cells.[51] This method has recently been used to support market authorization of gene therapy for lipoprotein lipase deficiency.

AFFORDABILITY OF GENE THERAPY

It is likely that gene therapy will command a high price, at least initially, in order to recoup the development cost. However, successful gene therapy offers the advantage of continuous endogenous expression of clotting factor, which will eliminate breakthrough bleeding and microhemorrhages, thereby reducing comorbidities and the need for frequent medical interventions while improving quality of life, thus yielding significant savings for the health care system and society in general. Therefore, if appropriately managed, gene therapy has the potential to be affordable when all such factors are considered.

SUMMARY

The availability of convincing evidence of long-term expression of transgenic FIX at therapeutic levels resulting in amelioration of the bleeding diathesis following AAV-mediated gene transfer is an important step to the eventual licensure of gene therapy for hemophilia. Although several obstacles still remain, the current rate of progress in this field suggests that a licensed gene therapy product will be commercially available within the next decade. Such a product would change the treatment paradigm for patients with severe hemophilia and, in addition, facilitate the development of gene therapy for other disorders affecting the liver where the treatment options are limited or nonexistent.

REFERENCES

1. Nathwani AC, Tuddenham EG. Epidemiology of coagulation disorders. Baillieres Clin Haematol 1992;5:383–439.
2. den Uijl IE, Fischer K, Van Der Bom JG, et al. Clinical outcome of moderate haemophilia compared with severe and mild haemophilia. Haemophilia 2009;15: 83–90.
3. Saldanha J, Minor P. Detection of human parvovirus B19 DNA in plasma pools and blood products derived from these pools: implications for efficiency and consistency of removal of B19 DNA during manufacture. Br J Haematol 1996;93: 714–9.
4. Lawlor E, Graham S, Davidson E, et al. Hepatitis A transmission by factor IX concentrates [see comments]. Vox Sang 1996;71:126–8.
5. Baxter T, Black D, Birks D. New-variant Creutzfeldt-Jakob disease and treatment of haemophilia [letter; see comment]. Lancet 1998;351:600–1.
6. Pipe SW. The hope and reality of long-acting hemophilia products. Am J Hematol 2012;87(Suppl 1):S33–9.
7. Shima M, Hanabusa H, Taki M, et al. Factor VIII-mimetic function of humanized bispecific antibody in hemophilia A. N Engl J Med 2016;374:2044–53.
8. Sehgal A, Barros S, Ivanciu L, et al. An RNAi therapeutic targeting antithrombin to rebalance the coagulation system and promote hemostasis in hemophilia. Nat Med 2015;21:492–7.
9. Kundu RK, Sangiorgi F, Wu LY, et al. Targeted inactivation of the coagulation factor IX gene causes hemophilia B in mice. Blood 1998;92:168–74.
10. Bi L, Lawler AM, Antonarakis SE, et al. Targeted disruption of the mouse factor VIII gene produces a model of haemophilia A [letter]. Nat Genet 1995;10:119–21.
11. Wang L, Zoppè M, Hackeng TM, et al. A factor IX-deficient mouse model for hemophilia B gene therapy. Proc Natl Acad Sci U S A 1997;94:11563–6.
12. Giles AR, Tinlin S, Hoogendoorn H, et al. Development of factor VIII: C antibodies in dogs with hemophilia A. Blood 1984;63:451–6.
13. Evans JP, Brinkhous KM, Brayer GD, et al. Canine hemophilia B resulting from a point mutation with unusual consequences. Proc Natl Acad Sci U S A 1989;86: 10095–9.
14. Roth DA, Tawa NE Jr, O'Brien JM, et al. Nonviral transfer of the gene encoding coagulation factor VIII in patients with severe hemophilia A. N Engl J Med 2001;344:1735–42.
15. Roth DA, Tawa NE, Proper J, et al. Implantation of non-viral ex vivo genetically modified autologous dermal fibroblasts that express B-domain deleted human factor VIII in 12 severe hemophilia A study subjects. Blood 2002;100:116a.
16. Qiu X, Lu D, Zhou J, et al. Implantation of autologous skin fibroblast genetically modified to secrete clotting factor IX partially corrects the hemorrhagic tendencies in two hemophilia B patients. Chin Med J (Engl) 1996;109:832–9.
17. Mannucci PM. Ham-Wasserman lecture: hemophilia and related bleeding disorders: a story of dismay and success. Hematology 2002;2002:1–9.
18. Manno CS, Chew AJ, Hutchison S, et al. AAV-mediated factor IX gene transfer to skeletal muscle in patients with severe hemophilia B. Blood 2003;101:2963–72.

19. Manno CS, Pierce GF, Arruda VR, et al. Successful transduction of liver in hemophilia by AAV-Factor IX and limitations imposed by the host immune response. Nat Med 2006;12:342–7.
20. Nathwani AC, Gray JT, Ng CY, et al. Self complementary adeno-associated virus vectors containing a novel liver-specific human factor IX expression cassette enable highly efficient transduction of murine and nonhuman primate liver. Blood 2006;107:2653–61.
21. Nathwani AC, Gray JT, McIntosh J, et al. Safe and efficient transduction of the liver after peripheral vein infusion of self complementary AAV vector results in stable therapeutic expression of human FIX in nonhuman primates. Blood 2007;109: 1414–21.
22. Thomas CE, Storm TA, Huang Z, et al. Rapid uncoating of vector genomes is the key to efficient liver transduction with pseudotyped adeno-associated virus vectors. J Virol 2004;78:3110–22.
23. Gao GP, Alvira MR, Wang L, et al. Novel adeno-associated viruses from rhesus monkeys as vectors for human gene therapy. Proc Natl Acad Sci U S A 2002; 99:11854–9.
24. Nathwani AC, Tuddenham EG, Rangarajan S, et al. Adenovirus-associated virus vector-mediated gene transfer in hemophilia B. N Engl J Med 2011;365:2357–65.
25. Nathwani AC, Rosales C, McIntosh J, et al. Long-term safety and efficacy following systemic administration of a self-complementary AAV vector encoding human FIX pseudotyped with serotype 5 and 8 capsid proteins. Mol Ther 2011;19:876–85.
26. Miao HZ, Sirachainan N, Palmer L, et al. Bioengineering of coagulation factor VIII for improved secretion. Blood 2004;103:3412–9.
27. Pittman DD, Alderman EM, Tomkinson KN, et al. Biochemical, immunological, and in vivo functional characterization of B-domain-deleted factor VIII. Blood 1993;81:2925–35.
28. Kaufman RJ, Pipe SW, Tagliavacca L, et al. Biosynthesis, assembly and secretion of coagulation factor VIII. Blood Coagul Fibrinolysis 1997;8(Suppl 2):S3–14.
29. Miao HZ, Sirachainan N, Palmer L, et al. Blood 2004;103:3412–9.
30. Malhotra JD, Miao H, Zhang K, et al. Antioxidants reduce endoplasmic reticulum stress and improve protein secretion. Proc Natl Acad Sci U S A 2008;105: 18525–30.
31. Davidson CJ, Hirt RP, Lal K, et al. Molecular evolution of the vertebrate blood coagulation network. Thromb Haemost 2003;89:420–8.
32. Burton M, Nakai H, Colosi P, et al. Coexpression of factor VIII heavy and light chain adeno-associated viral vectors produces biologically active protein. Proc Natl Acad Sci U S A 1999;96:12725–30.
33. Jiang H, Pierce GF, Ozelo MC, et al. Evidence of multiyear factor IX expression by AAV-mediated gene transfer to skeletal muscle in an individual with severe hemophilia B. Mol Ther 2006;14:452–5.
34. Chao H, Mao L, Bruce AT, et al. Sustained expression of human factor VIII in mice using a parvovirus-based vector. Blood 2000;95:1594–9.
35. Chao H, Sun L, Bruce A, et al. Expression of human factor VIII by splicing between dimerized AAV vectors. Mol Ther 2002;5:716–22.
36. Chen L, Zhu F, Li J, et al. The enhancing effects of the light chain on heavy chain secretion in split delivery of factor VIII gene. Mol Ther 2007;15:1856–62.
37. Chen L, Lu H, Wang J, et al. Enhanced factor VIII heavy chain for gene therapy of hemophilia A. Mol Ther 2009;17:417–24.

38. Ward NJ, Buckley SM, Waddington SN, et al. Codon optimization of human factor VIII cDNAs leads to high-level expression. Blood 2011;117:798–807.

39. Radcliffe PA, Sion CJ, Wilkes FJ, et al. Analysis of factor VIII mediated suppression of lentiviral vector titres. Gene Ther 2008;15:289–97.

40. McIntosh J, Lenting PJ, Rosales C, et al. Therapeutic levels of FVIII following a single peripheral vein administration of rAAV vector encoding a novel human factor VIII variant. Blood 2013;121:3335–44.

41. Gringeri A, Tagliaferri A, Tagariello G, et al. Efficacy and inhibitor development in previously treated patients with haemophilia A switched to a B domain-deleted recombinant factor VIII. Br J Haematol 2004;126:398–404.

42. Lusher JM, Lee CA, Kessler CM, et al. The safety and efficacy of B-domain deleted recombinant factor VIII concentrate in patients with severe haemophilia A. Haemophilia 2003;9:38–49.

43. Pollmann H, Externest D, Ganser A, et al. Efficacy, safety and tolerability of recombinant factor VIII (REFACTO) in patients with haemophilia A: interim data from a postmarketing surveillance study in Germany and Austria. Haemophilia 2007;13:131–43.

44. Lavigne-Lissalde G, Lacroix-Desmazes S, Wootla B, et al. Molecular characterization of human B domain-specific anti-factor VIII monoclonal antibodies generated in transgenic mice. Thromb Haemost 2007;98:138–47.

45. Manno CS, Pierce GF, Arruda VR, et al. Successful transduction of liver in hemophilia by AAV-Factor IX and limitations imposed by the host immune response. Nat Med 2006;12:342–7.

46. Arruda VR, Fields PA, Milner R, et al. Lack of germline transmission of vector sequences following systemic administration of recombinant AAV-2 vector in males. Mol Ther 2001;4:586–92.

47. Nowrouzi A, Penaud-Budloo M, Kaeppel C, et al. Integration frequency and intermolecular recombination of rAAV vectors in non-human primate skeletal muscle and liver. Mol Ther 2012;20:1177–86.

48. Li H, Malani N, Hamilton SR, et al. Assessing the potential for AAV vector genotoxicity in a murine model. Blood 2011;117:3311–9.

49. Nault JC, Datta S, Imbeaud S, et al. Recurrent AAV2-related insertional mutagenesis in human hepatocellular carcinomas. Nat Genet 2015;47:1187–93.

50. Grieger JC, Samulski RJ. Adeno-associated virus vectorology, manufacturing, and clinical applications. Methods Enzymol 2012;507:229–54.

51. Cecchini S, Negrete A, Kotin RM. Toward exascale production of recombinant adeno-associated virus for gene transfer applications. Gene Ther 2008;15: 823–30.

Hematopoietic Gene Therapies for Metabolic and Neurologic Diseases

Alessandra Biffi, MD

KEYWORDS

- Hematopoietic stem cells • Gene therapy • Nervous system • Storage
- Degeneration

KEY POINTS

- Hematopoietic stem cells can generate upon transplantation a myeloid cell progeny in the brain that is endowed with the potential to release therapeutic molecules.
- Genetic engineering of the cells to be transplanted can instruct their progeny for alleviating neurometabolic and neurodegenerative disorders.
- A deep understanding of microglia origin and maintenance during adulthood will allow more extensive exploiting of these events.

INTRODUCTION

An increasing number of patients affected by metabolic diseases affecting the central nervous system (CNS), such as adrenoleukodystrophy or Hurler syndrome, and neuroinflammatory disorders, such as multiple sclerosis (MS) or amyotrophic lateral sclerosis (ALS), receive hematopoietic cell transplantation (HCT) from healthy compatible donors or in the context of an autologous procedure in the attempt to slow the course of their disease, delay the onset of new clinical symptoms or attenuate their manifestations, and improve some pathologic findings. New indications are also hypothesized that include classic neurodegenerative diseases, such as Alzheimer disease (AD). The rationale for the use of HCT to treat these disorders is complex and based on multiple mechanisms, most of which relate to the possible replacement of brain-resident myeloid cells by the transplanted cell progeny. Indeed, microglia and, to a minor extent, brain-associated macrophages play a central role in these pathologic conditions and their replacement by cells novel to the patients' pathologic brain environment may interrupt or mitigate disease-associated pathologic cascades by modulation of local inflammation, establishment of proper metabolism, and induction of

Gene Therapy Program, Dana-Farber/Boston Children's Cancer and Blood Disorders Center, Harvard Medical School, Smith 1158, 450 Brookline Avenue, Boston, MA 02115, USA
E-mail address: Alessandra.Biffi@childrens.harvard.edu

Hematol Oncol Clin N Am 31 (2017) 869–881
http://dx.doi.org/10.1016/j.hoc.2017.06.004
0889-8588/17/© 2017 Elsevier Inc. All rights reserved.

hemonc.theclinics.com

neuroprotective effects. Genetic engineering of the hematopoietic stem cells (HSCs) to be transplanted (HSC gene therapy) may endow the brain myeloid progeny of these cells with enhanced or novel functions contributing to these therapeutic effects. However, an intense debate questions the actual contribution of HCT to microgliosis.

MICROGLIA

The CNS is composed of 2 major cell types, nerve cells and glial cells. Glial cells consist of astrocytes, oligodendrocytes, and microglia. Microglia account for approximately 10% of the total glial cell population within the CNS and are commonly referred to as the brain-resident immune cells or tissue-resident macrophages.[1] Indeed, microglia belongs to the mononuclear phagocyte lineage, related to other organ-specific macrophage populations, such as Kupffer cells of the liver and bone osteoclasts. Microglia was first recognized as a distinct cell type by Nissl who named them Staebchenzellen (rod cells) for their rod-shaped nuclei and considered them as reactive neuroglia. According to the classic morphologic studies based on silver carbonate staining, microglia cells were originally divided into ameboid, ramified, and intermediate forms. Interestingly, depending on their localization in the CNS, microglia present major morphologic differences with regard to the size and orientation of their ramifications. In this way, the shape of the ramified microglia is well adapted to the architecture of the CNS region they populate. Similarly, the density of microglia cells seems to be determined by region-specific cues in both rodents and humans. Such heterogeneity of microglia density and morphology might be linked to a functional heterogeneity. In support of this view, among the most remarkable features of microglia is their high level of morphologic and functional plasticity in response to activating stimuli. They respond not only to changes in the brain parenchymal integrity but also to very small alterations in their microenvironment, such as imbalances in ion homeostasis that precede pathologic changes.[2] In this context, classification of microglia can also describe their activation status, distinguishing between resting, activated, and ameboid phagocytic microglia.[3,4] Importantly, under multiple pathologic conditions, activation of microglia is coupled with their proliferation, which leads to the focal accumulation of activated cells, a process termed microgliosis.[2,5] Moreover, the expression of biological and biochemical microglial markers may vary according to different parameters, including interspecies variations and maturation or activation state. For example, neonatal microglia, differently from adult microglia, share some phenotypic and functional features with neural stem or progenitor cells, such as the in vitro and in vivo expression of nestin, a neural stem cell marker,[6–8] and the ability to express oligodendrocyte or neuronal markers under appropriate in vitro conditions.[7,9] Such neural stem cell-like features, whose functional relevance remains uncertain, were not evidenced in other populations of tissue-resident macrophages.

Microglia in Neurodegenerative Diseases

Microglia activation is present in diverse neurodegenerative diseases and is closely associated with pathologic condition, being crucial to the cause and the progressive nature of most of these disorders. For this reason, in a large variety of diseases, microglia is thought to be a promising target for therapeutic intervention.

Microglia and metabolic storage disorders

Metabolic storage disorders (SDs) are a group of inherited disorders caused by defects in the genes, which determine accumulation of undegraded material within cellular organelles. The most known examples include lysosomal SDs (LSDs) and peroxisomal disorders, such as X-linked adrenoleukodystrophy (X-ALD). The phenotype of these disorders is complex and frequently characterized by the variable association of visceral, hematologic, skeletal, and neurologic manifestations. These manifestations are, in most instances, responsible for physical and neurologic impairments. In particular, those related to the involvement of the CNS may cause progressive neurodegeneration and severe cognitive deficit.

The understanding of LSD pathophysiology has evolved during the past decade. For many years, the leading theory explaining tissue damage in LSDs has been that the pathologic phenotype was caused solely by the massive storage of the substrate. Currently, it is recognized that tissue damage and disease result from the perturbation of complex cell signaling mechanisms, which give rise to secondary structural and biochemical changes. According to this theory, substrate storage acts as a primary stimulus that leads to the alteration of housekeeping cellular functions and pathways, including receptor activation by nonphysiologic ligands, modulation of receptor responses and signal transduction cascades, activation of inflammatory responses, impaired intracellular trafficking of vesicles, impairment of autophagy, and others.[10] In this context, macrophage and microglia activation, which is seen in many SDs and is likely due to raised concentrations of cytokines and chemokines consequent to the primary defect,[11–13] may cause damage to the nervous system in terms of neuronal death[14] and compromise the blood brain barrier (BBB) functionality.[15] Microglia activation may also be induced by the primary storage and by the accumulation of debris due to their scavenger activity, triggering focal inflammation and secondary neurodegeneration.[12–17] In the case of X-ALD the mutation in the ABCD1 gene determines the accumulation of unbranched saturated very long chain fatty acids (VLCFAs) within phospholipid fractions, such as lysophatidylcholine, particularly in brain and adrenal cortex.[18] The initiation of the cerebral damage, which is demyelinating in nature, could be directly linked to the amount of VLCFA in complex lipids and to their inefficient degradation by microglia cells.[19] The loss of microglia and/or microglia dysfunction may play an important role in the early phases of demyelination, mainly due to the production of proinflammatory cytokines (CCL2, CCL4, IL-1a, and CXCL8) and to the altered ability to provide neuroprotective factors to defective oligodendrocytes.

In this scenario, microglia cells represent a key target for intervention. In this perspective, both allogeneic HSC transplantation,[20,21] as well as HSC gene therapy,[22–24] have been proposed as treatment of these diseases with the rationale to

1. Compensate the defective catalytic function
2. Modulate the activated and apoptotic phenotype of resident microglia, favoring their turnover with gene-corrected or donor-derived cells
3. In the case of LSDs, generate a local source of functional lysosomal enzyme for correction of the metabolic defect also in resident neural and glial cells.

Microglia and other neurodegenerative diseases
Microglia activation and dysfunction also play a central role in adult multifactorial neurodegenerative diseases. AD is the most common neurodegenerative disorder affecting older people worldwide. It is a progressive disorder mainly characterized by the presence of β-amyloid plaques and intraneuronal neurofibrillary tangles of hyperphosphorylated tau filament.[25] The cause of neurodegeneration in AD has yet to be elucidated, though several pathogenic mechanisms have been proposed, including mitochondrial dysfunction and the accumulation of β-amyloid in extracellular insoluble plaques. It is also well accepted that neuroinflammation constitutes an important feature in AD. Many studies have provided evidence that microglial cells

are attracted to amyloid deposits both in human samples and in rodent transgenic AD models. Microglia could become activated in the presence of β-amyloid and secrete neurotoxic molecules[26–31] or could exert a neuroprotective action by secreting neurotropic agents and eliminating β-amyloid by phagocytosis.[32–34] According to these hypotheses, the development of a strategy to target the recruitment of new and engineered microglia cells toward regions of β-amyloid deposits could lead to

1. Elimination of toxic plaques
2. Modulation of the local environment toward neuroprotection
3. Compensation of the defective function of senescent resident microglia.

Also in the case of ALS, a fatal neurodegenerative disease characterized by the progressive loss of both upper (brain) and lower (brain stem and spinal cord) motor neurons, multiple intracellular pathways have been proposed as relevant: the regulation of RNA transcription and editing, protein modification, folding and clearance, axonal transport, organelles maintenance, and cell death mechanisms.[35–37] Neuropathology in ALS is accompanied by robust microglial activation, which could be associated with either neuronal damage or neuroprotection according to the stage of the diseases.[38] Indeed, recent studies have shown evolution of microglia phenotype along with disease progression in the most used ALS animal model (mSOD mice[39]), with cells exhibiting a neurotrophic phenotype at disease onset and a potentially neurotoxic phenotype by end-stage disease.[40] Thus, as for other neurodegenerative diseases, microglia could either delay or exacerbate neurodegeneration depending on the balance between the production of trophic versus toxic factors. Skewing this balance in favor of a neurotrophic phenotype may be a site for therapeutic intervention. Interestingly, when the microglial compartment of mSOD mice was reconstituted with wild-type microglia, a significant delay in the progression of the disease and extended lifespan of the animals were observed.[41]

The observation that microglial activation occurs early during disease suggested that, although it may not be responsible for most inflammatory damage, it might initiate a cascade of events eventually leading to the entry of deleterious inflammatory monocytes into the CNS of patients or mice affected by MS or experimental autoimmune encephalomyelitis (EAE). The development of localized vascular permeability in the CNS observed in the early stages of the diseases could allow the extravasation of plasma components such as fibrinogen, which contributes to the induction of microglia expansion.[42] In this context, microglia could play a role in attracting circulating inflammatory monocytes, possibly by the expression of chemokines such as CCL2/MCP1. Infiltration of inflammatory monocytes in the CNS parenchyma exacerbates the damage and triggers progression toward severe disease through a variety of mechanisms likely involving myelin stripping and secretion of neurotoxic cytokines. Bone marrow chimera experiments demonstrated that microglia activation and proliferation precedes the onset of EAE, and that inhibition of their activation suppresses the development and maintenance of inflammatory lesions in the CNS.[43] Thus, in MS, microglia also represents a key target and its potential replacement with nonactivated cells may eventually secrete locally factors favorably modulating local inflammation.

Overall, modulation of local brain environment through microglia is highly desirable in many neurodegenerative diseases and could be obtained by replacing pathologic and activated microglia cells with hematopoietic lineage cells of donor origin or autologous cells engineered to express therapeutic molecules. However, studies on the developmental origin and maintenance of microglia cells in adulthood have challenged this concept.

Microglia Origin in the Developing Brain

Del Rio Hortega identified microglia as a distinct cell type apart from astrocytes and oligodendrocytes, originating from mononuclear cells of the circulating blood, and having the ability to transform from resting ramified cells into ameboid macrophages. Despite these early speculations regarding microglia ontogeny, for the better part of a century the identity of the cellular precursors of microglia remained a controversial topic with the generation of conflicting hypothesis. Currently, microglia are believed to originate from primitive yolk sac (YS) myeloid progenitors that colonize the brain rudiment during embryogenesis, and then transform into the resting ramified microglia of the normal mature CNS.[44–46] In their seminal work, Ginhoux and colleagues[45] clearly showed appearance of YS-derived macrophages in the CNS before definitive hematopoiesis in the embryo was established. Confirmation subsequently came from Schulz and colleagues[47] who demonstrated that, in the absence of definitive hemato-poiesis in the embryo, microglial development is not affected and primitive macro-phages originating in the YS give rise to microglia, thus underlining that YS-derived macrophages constitute an independent lineage, distinct from the progeny of defini-tive HSCs.[47] More recently, CD45-c-kit + cells within the YS have been identified as the source of immigrating macrophages in the developing mouse brain. These cells thus constitute the direct precursors of the definitive microglia population in the CNS.[46] These cells also generate Ter119 expressing erythrocytes, indicating the exis-tence of a common erythromyeloid progenitor in the YS for both lineages. The devel-opmental process is characterized by a concomitant maturation and differentiation of microglia progenitors via CX3CR1-and CX3CR1+ stages.

Microglia Maintenance in Adulthood

The observation that the microglia fate is established during early embryogenesis rai-ses several questions. Of particular interest is the understanding of how these cells are maintained in adulthood, turn over, and adapt to changes in the brain microenviron-ment. During the last decades, several in vitro[48,49] and in vivo studies,[50,51] by means of different techniques, have tried to address this issue. Parapsilosis and/or irradiation-based hematopoietic chimerism were often used to address central questions regarding the turnover and proliferative capacity of microglia and perivascular cells.[48,52–54] These approaches have shown that both in basal conditions and in the presence of a neurologic disease, circulating monocytes do not substantially contribute to the adult microglial pool, despite high rates of colonization of other extra-CNS or-gans, such as the liver and the bone marrow.[55,56] Other studies showed the recruitment of bone marrow-derived cells, to some extent, to the brain of chimeric animals charac-terized by pathologic conditions affecting the CNS, suggesting a possible contribution of these elements to the postnatal microglial populations. A recent study conducted in EAE mice demonstrated that monocytes could infiltrate the brain parenchyma through the BBB and participate in disease progression. Moreover, the investigators interest-ingly showed that circulating cells do not contribute to the microglial pool because blood-derived monocytes finally disappear once the inflammation resolves.[57] Based on these original studies, microglia maintenance during adulthood has been attributed to local, CNS-resident precursor cells, likely derived from YS early progenitors.

However, by using optimized protocols based on hematopoietic stem and progen-itor cell (HSPC) transplantation and pretransplant myeloablative chemoconditioning, researchers observed that (1) a considerable number of HSPC–derived cells can cross the BBB to populate the brain parenchyma, particularly in presence of external injuries and neuropathology, and (2) perivascular macrophages and microglia-like cells can be renewed, to some extent, by HSPC-derived cells,[53,54,58–60] establishing the basis for clinical translation of these concepts in different CNS disorders. The pre-transplant use of a proper conditioning regimen based on the alkylating agent busulfan was essential for this happening reproducibly and at high rates. Indeed, conditioning regimens acting on the CNS could modulate the local brain environment in a favorable manner, likely by creating opportunity and space for the engraftment of donor-derived cells.[54] In particular, a role of busulfan conditioning was postulated in ablating functionally defined brain-resident microglia precursors. In this setting, the cells of donor origin found in the brain of transplanted animals were shown to derive from the local proliferation and differentiation of HSPCs migrated to the brain shortly after transplant.

The observation that infiltrating cells can contribute to parenchymal cells has significant bearing from a therapeutic perspective. Indeed, these finding offer the possibility that circulating cells can be guided, for example, to the lesion site to control the progression of microgliosis and/or used as vehicle cells for the treatment of CNS disorders, if properly engineered.

REPLACING MICROGLIA BY HEMATOPOIETIC STEM CELL TRANSPLANTATION: THE CASE OF STORAGE DISORDERS

Although it is recognized that microglia cells have a different developmental origin compared with bone marrow-derived myeloid cells, many in vivo studies performed in myeloablated mice reconstituted with genetically labeled cells showed that, in specific situations, microglia-like cells could be replaced to some extent by the progeny of HSCs or HSPCs.[53–56]

Transplantation of HSCs has been extensively used to repopulate the recipient myeloid compartment, including brain microglia, with cells of donor origin in LSDs.[61] Because macrophages and microglia represent major effectors of the catabolism of the storage material, their replacement by normal cells has the potential to restore a critical scavenger function, contributing to the reduction of microglia activation and of proinflammatory cytokines release, factors both involved in the pathogenesis of CNS damage.[14,16,17,62] Moreover, by acting as mini-pumps, these cells could synthesize and secrete a portion of their lysosomal enzymes, which in turn could be taken up by neighboring cells with the cross-correction mechanism (**Fig. 1**).[59,61] Current therapeutic approaches take advantage of this secretion or uptake system to provide an exogenous supply of the missing enzyme that can be taken up by target cells and thus correct the metabolic defect.

Based on this rationale, over the past 3 decades, allogeneic HCT has been applied worldwide for patients with a wide range of different LSDs in the attempt to slow the course of the disease, prevent the onset of clinical symptoms, and improve some pathologic findings.[21,58,63–65] The first proof of efficacy of HSC transplantation in humans to arrest the evolution of LSDs was obtained in Hurler syndrome.[21] Results obtained in these patients provided the first indication that the transplant of donor hematopoietic cells could contribute to enzyme delivery to multiple disease sites, including the brain, thus overcoming the BBB penetrance issue. From the impressive clinical outcome observed in Hurler-transplanted children, it was expected that most SDs could be alleviated by HCT.[21,66] However, HCT provides diverse degrees of benefit according to the disease, the involvement of the CNS, and its stage at time of transplant. In particular, HCT was proven to be ineffective in patients with overt neurologic symptoms or in those with early onset of aggressive infantile forms. The likely reason for this limited efficacy is related to the slow pace of replacement of fixed

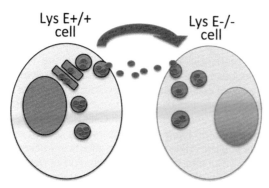

Fig. 1. Cross-correction. The cross-correction phenomenon is unique of lysosomal enzymes (Lys E) because mannose 6 phosphate (MP6) groups are added exclusively to the N-linked oligosaccharides of these soluble enzymes as they pass through the cis-Golgi network. After being modified, the Lys E binds the M6P receptor in the trans-Golgi network and is sorted to the late endosomes to reach the lysosome. About 40% of the enzyme escapes this pathway and is secreted in the extracellular space by enzymatically competent cells (Lys E+/+). This enzyme can then bind the M6P receptor on the membrane of the producer cell or surrounding cells, including Lys E−/− cells, and can be endocytosed and sorted to the lysosome.

tissue macrophages or histiocytes and microglial populations by the transplanted hematopoietic cell progeny compared with the rapid progression of the primary disease. Due to this lag period, which is expected to be in the range of 12 to 24 months before initial disease stabilization, the more severe the phenotype is and the longer the interval from onset of first obvious symptoms to HCT, the worse the outcome is. For this reason, the most promising results were obtained when HCT was performed in presymptomatic patients, identified in the uterus or at birth because of family history.

Very similar considerations apply to X-ALD. In practice, allogeneic HCT can arrest the neuroinflammatory demyelinating process of the disease, provided the procedure is performed at an early stage when the patients have minimal neurologic and neuropsychological deficits and limited extension of demyelinating lesions at brain MRI. After the transplantation procedure, demyelinating lesions usually continue to extend for 12 to 18 months; then they stop progressing. As for LSDs, this delay in the benefit of HCT is likely due to the slow replacement of brain microglia from transplant-derived cells. The mechanism by which allogeneic HCT benefits the disease may depend on the correction of the abnormal function of brain microglia, providing a population of efficient scavenger cells within the CNS with the potential to clear some of the accumulated substrate and cellular debris, as well as reversing the detrimental effects of the microglia activation response on other CNS cell types.

In addition to the stage of the disease, HCT effectiveness in SDs could be overshadowed by some serious transplant-related issues, such as identification of suitable matched-related donors, absence of standardized conditioning protocols, specific transplant-related complications (eg, graft-versus-host disease [GvHD] and incomplete engraftment), and the mortality rate.[67–69]

Hematopoietic Stem Cell Gene Therapy: Improving Safety and Enhancing Benefits of Allogeneic Hematopoietic Cell Transplantation

Gene therapy strategies aimed at the correction of the genetic defect in patients' HSCs could represent a significant improvement compared with conventional allogeneic HCT. Autologous cells can be genetically modified to constitutively express the therapeutic molecule compensating patients' genetic defect. Importantly, in the case of LSDs, the lysosomal enzyme could be not only restored in its function but also expressed at supranormal levels, thus rendering the tissue progeny of the gene-corrected autologous HSCs a quantitatively more effective source of functional enzyme than healthy donor cells, possibly also within the nervous system. Moreover, the autologous procedure is associated with a significantly reduced transplant-related morbidity and mortality, and avoids the risks of GvHD.

HSC gene therapy based on integrating vectors was proven effective in restoring the functional enzyme and providing therapeutic effects in visceral organs of different LSD animal models.[70,71] Subsequently, the contribution of gene-corrected HSCs to phenotypic amelioration of LSDs with CNS involvement was demonstrated in the animal disease models.[54,72–75] Importantly, in these experimental settings, HSC gene therapy had a significantly better therapeutic impact than wild-type HSC transplantation. Moreover, the degree of efficacy of gene therapy was demonstrated to mostly depend on the high frequency of HSC transduction and on the levels of enzyme activity in their differentiated in vivo progeny. The use of lentiviral vectors (LVs), with their capability to efficiently transduce HSCs,[76] contributed to the achievement of these results. Recently, therapeutic efficacy of LV-based HSC gene therapy in controlling LSD disease manifestations has been shown in patients with early forms of the demyelinating LSD metachromatic leukodystrophy (MLD).[23,24] Importantly, experience in the context of this clinical trial provided relevant insights on the therapeutic potential of strategies based on HSCs for microglia reconstitution and brain delivery of therapeutic molecules. Indeed, even if it was not possible to directly probe patients for the migration of gene-modified cells into the CNS, substantial levels of the therapeutic arylsulphatase A enzyme, whose expression was induced by LVs into the patients HSCs, were documented in cerebrospinal fluid samples collected from the patients long-term after treatment,[23,24] formally proving that the CNS was seeded by gene-corrected myeloid cells on HSC gene therapy. These findings were associated with marked clinical benefit in the patients treated in presymptomatic stage.

Similarly, lentiviral-mediated gene therapy for HSCs provided benefits in X-ALD patients. Indeed, on infusion of the genetically corrected cells, progressive cerebral demyelination in the treated patients was interrupted, without further progression up to the last follow-up, with a clinical outcome comparable to that achieved after allogeneic HCT.[22,77] Long-term follow-up demonstrated stable expression of the lentivirally encoded ALD protein in both myeloid and lymphoid cells in the hematopoietic compartment despite a limited percentage of their correction. Also, in the case of X-ALD, the efficacy of HSC gene therapy likely derives from the ability of transplanted cells or their progeny to infiltrate in the affected CNS tissue. Interestingly, clinical benefit comparable to that observed following donor HCT was observed in X-ALD children in the presence of a partial transduced cell engraftment. This finding could be interpreted in different ways, including by hypothesizing a role for overexpression of the ALD protein in corrected myeloid brain cells or the existence of a different chimerism in the brain myeloid populations compared with the bone marrow and other hematopoietic tissues.

Overall, the experience with MLD and X-ALD demonstrates that the recruitment in the CNS of HSCs or HSC-derived cells contributing to myeloid cell populations may provide an important therapeutic hint that could be extended for adequately designed cell-based therapies for other genetic and multifactorial CNS diseases characterized by prominent microglia role, such as ALS, AD, and MS. Of course, the possibility of addressing these multifactorial adult onset diseases by this kind of strategy is based on the following:

1. Proper target pathways must be identified that could be modulated either by the generation of new microglia cells novel to or not primed by the pathologic brain microenvironment, or by the engineering of the transplanted HSCs and their microglia progeny cells. Engineering could endow these cells with novel functions, such as production of molecules positively affecting disease mechanisms (ie, neuroprotective factors) or modulation and shaping of their phenotype.
2. Advanced engineering tools (ie, specific promoters) endowed with potential for precise regulation of therapeutic gene expression must be used to respond to disease progression, local damage, and inflammation
3. Advanced transplant protocols must be developed to reduce the overall transplant burden for patients and the risks associated with HSC gene therapy, including innovative conditioning regimens preferentially targeting the CNS or novel modalities of HSC transplantation favoring their contribution to myeloid brain cells rather than hematopoietic lineage replacement.
4. Different approaches must be combined to obtain the highest therapeutic efficacy and to personalize treatment protocols for each disorder.

REFERENCES

1. Pelvig DP, Pakkenberg H, Stark AK, et al. Neocortical glial cell numbers in human brains. Neurobiol Aging 2008;29:1754–62.
2. Gehrmann J, Banati RB. Microglial turnover in the injured CNS: activated microglia undergo delayed DNA fragmentation following peripheral nerve injury. J Neuropathol Exp Neurol 1995;54:680–8.
3. Streit WJ, Graeber MB, Kreutzberg GW. Expression of Ia antigen on perivascular and microglial cells after sublethal and lethal motor neuron injury. Exp Neurol 1989;105:115–26.
4. Sasaki A, Hirato J, Nakazato Y. Immunohistochemical study of microglia in the Creutzfeldt-Jakob diseased brain. Acta Neuropathol 1993;86:337–44.
5. Streit WJ, Walter SA, Pennell NA. Reactive microgliosis. Prog Neurobiol 1999;57:563–81.
6. Davoust N, Vuaillat C, Cavillon G, et al. Bone marrow CD34+/B220+ progenitors target the inflamed brain and display in vitro differentiation potential toward microglia. FASEB J 2006;20:2081–92.
7. Yokoyama A, Yang L, Itoh S, et al. Microglia, a potential source of neurons, astrocytes, and oligodendrocytes. Glia 2004;45:96–104.
8. Nataf S, Anginot A, Vuaillat C, et al. Brain and bone damage in KARAP/DAP12 loss-of-function mice correlate with alterations in microglia and osteoclast lineages. Am J Pathol 2005;166:275–86.
9. Butovsky O, Bukshpan S, Kunis G, et al. Microglia can be induced by IFN-gamma or IL-4 to express neural or dendritic-like markers. Mol Cell Neurosci 2007;35:490–500.
10. Ballabio A, Gieselmann V. Lysosomal disorders: from storage to cellular damage. Biochim Biophys Acta 2009;1793:684–96.
11. Allen MJ, Myer BJ, Khokher AM, et al. Pro-inflammatory cytokines and the pathogenesis of Gaucher's disease: increased release of interleukin-6 and interleukin-10. QJM 1997;90:19–25.

12. Wu YP, McMahon E, Kraine MR, et al. Distribution and characterization of GFP(+) donor hematogenous cells in Twitcher mice after bone marrow transplantation. Am J Pathol 2000;156:1849–54.

13. Jeyakumar M, Thomas R, Elliot-Smith E, et al. Central nervous system inflammation is a hallmark of pathogenesis in mouse models of GM1 and GM2 gangliosidosis. Brain 2003;126:974–87.

14. Wada R, Tifft CJ, Proia RL. Microglial activation precedes acute neurodegeneration in Sandhoff disease and is suppressed by bone marrow transplantation. Proc Natl Acad Sci U S A 2000;97:10954–9.

15. Zenker D, Begley D, Bratzke H, et al. Human blood-derived macrophages enhance barrier function of cultured primary bovine and human brain capillary endothelial cells. J Physiol 2003;551:1023–32.

16. Hess B, Saftig P, Hartmann D, et al. Phenotype of arylsulfatase A-deficient mice: relationship to human metachromatic leukodystrophy. Proc Natl Acad Sci U S A 1996;93:14821–6.

17. Ohmi K, Greenberg DS, Rajavel KS, et al. Activated microglia in cortex of mouse models of mucopolysaccharidoses I and IIIB. Proc Natl Acad Sci U S A 2003;100:1902–7.

18. Bezman L, Moser AB, Raymond GV, et al. Adrenoleukodystrophy: incidence, new mutation rate, and results of extended family screening. Ann Neurol 2001;49:512–7.

19. Eichler FS, Ren JQ, Cossoy M, et al. Is microglial apoptosis an early pathogenic change in cerebral X-linked adrenoleukodystrophy? Ann Neurol 2008;63:729–42.

20. Aubourg P, Blanche S, Jambaqué I, et al. Reversal of early neurologic and neuroradiologic manifestations of X-linked adrenoleukodystrophy by bone marrow transplantation. N Engl J Med 1990;322:1860–6.

21. Staba SL, Escolar ML, Poe M, et al. Cord-blood transplants from unrelated donors in patients with Hurler's syndrome. N Engl J Med 2004;350:1960–9.

22. Cartier N, Hacein-Bey-Abina S, Bartholomae CC, et al. Hematopoietic stem cell gene therapy with a lentiviral vector in X-linked adrenoleukodystrophy. Science 2009;326:818–23.

23. Biffi A, Montini E, Lorioli L, et al. Lentiviral hematopoietic stem cell gene therapy benefits metachromatic leukodystrophy. Science 2013;341:1233158.

24. Sessa M, Lorioli L, Fumagalli F, et al. Lentiviral haemopoietic stem-cell gene therapy in early-onset metachromatic leukodystrophy: an ad-hoc analysis of a non-randomised, open-label, phase 1/2 trial. Lancet 2016;388:476–87.

25. Mott RT, Hulette CM. Neuropathology of Alzheimer's disease. Neuroimaging Clin N Am 2005;15:755–65, ix.

26. Combs CK, Johnson DE, Karlo JC, et al. Inflammatory mechanisms in Alzheimer's disease: inhibition of beta-amyloid-stimulated proinflammatory responses and neurotoxicity by PPARgamma agonists. J Neurosci 2000;20:558–67.

27. Qin L, Liu Y, Cooper C, et al. Microglia enhance beta-amyloid peptide-induced toxicity in cortical and mesencephalic neurons by producing reactive oxygen species. J Neurochem 2002;83:973–83.

28. Cotter RL, Burke WJ, Thomas VS, et al. Insights into the neurodegenerative process of Alzheimer's disease: a role for mononuclear phagocyte-associated inflammation and neurotoxicity. J Leukoc Biol 1999;65:416–27.

29. Giulian D. Microglia and the immune pathology of Alzheimer disease. Am J Hum Genet 1999;65:13–8.

30. Meyer-Luehmann M, Spires-Jones TL, Prada C, et al. Rapid appearance and local toxicity of amyloid-beta plaques in a mouse model of Alzheimer's disease. Nature 2008;451:720–4.
31. Kim SU, de Vellis J. Microglia in health and disease. J Neurosci Res 2005;81: 302–13.
32. Simard AR, Soulet D, Gowing G, et al. Bone marrow-derived microglia play a critical role in restricting senile plaque formation in Alzheimer's disease. Neuron 2006;49:489–502.
33. Stalder AK, Ermini F, Bondolfi L, et al. Invasion of hematopoietic cells into the brain of amyloid precursor protein transgenic mice. J Neurosci 2005;25: 11125–32.
34. Qiu WQ, Walsh DM, Ye Z, et al. Insulin-degrading enzyme regulates extracellular levels of amyloid beta-protein by degradation. J Biol Chem 1998;273:32730–8.
35. Robberecht W, Philips T. The changing scene of amyotrophic lateral sclerosis. Nat Rev Neurosci 2013;14:248–64.
36. Bucchia M, Ramirez A, Parente V, et al. Therapeutic development in amyotrophic lateral sclerosis. Clin Ther 2015;37:668–80.
37. Cozzolino M, Rossi S, Mirra A, et al. Mitochondrial dynamism and the pathogenesis of amyotrophic lateral sclerosis. Front Cell Neurosci 2015;9:31.
38. Boillee S, Yamanaka K, Lobsiger CS, et al. Onset and progression in inherited ALS determined by motor neurons and microglia. Science 2006;312:1389–92.
39. Grieb P. Transgenic models of amyotrophic lateral sclerosis. Folia Neuropathol 2004;42:239–48.
40. Liao B, Zhao W, Beers DR, et al. Transformation from a neuroprotective to a neurotoxic microglial phenotype in a mouse model of ALS. Exp Neurol 2012; 237:147–52.
41. Beers DR, Henkel JS, Xiao Q, et al. Wild-type microglia extend survival in PU.1 knockout mice with familial amyotrophic lateral sclerosis. Proc Natl Acad Sci U S A 2006;103:16021–6.
42. Ramaglia V, Hughes TR, Donev RM, et al. C3-dependent mechanism of microglial priming relevant to multiple sclerosis. Proc Natl Acad Sci U S A 2012;109:965–70.
43. Heppner FL, Greter M, Marino D, et al. Experimental autoimmune encephalomyelitis repressed by microglial paralysis. Nat Med 2005;11:146–52.
44. Alliot F, Godin I, Pessac B. Microglia derive from progenitors, originating from the yolk sac, and which proliferate in the brain. Brain Res Dev Brain Res 1999;117: 145–52.
45. Ginhoux F, Greter M, Leboeuf M, et al. Fate mapping analysis reveals that adult microglia derive from primitive macrophages. Science 2010;330:841–5.
46. Kierdorf K, Erny D, Goldmann T, et al. Microglia emerge from erythromyeloid precursors via Pu.1- and Irf8-dependent pathways. Nat Neurosci 2013;16:273–80.
47. Schulz C, Gomez Perdiguero E, Chorro L, et al. A lineage of myeloid cells independent of Myb and hematopoietic stem cells. Science 2012;336:86–90.
48. Ponomarev ED, Shriver LP, Maresz K, et al. Microglial cell activation and proliferation precedes the onset of CNS autoimmunity. J Neurosci Res 2005;81:374–89.
49. Boucsein C, Zacharias R, Färber K, et al. Purinergic receptors on microglial cells: functional expression in acute brain slices and modulation of microglial activation in vitro. Eur J Neurosci 2003;17:2267–76.
50. Davalos D, Grutzendler J, Yang G, et al. ATP mediates rapid microglial response to local brain injury in vivo. Nat Neurosci 2005;8:752–8.
51. Nimmerjahn A, Kirchhoff F, Helmchen F. Resting microglial cells are highly dynamic surveillants of brain parenchyma in vivo. Science 2005;308:1314–8.

52. Flugel A, Bradl M, Kreutzberg GW, et al. Transformation of donor-derived bone marrow precursors into host microglia during autoimmune CNS inflammation and during the retrograde response to axotomy. J Neurosci Res 2001;66:74–82.

53. Capotondo A, Milazzo R, Politi LS, et al. Brain conditioning is instrumental for successful microglia reconstitution following hematopoietic stem cell transplantation. Proc Natl Acad Sci U S A 2012;109:15018–23.

54. Biffi A, De Palma M, Quattrini A, et al. Correction of metachromatic leukodystrophy in the mouse model by transplantation of genetically modified hematopoietic stem cells. J Clin Invest 2004;113:1118–29.

55. Ajami B, Bennett JL, Krieger C, et al. Local self-renewal can sustain CNS microglia maintenance and function throughout adult life. Nat Neurosci 2007;10: 1538–43.

56. Mildner A, Schmidt H, Nitsche M, et al. Microglia in the adult brain arise from Ly-6ChiCCR2+ monocytes only under defined host conditions. Nat Neurosci 2007; 10:1544–53.

57. Ajami B, Bennett JL, Krieger C, et al. Infiltrating monocytes trigger EAE progression, but do not contribute to the resident microglia pool. Nat Neurosci 2011;14: 1142–9.

58. Asheuer M, Pflumio F, Benhamida S, et al. Human CD34+ cells differentiate into microglia and express recombinant therapeutic protein. Proc Natl Acad Sci U S A 2004;101:3557–62.

59. Eglitis MA, Mezey E. Hematopoietic cells differentiate into both microglia and macroglia in the brains of adult mice. Proc Natl Acad Sci U S A 1997;94:4080–5.

60. Priller J, Flügel A, Wehner T, et al. Targeting gene-modified hematopoietic cells to central nervous system; use of green fluorescent protein uncovers microglial engraftment. Nat Med 2001;7:1356–61.

61. Krivit W, Sung JH, Shapiro EG, et al. Microglia: the effector cell for reconstitution of the central nervous system following bone marrow transplantation for lysosomal and peroxisomal storage diseases. Cell Transplant 1995;4:385–92.

62. German DC, Liang CL, Song T, et al. Neurodegeneration in the Niemann-Pick C mouse: glial involvement. Neuroscience 2002;109:437–50.

63. Peters C, Steward CG. Hematopoietic cell transplantation for inherited metabolic diseases: an overview of outcomes and practice guidelines. Bone Marrow Transplant 2003;31:229–39.

64. Krivit W, Aubourg P, Shapiro E, et al. Bone marrow transplantation for globoid cell leukodystrophy, adrenoleukodystrophy, metachromatic leukodystrophy, and Hurler syndrome. Curr Opin Hematol 1999;6:377–82.

65. Escolar ML, Poe MD, Provenzale JM, et al. Transplantation of umbilical-cord blood in babies with infantile Krabbe's disease. N Engl J Med 2005;352:2069–81.

66. Krivit W. Stem cell bone marrow transplantation in patients with metabolic storage diseases. Adv Pediatr 2002;49:359–78.

67. Orchard PJ, Tolar J. Transplant outcomes in leukodystrophies. Semin Hematol 2010;47:70–8.

68. Martin HR, Poe MD, Provenzale JM, et al. Neurodevelopmental outcomes of umbilical cord blood transplantation in metachromatic leukodystrophy. Biol Blood Marrow Transplant 2013;19:616–24.

69. Gaipa G, Dassi M, Perseghin P, et al. Allogeneic bone marrow stem cell transplantation following CD34+ immunomagnetic enrichment in patients with inherited metabolic storage diseases. Bone Marrow Transplant 2003;31:857–60.

70. Leiming T, Mann L, Martin Mdel P, et al. Functional amelioration of murine galactosialidosis by genetically modified bone marrow hematopoietic progenitor cells. Blood 2002;99:3169–78.
71. Zheng Y, Ryazantsev S, Ohmi K, et al. Retrovirally transduced bone marrow has a therapeutic effect on brain in the mouse model of mucopolysaccharidosis IIIB. Mol Genet Metab 2004;82:286–95.
72. Biffi A, Naldini L. Gene therapy of storage disorders by retroviral and lentiviral vectors. Hum Gene Ther 2005;16:1133–42.
73. Gentner B, Visigalli I, Hiramatsu H, et al. Identification of hematopoietic stem cell-specific miRNAs enables gene therapy of globoid cell leukodystrophy. Sci Transl Med 2010;2:58ra84.
74. Matzner U, Hartmann D, Lüllmann-Rauch R, et al. Bone marrow stem cell-based gene transfer in a mouse model for metachromatic leukodystrophy: effects on visceral and nervous system disease manifestations. Gene Ther 2002;9:53–63.
75. Visigalli I, Ungari S, Martino S, et al. The galactocerebrosidase enzyme contributes to the maintenance of a functional hematopoietic stem cell niche. Blood 2010;116:1857–66.
76. Vigna E, Naldini L. Lentiviral vectors: excellent tools for experimental gene transfer and promising candidates for gene therapy. J Gene Med 2000;2:308–16.
77. Cartier N, Hacein-Bey-Abina S, Bartholomae CC, et al. Lentiviral hematopoietic cell gene therapy for X-linked adrenoleukodystrophy. Methods Enzymol 2012;507:187–98.

Gene Therapy Approaches to Human Immunodeficiency Virus and Other Infectious Diseases

Geoffrey L. Rogers, PhD, Paula M. Cannon, PhD*

KEYWORDS

- Gene therapy • HIV • Gene editing • Targeted nuclease • Cas9 • AAV

KEY POINTS

- Recent innovations and clinical successes in gene therapy have provided the impetus to apply these techniques toward the treatment of infectious diseases, particularly human immunodeficiency virus (HIV).
- One significant gene therapy for HIV currently in translation involves the use of zinc finger nucleases to disrupt the HIV coreceptor CCR5, rendering T cells resistant to HIV infection.
- Targeted nucleases are being developed to disrupt or excise proviral DNA in HIV and hepatitis B virus infection, directly targeting latent viral reservoirs that are invisible to the immune system.
- Gene transfer using adeno-associated virus vectors allows systemic expression of broadly neutralizing antibodies against HIV, influenza, and respiratory syncytial virus, representing an approach for long-lived passive immunization.
- Gene therapy also allows for combinatorial approaches, targeting multiple aspects of a pathogen, and potentially paving the path toward long-term suppression or cure for HIV and other pernicious infections.

INTRODUCTION

Gene therapy has experienced a significant revival in recent years, with several successes in the treatment of monogenetic disorders[1] and cancer.[2] Gene therapy is now also being considered for serious infectious diseases, led by a focus on the human immunodeficiency virus (HIV). Although antiretroviral therapy (ART) can control

Disclosure Statement: The authors have nothing to disclose.
Department of Molecular Microbiology and Immunology, Keck School of Medicine, University of Southern California, 2011 Zonal Avenue, HMR 413A, Los Angeles, CA 90033, USA
* Corresponding author. Department of Molecular Microbiology and Immunology, Keck School of Medicine, University of Southern California, 2011 Zonal Avenue, HMR 413A, Los Angeles, CA 90033.
E-mail address: pcannon@usc.edu

HIV infection in most patients, there is currently no vaccine or cure for the virus due to its high mutagenic rate, subversion of the host immune system, and ability to remain latent for extended periods of time in long-lived T cells.[3,4] The lone exception to this stark reality is the so-called Berlin patient, who seems to have been cured of HIV following a bone marrow transplant from a donor with 2 copies of a defective CCR5 gene, CCR5Δ32, which is a commonly used coreceptor for HIV.[5] This case renewed excitement for the potential of gene therapy to be used against HIV and, in particular, by using the new tools available in the field.[6,7]

GENE EDITING: ENGINEERING RESISTANCE TO VIRUSES

In addition to classic gene therapies mediated by viral vectors, targeted nucleases such as the CRISPR/Cas9 system have sparked a revolution in gene therapy by making possible site-specific gene editing.[8] Although CRISPR/Cas9 is similar in action and efficacy to protein-based targeted nucleases, such as zinc finger nucleases (ZFNs) and transcription activator-like effector nucleases (TALENs),[9] the ease of design and testing of these reagents through the construction of single-guide RNAs (sgRNAs) has made gene editing available for a wider variety of users and applications.

Targeted nucleases can cut, nick, or bind DNA in a sequence-specific manner, and have thereby made possible several novel applications that were not previously feasible in humans.[10] One notable application of these reagents is to achieve permanent gene disruption. Following the creation of a double-stranded break (DSB) within the coding sequence of a gene, error-prone nonhomologous end-joining (NHEJ) DNA repair can result in insertions and deletions (indels) that result in frameshift or nonsense mutations that inactivate the gene. Much of the groundwork for using these types of strategies was developed or considered using therapeutic RNA interference (RNAi),[11–13] but nuclease-mediated gene disruption has the advantage of providing permanent and more complete gene knockdown, with the possibility of engineering long-lived resistance to pathogenic organisms.

In addition to the NHEJ repair pathway, DSBs can also be repaired by homology-directed repair (HDR) pathways.[14] By providing a DNA homology template along with a targeted nuclease, it is possible to exploit these pathways to either insert a gene into a specific site within the host DNA or to mutate a gene to create a more desirable variant.[10] The homology templates can be introduced using plasmids or single-stranded DNA oligonucleotides, but more success has been achieved in sensitive primary cells using viral vectors based on adeno-associated virus (AAV) or integrase-deficient lentivirus.[15–17]

These techniques, along with more classic gene therapy approaches using viral vectors to express genes or RNA regulators, provide a variety of approaches for the treatment of HIV and other infectious diseases. This article discusses several different gene therapy strategies that take advantage of these various platforms and approaches (**Fig. 1**).

ELIMINATING VIRAL ENTRY RECEPTORS

In the context of HIV infection, gene disruption technologies provide the potential to replicate the case of the Berlin patient, who received a CCR5Δ32 bone marrow transplant, by introducing CCR5 mutations into autologous lymphocytes or the precursor hematopoietic stem and progenitor cells (HSPCs).[18] The CCR5Δ32 mutation is relatively common in European populations and has not been associated with any major deleterious phenotype.[19] By packaging engineered ZFNs targeting CCR5 into

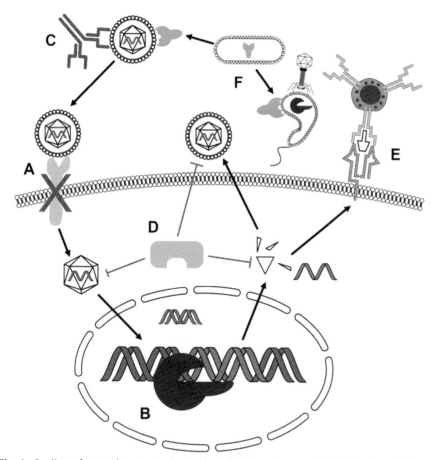

Fig. 1. Outline of gene therapy strategies for infectious diseases. (*A*) Eliminating viral entry receptors: gene editing can be used to disrupt genes encoding receptors used by viruses to enter target cells. (*B*) Directly targeting viral genomes: Cas9 or other nucleases can be expressed to disrupt integrated or free viral genomes. (*C*) Systemic expression of antiviral factors: antibodies or other circulating factors that neutralize pathogens can be constitutively expressed as a passive immunization approach. (*D*) Introducing other viral resistance factors: proteins that interfere with other aspects of the viral life cycle, including entry or uncoating, synthesis of viral proteins and genome incorporation, and release of new virions can be expressed to provide cells with additional resistance to viral infection. (*E*) Engineering immunity: antigen-specific CD8+ T cells can be generated by ex vivo gene modification or engineered vaccination to target infected cells. (*F*) Antibacterial strategies: commensal bacteria can be gene-modified to express soluble factors that inhibit pathogenic organisms; virulent bacteria can also be targeted with engineered bacteriophages.

adenovirus (Ad5/35) vectors, Perez and colleagues[20] first demonstrated that gene editing could protect human CD4+ T cells from HIV infection in culture and in humanized mice. In a clinical trial of this strategy in HIV-positive patients, autologous T cells could be modified and expanded ex vivo, leading to safe and efficient engraftment on reinfusion.[21] Encouragingly, when patients were withdrawn from ART therapy, depletion of the modified CD4+ T cells was observed to be slower than for unmodified cells.

Beyond these initial trials, other CCR5 editing strategies under development include using ZFNs to target alternative sites in CCR5 or using Cas9–sgRNA constructs, alternative delivery systems, such as nonintegrating lentiviral vectors or electroporation of in vitro transcribed mRNA,[16,22–24] and alternative target cells by modifying autologous HSPCs.[18] The anti-HIV potential of engineered HSPCs was initially demonstrated using CCR5-targeted ZFNs; selection for HIV-resistant CD4[+] T cell progeny was observed following engraftment into immunodeficient mice and HIV challenge.[25] More recent methods involve electroporation of ZFN mRNA for efficient disruption of CCR5 in mobilized peripheral blood and fetal liver-derived HSPCs.[15,26] In similar experiments using pigtailed macaques, ZFN mRNA electroporation of HSPCs resulted in approximately 3% to 5% CCR5 disruption in both lymphoid and myeloid lineages in peripheral blood for at least 6 months after reinfusion of autologous modified cells.[27]

Other emerging strategies for HSPC gene editing have focused on development of the CRISPR/Cas9 system. Chemically modified sgRNAs, when combined with electroporation of Cas9 mRNA or delivered as preformed Cas9-sgRNA ribonucleoprotein complexes, were shown to facilitate efficient gene disruption in mobilized human CD34[+] HSPCs.[28]

One potential drawback of CCR5 disruption strategies is the lack of impact against strains of HIV that can use alternate coreceptors, such as CXCR4.[29] Although CXCR4 disruption is not considered feasible in HSPCs due to its role in stem cell engraftment,[30] CXCR4-targeted ZFNs are being deployed in T cells to protect against X4-tropic HIV, including simultaneous disruption of both coreceptors.[31–33]

Gene editing technologies could also be used to disrupt entry receptors for other viruses. Experiments with RNAi or soluble inhibitors have suggested that entry receptor disruption could be a viable strategy against other viruses such as HCV[34] and dengue virus,[35,36] though more research will likely be required to verify that such targets can be safely disrupted.

DIRECTLY TARGETING VIRAL GENOMES

Targeted nucleases can also be engineered to directly recognize viral genetic material.[37] This approach is particularly appealing in HIV cure research because it provides a pathway to disrupt even latent HIV proviruses. Nucleases can be targeted to coding regions in the viral genome, to inactivate essential viral genes, or to the flanking long terminal repeats (LTRs) that control viral transcription and replication.[38] HIV inactivation can then occur as a result of indel formation that disrupts the targeted region, or alternatively because nucleases targeted to the LTRs can excise most of the HIV genome by creating DSBs at both ends of the proviral genome.[39–41] Sarkar and colleagues[42] pioneered this strategy in 2007 using directed evolution to generate a mutated Cre recombinase that could recognize a sequence within the LTR of an integrated HIV provirus. Similar methodologies have since been reported using ZFNs,[43] TALENs,[44,45] and the CRISPR/Cas9 system.[39–41,46,47] Beyond nuclease activity, Cas9 variants have also been directed to the LTRs to cause transcriptional activation and thereby activate latent viruses. Such approaches could facilitate viral eradication in conjunction with other strategies that target actively replicating viruses.[48,49]

Although indel formation resulting from the action of targeted nucleases can lead to HIV proviral inactivation, evidence suggests that HIV can also mutate and escape from such sequence-specific nucleases.[50–52] Resistance can occur either because of HIV's naturally high rate of mutagenesis, or because indels generated during NHEJ repair can themselves destroy the nuclease recognition sequence. This is likely to be a major mechanism of viral escape, particularly if the edited sequence can be tolerated.[50,51] For LTR-targeted nucleases, the ratios of proviral inactivation due to indels versus whole genome dropout may vary depending on the cell type and nuclease type, but skewing the ratio toward excision could reduce the risks of such escape mutations developing. In addition, because the LTR is among of the most conserved regions in the HIV genome, small sequence variations that would be tolerated could be addressed by using multiplex guide RNA strategies with Cas9 to target all circulating viral quasispecies.[53]

Like HIV, chronic hepatitis B virus (HBV) infection can currently be controlled by drugs that inhibit viral replication. However, these do not clear the covalently closed circular DNA (cccDNA) genomes, which can remain within infected hepatocytes. Numerous investigators have demonstrated the ability of CRISPR/Cas9, ZFNs, or TALENs to clear HBV cccDNA from infected cells in vitro, as well as in vivo models based on the codelivery of HBV DNA and CRISPR/Cas9 to hepatocytes via hydrodynamic injection of plasmids.[54] Other viruses in which DNA genomes have been targeted by CRISPR/Cas9 include human papillomavirus, Epstein-Barr virus, herpes simplex virus, and John Cunningham virus.[55] Of note, these are all latent or persistent infections, continuing the theme of targeting genetic material that the immune system cannot eradicate.

Although most efforts to date to disrupt viral genomes have focused on DNA viruses, it is also possible to cleave RNA genomes. The prototypical *Streptococcus pyogenes* Cas9 requires a protospacer adjacent motif (PAM) sequence on the nontarget DNA strand.[56] However, by providing the PAM in trans as a DNA oligonucleotide, it is possible to also target RNA molecules, which is opening up these approaches to other virus families.[57,58] Alternatively, other members of the CRISPR/Cas9 family have been identified that possess RNA-targeting capability and can target the hepatitis C virus (+ssRNA genome) in eukaryotic cells.[59,60]

Finally, expression of nucleases targeting viral genetic material can also be envisioned as a mechanism to prevent infection rather than by eliminating an entrenched infection.[47] In HIV infection, expression of such nucleases could be limited to HIV-infected cells by using the HIV LTR promoter to drive expression,[61] which may increase the safety profile of such approaches.

SYSTEMIC EXPRESSION OF ANTIVIRAL FACTORS

Long-term passive immunization using circulating antiviral factors such as antibodies is another strategy that can be made more practicable using gene therapy approaches. Broadly neutralizing antibodies (bNABs) are one interesting category of anti-HIV factors. These antibodies, which are only present in a small fraction of patients, are effective against a wide variety of HIV isolates, and their emergence requires long periods of coevolution between the virus and the antibody response.[62,63] For these reasons, bNABs are excellent candidates for passive immunization. Indeed, clinical trials of injections of the bNAB 3BNC117 have already commenced in human subjects and have shown promise for HIV control through multiple mechanisms, albeit with the ever-present risk of viral escape mutations.[64–67]

To achieve sustained, intrinsic production of antiviral factors, investigators have used muscle-directed gene transfer using AAV vectors. The vectors have been used to express bNABs or immunoadhesin constructs in mice and macaques, and have been shown to provide protection from HIV or simian immunodeficiency virus.[68–70] A phase I clinical trial is currently underway using AAV1 vectors to deliver the bNAB

PG9 to skeletal muscle in healthy adults (NCT01937455). However, recent reports have identified a confounding immune response in macaques receiving intramuscular AAV-bNABs, in which anti-antibodies developed that were directed against the antigen-binding regions of the therapeutic antibodies. These anti-antibodies impaired the functionality of this strategy, and developed against even fully rhesusized antibody constructs.[71-73] Immunosuppression with cyclophosphamide was able to transiently suppress anti-antibodies, but circulating transgene product levels declined following withdrawal of immunosuppression.[73] It remains to be seen whether this immune reaction will also occur in human subjects.

As an alternative to bNABs, soluble receptors capable of neutralizing HIV are also being considered for intrinsic expression. One such construct, an immunoadhesin called "eCD4-Ig", incorporates extracellular domains of the primary HIV receptor, CD4, together with an IgG-Fc region and a CCR5 mimetic peptide.[74] Due to the presence of the domains that HIV recognizes in its primary and coreceptors, eCD4-Ig possesses broad neutralizing capacity, including activity against CXCR4-tropic viruses. Muscle-directed gene transfer using AAV vectors expressing a rhesusized eCD4-Ig construct protected macaques from simian-human immunodeficiency virus (SHIV) challenge, while exhibiting reduced immunogenicity relative to bNABs.[74]

Antibody expression from AAV vectors is also being explored as protection against respiratory viral infections that can be dangerous in high-risk populations, such as infants, the elderly, and immunocompromised individuals.[75,76] Intrapleural administration of AAV vectors expressing a monoclonal antibody (palivizumab), which is currently used prophylactically, achieved sustained expression and protection from respiratory syncytial virus infection.[77] Similarly, AAV-mediated expression of broadly neutralizing influenza antibodies in skeletal muscle or lungs protected mice (including immunodeficient ones) from a variety of influenza stains.[78,79]

As an alternate strategy to achieve long-term expression, HDR-mediated gene insertion could also be used to integrate cassettes into specific sites in the genome and thereby express secreted antiviral factors. One such target is the albumin locus in hepatocytes,[80,81] which is being developed as a universal platform to facilitate expression of proteins in circulation[82] and could also be envisioned as a strategy to express secreted antiviral factors. Finally, immune cells themselves could also be modified to express such molecules. This includes their use in combinatorial therapies, in which the insertion of an expression cassette into a locus such as CCR5 would result in a simultaneous gene disruption event that could itself enhance resistance.[83]

INTRODUCING OTHER VIRAL RESISTANCE FACTORS

There are many antiviral factors that have been suggested as potential candidates for expression via gene therapy-based approaches. In HIV, these include fusion inhibitors, gene decoys or *trans*-dominant variants, as well as endogenous factors that act after HIV entry to prevent viral replication (ie, TRIM5α, tetherin, and APOBEC3G).[18] For these endogenous factors, the virus has evolved mechanisms to avoid their actions in human hosts, though variants with elevated anti-HIV activity have been identified.[84] Similarly, genome-wide association studies have identified dependency factors that enhance HIV infectivity, or variants of genes associated with greater control of HIV.[85] Together, these provide targets that could be introduced into cells or manipulated to enhance HIV resistance.[86] Gene editing provides additional opportunities for using these factors, including site-specific insertion at loci already being disrupted (eg, CCR5),[83] or by the conversion of endogenous genes to more effective antiviral variants.[6] Although not discussed in detail, some of these outcomes could also be achieved using RNAi therapies, which share many commonalities with gene editing as an alternative method to prevent expression of host or viral genes.[13,87]

ENGINEERING IMMUNITY

Gene therapies designed to enhance immune function are another intriguing area being considered for the treatment of infectious disease. One particularly interesting strategy involves redirecting CD8$^+$ T cells to target HIV-infected cells through ex vivo modifications that lead to the expression of pathogen-specific T cell receptors or chimeric antigen receptors (CARs).[88] CAR T cells with HIV-specificity have been generated using bNABs[89] or CD4[90,91] to provide the recognition domain, and similar technologies are being used to modify HSPCs, which can then differentiate into functional HIV-specific T and natural killer cells that are able to suppress HIV replication in humanized mice.[92] However, given the role that immune exhaustion plays in HIV pathogenesis,[93] these strategies may need to also incorporate strategies developed in cancer research, in which CAR T cell antitumor activity can be enhanced through Cas9-mediated disruption of the exhaustion receptor, programmed cell death protein 1 (PD-1).[94,95] Finally, new generations of engineered viral vectors expressing viral proteins are emerging as a potential next frontier in HIV vaccine research,[96] with the potential to prime uniquely broad immune responses that cannot be achieved with classic vaccination approaches.[97]

ANTIBACTERIAL STRATEGIES

Although most gene therapies to date have targeted viral infections, the increase of antibiotic-resistance means that there is also growing interest in using gene therapy to target bacterial infections.[98] One approach is that bacterial viruses (bacteriophages) can be modified to infect specific bacteria using restrictions in their tropism and can be engineered to express CRISPR/Cas9 constructs that are toxic to pathogenic but not commensal bacteria.[99–101] Alternatively, nonpathogenic bacteria have been gene-modified for a variety of purposes, including the expression of heterologous antigens for vaccination, to disrupt communication among pathogenic bacteria, or as factories to secrete antitoxins or antimicrobial agents.[98] The potential of such bacterially secreted factors is not limited to bacterial infections[98] because the introduction of lactobacilli engineered to secrete an HIV entry inhibitor into macaques provided partial protection from intravaginal SHIV challenge.[102]

SUMMARY

Increasingly, gene therapy is being considered for novel treatments of chronic and serious infectious diseases, with anti-HIV approaches leading the way. Recent developments in gene editing capabilities are allowing the opportunity to engineer host resistance to infections, as well as directly target viral genomes for degradation. Compared with other gene therapy strategies, gene editing has the potential to provide longer-lasting effects, and provides opportunities for combinatorial therapies using either CRISPR/Cas9 multiplexing capabilities or inserting antiviral factors into the CCR5 locus. This is still a relatively new technology. Concerns not addressed in this article that may be barriers to practical implementation include ethical, safety, and efficacy considerations, as well as the challenge of gene delivery to the appropriate cell type for any desired application.[55,103,104] However, once the technology breaks through into mainstream usage, gene therapies have the potential to revolutionize the treatment of human infectious disease in ways not previously (or perhaps not yet) imagined.

REFERENCES

1. Kumar SR, Markusic DM, Biswas M, et al. Clinical development of gene therapy: results and lessons from recent successes. Mol Ther Methods Clin Dev 2016;3: 16034.
2. Jackson HJ, Rafiq S, Brentjens RJ. Driving CAR T-cells forward. Nat Rev Clin Oncol 2016;13(6):370–83.
3. Haynes BF, Shaw GM, Korber B, et al. HIV-Host interactions: implications for vaccine design. Cell Host Microbe 2016;19(3):292–303.
4. Miles B, Connick E. TFH in HIV latency and as sources of replication-competent virus. Trends Microbiol 2016;24(5):338–44.
5. Allers K, Hutter G, Hofmann J, et al. Evidence for the cure of HIV infection by CCR5Delta32/Delta32 stem cell transplantation. Blood 2011;117(10):2791–9.
6. Wang CX, Cannon PM. The clinical applications of genome editing in HIV. Blood 2016;127(21):2546–52.
7. Santa-Marta M, de Brito PM, Godinho-Santos A, et al. Host factors and HIV-1 replication: clinical evidence and potential therapeutic approaches. Front Immunol 2013;4:343.
8. Wang H, La Russa M, Qi LS. CRISPR/Cas9 in genome editing and beyond. Annu Rev Biochem 2016;85:227–64.
9. Gaj T, Gersbach CA, Barbas CF 3rd. ZFN, TALEN, and CRISPR/Cas-based methods for genome engineering. Trends Biotechnol 2013;31(7):397–405.
10. Porteus M. Genome editing: a new approach to human therapeutics. Annu Rev Pharmacol Toxicol 2016;56:163–90.
11. Huang DD. The potential of RNA interference-based therapies for viral infections. Curr HIV/AIDS Rep 2008;5(1):33–9.
12. Grimm D, Kay MA. RNAi and gene therapy: a mutual attraction. Hematol Am Soc Hematol Educ Program 2007;473–81.
13. Bobbin ML, Rossi JJ. RNA interference (RNAi)-based therapeutics: delivering on the promise? Annu Rev Pharmacol Toxicol 2016;56:103–22.
14. Jasin M, Rothstein R. Repair of strand breaks by homologous recombination. Cold Spring Harb Perspect Biol 2013;5(11):a012740.
15. Wang J, Exline CM, DeClercq JJ, et al. Homology-driven genome editing in hematopoietic stem and progenitor cells using ZFN mRNA and AAV6 donors. Nat Biotechnol 2015;33(12):1256–63.
16. Wang J, DeClercq JJ, Hayward SB, et al. Highly efficient homology-driven genome editing in human T cells by combining zinc-finger nuclease mRNA and AAV6 donor delivery. Nucleic Acids Res 2016;44(3):e30.
17. Genovese P, Schiroli G, Escobar G, et al. Targeted genome editing in human repopulating haematopoietic stem cells. Nature 2014;510(7504):235–40.
18. Kiem HP, Jerome KR, Deeks SG, et al. Hematopoietic-stem-cell-based gene therapy for HIV disease. Cell Stem Cell 2012;10(2):137–47.
19. Galvani AP, Novembre J. The evolutionary history of the CCR5-Delta32 HIV-resistance mutation. Microbes Infect 2005;7(2):302–9.
20. Perez EE, Wang J, Miller JC, et al. Establishment of HIV-1 resistance in CD4+ T cells by genome editing using zinc-finger nucleases. Nat Biotechnol 2008; 26(7):808–16.
21. Tebas P, Stein D, Tang WW, et al. Gene editing of CCR5 in autologous CD4 T cells of persons infected with HIV. N Engl J Med 2014;370(10):901–10.

22. Badia R, Riveira-Munoz E, Clotet B, et al. Gene editing using a zinc-finger nuclease mimicking the CCR5Delta32 mutation induces resistance to CCR5-using HIV-1. J Antimicrob Chemother 2014;69(7):1755–9.

23. Wang W, Ye C, Liu J, et al. CCR5 gene disruption via lentiviral vectors expressing Cas9 and single guided RNA renders cells resistant to HIV-1 infection. PLoS One 2014;9(12):e115987.

24. Yi G, Choi JG, Bharaj P, et al. CCR5 gene editing of resting CD4(+) T cells by transient ZFN expression from HIV Envelope pseudotyped nonintegrating lentivirus confers HIV-1 resistance in humanized mice. Mol Ther Nucleic Acids 2014; 3:e198.

25. Holt N, Wang J, Kim K, et al. Human hematopoietic stem/progenitor cells modified by zinc-finger nucleases targeted to CCR5 control HIV-1 in vivo. Nat Biotechnol 2010;28(8):839–47.

26. DiGiusto DL, Cannon PM, Holmes MC, et al. Preclinical development and qualification of ZFN-mediated CCR5 disruption in human hematopoietic stem/progenitor cells. Mol Ther Methods Clin Dev 2016;3:16067.

27. Peterson CW, Wang J, Norman KK, et al. Long-term multilineage engraftment of autologous genome-edited hematopoietic stem cells in nonhuman primates. Blood 2016;127(20):2416–26.

28. Hendel A, Bak RO, Clark JT, et al. Chemically modified guide RNAs enhance CRISPR-Cas genome editing in human primary cells. Nat Biotechnol 2015; 33(9):985–9.

29. Connor RI, Sheridan KE, Ceradini D, et al. Change in coreceptor use correlates with disease progression in HIV-1–infected individuals. J Exp Med 1997;185(4): 621–8.

30. Peled A, Petit I, Kollet O, et al. Dependence of human stem cell engraftment and repopulation of NOD/SCID mice on CXCR4. Science 1999;283(5403):845–8.

31. Yuan J, Wang J, Crain K, et al. Zinc-finger nuclease editing of human cxcr4 promotes HIV-1 CD4(+) T cell resistance and enrichment. Mol Ther 2012;20(4): 849–59.

32. Wilen CB, Wang J, Tilton JC, et al. Engineering HIV-resistant human CD4+ T cells with CXCR4-specific zinc-finger nucleases. PLoS Pathog 2011;7(4): e1002020.

33. Didigu CA, Wilen CB, Wang J, et al. Simultaneous zinc-finger nuclease editing of the HIV coreceptors ccr5 and cxcr4 protects CD4+ T cells from HIV-1 infection. Blood 2014;123(1):61–9.

34. Jahan S, Samreen B, Khaliq S, et al. HCV entry receptors as potential targets for siRNA-based inhibition of HCV. Genet Vaccin Ther 2011;9:15.

35. Alhoot MA, Wang SM, Sekaran SD. Inhibition of dengue virus entry and multiplication into monocytes using RNA interference. PLoS Negl Trop Dis 2011;5(11): e1410.

36. Alhoot MA, Wang SM, Sekaran SD. RNA interference mediated inhibition of dengue virus multiplication and entry in HepG2 cells. PLoS One 2012;7(3): e34060.

37. White MK, Hu W, Khalili K. The CRISPR/Cas9 genome editing methodology as a weapon against human viruses. Discov Med 2015;19(105):255–62.

38. Karn J, Stoltzfus CM. Transcriptional and posttranscriptional regulation of HIV-1 gene expression. Cold Spring Harb Perspect Med 2012;2(2):a006916.

39. Kaminski R, Chen Y, Fischer T, et al. Elimination of HIV-1 genomes from human T-lymphoid cells by CRISPR/Cas9 gene editing. Sci Rep 2016;6:22555.

40. Hu W, Kaminski R, Yang F, et al. RNA-directed gene editing specifically eradicates latent and prevents new HIV-1 infection. Proc Natl Acad Sci U S A 2014;111(31):11461–6.

41. Ebina H, Misawa N, Kanemura Y, et al. Harnessing the CRISPR/Cas9 system to disrupt latent HIV-1 provirus. Sci Rep 2013;3:2510.

42. Sarkar I, Hauber I, Hauber J, et al. HIV-1 proviral DNA excision using an evolved recombinase. Science 2007;316(5833):1912–5.

43. Qu X, Wang P, Ding D, et al. Zinc-finger-nucleases mediate specific and efficient excision of HIV-1 proviral DNA from infected and latently infected human T cells. Nucleic Acids Res 2013;41(16):7771–82.

44. Strong CL, Guerra HP, Mathew KR, et al. Damaging the Integrated HIV Proviral DNA with TALENs. PLoS One 2015;10(5):e0125652.

45. Ebina H, Kanemura Y, Misawa N, et al. A high excision potential of TALENs for integrated DNA of HIV-based lentiviral vector. PLoS One 2015;10(3):e0120047.

46. Zhu W, Lei R, Le Duff Y, et al. The CRISPR/Cas9 system inactivates latent HIV-1 proviral DNA. Retrovirology 2015;12:22.

47. Liao HK, Gu Y, Diaz A, et al. Use of the CRISPR/Cas9 system as an intracellular defense against HIV-1 infection in human cells. Nat Commun 2015;6:6413.

48. Saayman SM, Lazar DC, Scott TA, et al. Potent and targeted activation of latent HIV-1 using the CRISPR/dCas9 activator complex. Mol Ther 2016;24(3):488–98.

49. Limsirichai P, Gaj T, Schaffer DV. CRISPR-mediated activation of latent HIV-1 expression. Mol Ther 2016;24(3):499–507.

50. Yoder KE, Bundschuh R. Host double strand break repair generates HIV-1 strains resistant to CRISPR/Cas9. Sci Rep 2016;6:29530.

51. Wang G, Zhao N, Berkhout B, et al. CRISPR-Cas9 can inhibit HIV-1 replication but NHEJ repair facilitates virus escape. Mol Ther 2016;24(3):522–6.

52. De Silva Feelixge HS, Stone D, Pietz HL, et al. Detection of treatment-resistant infectious HIV after genome-directed antiviral endonuclease therapy. Antiviral Res 2016;126:90–8.

53. Dampier W, Nonnemacher MR, Sullivan NT, et al. HIV excision utilizing CRISPR/Cas9 technology: attacking the proviral quasispecies in reservoirs to achieve a cure. MOJ Immunol 2014;1(4) [pii:00022].

54. Ely A, Moyo B, Arbuthnot P. Progress with developing use of gene editing to cure chronic infection with hepatitis B virus. Mol Ther 2016;24(4):671–7.

55. Stone D, Niyonzima N, Jerome KR. Genome editing and the next generation of antiviral therapy. Hum Genet 2016;135(9):1071–82.

56. Jinek M, Chylinski K, Fonfara I, et al. A programmable dual-RNA-guided DNA endonuclease in adaptive bacterial immunity. Science 2012;337(6096):816–21.

57. O'Connell MR, Oakes BL, Sternberg SH, et al. Programmable RNA recognition and cleavage by CRISPR/Cas9. Nature 2014;516(7530):263–6.

58. Nelles DA, Fang MY, O'Connell MR, et al. Programmable RNA tracking in live cells with CRISPR/Cas9. Cell 2016;165(2):488–96.

59. Abudayyeh OO, Gootenberg JS, Konermann S, et al. C2c2 is a single-component programmable RNA-guided RNA-targeting CRISPR effector. Science 2016;353(6299):aaf5573.

60. Price AA, Sampson TR, Ratner HK, et al. Cas9-mediated targeting of viral RNA in eukaryotic cells. Proc Natl Acad Sci U S A 2015;112(19):6164–9.

61. Hauber I, Hofmann-Sieber H, Chemnitz J, et al. Highly significant antiviral activity of HIV-1 LTR-specific tre-recombinase in humanized mice. PLoS Pathog 2013;9(9):e1003587.

62. Stamatatos L, Morris L, Burton DR, et al. Neutralizing antibodies generated during natural HIV-1 infection: good news for an HIV-1 vaccine? Nat Med 2009; 15(8):866–70.

63. Klein F, Diskin R, Scheid JF, et al. Somatic mutations of the immunoglobulin framework are generally required for broad and potent HIV-1 neutralization. Cell 2013;153(1):126–38.

64. Lu CL, Murakowski DK, Bournazos S, et al. Enhanced clearance of HIV-1-infected cells by broadly neutralizing antibodies against HIV-1 in vivo. Science 2016;352(6288):1001–4.

65. Scheid JF, Horwitz JA, Bar-On Y, et al. HIV-1 antibody 3BNC117 suppresses viral rebound in humans during treatment interruption. Nature 2016;535(7613): 556–60.

66. Caskey M, Klein F, Lorenzi JC, et al. Viraemia suppressed in HIV-1-infected humans by broadly neutralizing antibody 3BNC117. Nature 2015;522(7557): 487–91.

67. Schoofs T, Klein F, Braunschweig M, et al. HIV-1 therapy with monoclonal antibody 3BNC117 elicits host immune responses against HIV-1. Science 2016; 352(6288):997–1001.

68. Lewis AD, Chen R, Montefiori DC, et al. Generation of neutralizing activity against human immunodeficiency virus type 1 in serum by antibody gene transfer. J Virol 2002;76(17):8769–75.

69. Johnson PR, Schnepp BC, Zhang J, et al. Vector-mediated gene transfer engenders long-lived neutralizing activity and protection against SIV infection in monkeys. Nat Med 2009;15(8):901–6.

70. Balazs AB, Chen J, Hong CM, et al. Antibody-based protection against HIV infection by vectored immunoprophylaxis. Nature 2012;481(7379):81–4.

71. Fuchs SP, Martinez-Navio JM, Piatak M Jr, et al. AAV-delivered antibody mediates significant protective effects against SIVmac239 challenge in the absence of neutralizing activity. PLoS Pathog 2015;11(8):e1005090.

72. Martinez-Navio JM, Fuchs SP, Pedreno-Lopez S, et al. Host anti-antibody responses following adeno-associated virus-mediated delivery of antibodies against HIV and SIV in rhesus monkeys. Mol Ther 2016;24(1):76–86.

73. Saunders KO, Wang L, Joyce MG, et al. Broadly neutralizing human immunodeficiency virus type 1 antibody gene transfer protects nonhuman primates from mucosal simian-human immunodeficiency virus infection. J Virol 2015;89(16): 8334–45.

74. Gardner MR, Kattenhorn LM, Kondur HR, et al. AAV-expressed eCD4-Ig provides durable protection from multiple SHIV challenges. Nature 2015; 519(7541):87–91.

75. Hall CB. Respiratory syncytial virus and parainfluenza virus. N Engl J Med 2001; 344(25):1917–28.

76. Goodwin K, Viboud C, Simonsen L. Antibody response to influenza vaccination in the elderly: a quantitative review. Vaccine 2006;24(8):1159–69.

77. Skaricic D, Traube C, De B, et al. Genetic delivery of an anti-RSV antibody to protect against pulmonary infection with RSV. Virology 2008;378(1):79–85.

78. Limberis MP, Adam VS, Wong G, et al. Intranasal antibody gene transfer in mice and ferrets elicits broad protection against pandemic influenza. Sci Transl Med 2013;5(187):187ra172.

79. Balazs AB, Bloom JD, Hong CM, et al. Broad protection against influenza infection by vectored immunoprophylaxis in mice. Nat Biotechnol 2013;31(7):647–52.

80. Anguela XM, Sharma R, Doyon Y, et al. Robust ZFN-mediated genome editing in adult hemophilic mice. Blood 2013;122(19):3283–7.

81. Li H, Haurigot V, Doyon Y, et al. In vivo genome editing restores haemostasis in a mouse model of haemophilia. Nature 2011;475(7355):217–21.

82. Sharma R, Anguela XM, Doyon Y, et al. In vivo genome editing of the albumin locus as a platform for protein replacement therapy. Blood 2015;126(15): 1777–84.

83. Voit RA, McMahon MA, Sawyer SL, et al. Generation of an HIV resistant T-cell line by targeted "stacking" of restriction factors. Mol Ther 2013;21(4):786–95.

84. Malim MH, Bieniasz PD. HIV restriction factors and mechanisms of evasion. Cold Spring Harb Perspect Med 2012;2(5):a006940.

85. Chinn LW, Tang M, Kessing BD, et al. Genetic associations of variants in genes encoding HIV-dependency factors required for HIV-1 infection. J Infect Dis 2010;202(12):1836–45.

86. DiGiusto DL, Krishnan A, Li L, et al. RNA-based gene therapy for HIV with lentiviral vector-modified CD34(+) cells in patients undergoing transplantation for AIDS-related lymphoma. Sci Transl Med 2010;2(36):36ra43.

87. Lundstrom K. Special issue: gene therapy with emphasis on RNA interference. Viruses 2015;7(8):4482–7.

88. Leibman RS, Riley JL. Engineering T Cells to Functionally Cure HIV-1 Infection. Mol Ther 2015;23(7):1149–59.

89. Ali A, Kitchen SG, Chen IS, et al. HIV-1-specific chimeric antigen receptors based on broadly neutralizing antibodies. J Virol 2016;90(15):6999–7006.

90. Sahu GK, Sango K, Selliah N, et al. Anti-HIV designer T cells progressively eradicate a latently infected cell line by sequentially inducing HIV reactivation then killing the newly gp120-positive cells. Virology 2013;446(1–2):268–75.

91. Liu L, Patel B, Ghanem MH, et al. Novel CD4-based bispecific chimeric antigen receptor designed for enhanced anti-HIV potency and absence of HIV entry receptor activity. J Virol 2015;89(13):6685–94.

92. Zhen A, Kamata M, Rezek V, et al. HIV-specific immunity derived from chimeric antigen receptor-engineered stem cells. Mol Ther 2015;23(8):1358–67.

93. Porichis F, Kaufmann DE. Role of PD-1 in HIV pathogenesis and as target for therapy. Curr HIV/AIDS Rep 2012;9(1):81–90.

94. Ren J, Liu X, Fang C, et al. Multiplex genome editing to generate universal CAR T cells resistant to PD1 inhibition. Clin Cancer Res 2016;23(9):2255–66.

95. Su S, Hu B, Shao J, et al. CRISPR-Cas9 mediated efficient PD-1 disruption on human primary T cells from cancer patients. Sci Rep 2016;6:20070.

96. Stephenson KE, D'Couto HT, Barouch DH. New concepts in HIV-1 vaccine development. Curr Opin Immunol 2016;41:39–46.

97. Hansen SG, Wu HL, Burwitz BJ, et al. Broadly targeted CD8(+) T cell responses restricted by major histocompatibility complex E. Science 2016;351(6274): 714–20.

98. Braff D, Shis D, Collins JJ. Synthetic biology platform technologies for antimicrobial applications. Adv Drug Deliv Rev 2016;105(Pt A):35–43.

99. Pires DP, Cleto S, Sillankorva S, et al. Genetically engineered phages: a review of advances over the last decade. Microbiol Mol Biol Rev 2016;80(3):523–43.

100. Citorik RJ, Mimee M, Lu TK. Sequence-specific antimicrobials using efficiently delivered RNA-guided nucleases. Nat Biotechnol 2014;32(11):1141–5.

101. Bikard D, Euler CW, Jiang W, et al. Exploiting CRISPR-Cas nucleases to produce sequence-specific antimicrobials. Nat Biotechnol 2014;32(11):1146–50.

102. Lagenaur LA, Sanders-Beer BE, Brichacek B, et al. Prevention of vaginal SHIV transmission in macaques by a live recombinant Lactobacillus. Mucosal Immunol 2011;4(6):648–57.

103. Kohn DB, Porteus MH, Scharenberg AM. Ethical and regulatory aspects of genome editing. Blood 2016;127(21):2553–60.

104. Wang L, Li F, Dang L, et al. In vivo delivery systems for therapeutic genome editing. Int J Mol Sci 2016;17(5) [pii:E626].

Hematopoietic Stem Cell Approaches to Cancer

 CrossMark

Jennifer E. Adair, PhD, Sara P. Kubek, PhD, Hans-Peter Kiem, MD, PhD*

KEYWORDS

- Hematopoietic stem cells • In vivo selection and chemoprotection
- Methylguanine methyltransferase • Glioblastoma • CAR T cells
- Engineered TCRs

KEY POINTS

- Cancers with high expression of methlylguanine methyltransferase (MGMT) have a worse prognosis owing to resistance to temozolomide (TMZ) treatment, especially for glioblastoma.
- O^6-benzylguanine (O^6BG) is effective in reversing MGMT-mediated chemotherapy resistance but renders hematopoietic cells highly susceptible to TMZ-associated toxicities.
- The P140K mutant MGMT does not bind O^6BG and thus when expressed in blood cells can make them resistant to the combination therapy O^6BG and temozolomide.
- Combination O^6BG and TMZ treatment improves survival in glioblastoma and potentially other cancers with high expression of MGMT.
- Hematopoietic stem cells (HSCs) can also be targeted to produce T cells expressing engineered T-cell receptors and chimeric antigen receptors for immunotherapy.

INTRODUCTION
Hematopoietic Stem Cells

Hematopoietic stem cells (HSCs) and progenitor cells are particularly attractive for gene therapy. The ability to make all different kinds of blood cells for the life of a recipient is unique and could treat many diseases affecting the blood system from genetic disorders to human immunodeficiency virus and cancer. There are many different ways to genetically engineer HSCs, although lentiviral vectors are currently the most common method for gene transfer and gene modification

Disclosure Statement: Drs J.E. Adair and H.P. Kiem are consultants for Rocket Pharma.
Due to word limits, only essential references are included.
Funding Sources: U19AI096111, R01HL116217, R01AI080326.
Stem Cell and Gene Therapy Program, Fred Hutchison Cancer Research Center, 1100 Fairview Avenue N. D1-100 Seattle, WA 98109-1024, USA
* Corresponding author. Fred Hutchinson Cancer Research Center, 1100 Fairview Avenue North, D1-100, Seattle, WA 98109-1024.
E-mail address: hkiem@fredhutch.org

Hematol Oncol Clin N Am 31 (2017) 897–912
http://dx.doi.org/10.1016/j.hoc.2017.06.012
0889-8588/17/© 2017 Elsevier Inc. All rights reserved.

hemonc.theclinics.com

systems used owing to their versatility and ability to stably integrate into the genome. One critical limitation of HSC gene therapy has been the low level of engraftment of genetically modified HSCs. Engraftment of genetically modified HSCs and multilineage repopulating cells depends mainly on the number of genetically modified HSCs infused into patients and the level of conditioning and reduction of endogenous HSC competition. Herein we discuss how the number of gene-modified cells can be increased for use in HSC gene therapy for cancer. Once the cells are infused, the only other mechanism for increasing the level of gene marking is with in vivo selection. This selection can be accomplished 2 ways, either if the therapeutic transgene confers a natural, constitutive selective advantage on the genetic correction relative to the unmodified cells or if a conditionally selectable gene is introduced and an in vivo selection step can be applied

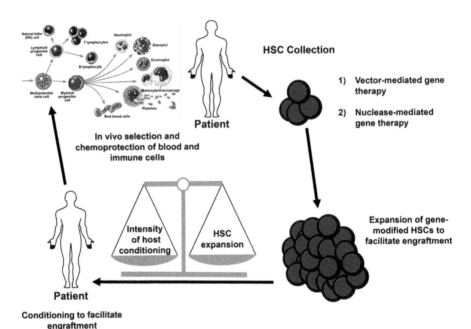

Fig. 1. Hematopoietic stem cell (HSC) therapy for cancer. HSCs are enriched from marrow or mobilized peripheral blood, usually using CD34 expression for the enrichment. CD34$^+$ cells can then be modified either with gammaretroviral or lentiviral vectors or with gene editing technology. The next step can include HSC expansion to increase cell numbers to facilitate engraftment. The balance indicates the relationship between the number of gene-modified HSCs available for transplant and the level of conditioning required to create space for the infused gene-modified cells. The more gene-modified HSCs are available for transplantation, the less host or patient conditioning will be required. Once infused, the cells will contribute to the reconstitution of the entire hematopoietic system. In genetic diseases, the disease phenotype can be corrected; human immunodeficiency virus (HIV) cells can be protected against HIV infection and, in the setting of cancer therapy, HSCs and the resulting gene-modified blood and immune cells can be rendered resistant to the chemotherapy used for the treatment of a particular cancer (eg, MGMTP140K) to protect blood and immune cells from the combination of O^{6}BG and N,N'-bis(2-chloroethyl)-N-ni-troso-urea or temozolomide. (*Adapted from* Kiem HP, Jerome KR, Deeks SG, et al. Hematopoietic-stem-cell-based gene therapy for HIV disease [review]. Cell Stem Cell 2012;10(2):138; with permission.)

to confer modified cells with a selective advantage (**Fig. 1**). There are several conditional selection technologies that have been explored including the F36VMpl-based system,[1,2] the methotrexate-resistance system,[3] and the P140K mutant methylguanine methyltransferase (MGMTP140K) system. The MGMTP140K system is the only system that has been shown to allow for HSC selection in large animal models as well as in patients. Herein we review how the number of HSCs can be increased with novel expansion technologies, and how the level of gene-corrected cells can be increased using the MGMTP140K mechanism, which render cells resistant to chemotherapy with TMZ or N,N′-bis(2-chloroethyl)-N-nitroso-urea (BCNU). This in turn can protect the hematopoietic system from the myeloablative or myelosuppressive effect of these alkylating chemotherapy agents. We review how this approach can be used in the treatment of patients with a poor prognosis brain tumor glioblastoma (glioblastoma multiforme [GBM]). Because HSCs will generate all the different blood lineages, modification of HSCs can also be used to generate blood cells expressing either chimeric antigen receptors (CARs) or engineered T-cell receptors (TCRs). Although this approach has also been discussed for many years, its clinical implementation is still in the beginning stages.

Improving Engraftment of Hematopoietic Stem Cells

Expansion of hematopoietic stem cells

An important variable for successful engraftment of gene-modified HSCs is the quality and quantity of these cells. Endogenous competition can be limited or reduced via different conditioning regimens at various levels of intensity or with more novel nongenotoxic conditioning regimens as discussed in the article "Opening Marrow Niches in Patients Undergoing Autologous Hematopoietic Stem Cell Gene Therapy" by Morton J. Cowan and colleagues and described by others.[4–6] Herein, we focus on the ability to expand the number of HSCs available for treatment. Recently, several compounds and technologies have been proposed. Prostaglandin E2 and StemRegenin-1, an aryl-hydrocarbon receptor antagonist, have shown promise within xenografts and in phase I clinical trials for expanding human umbilical cord blood (CB) HSCs.[7–10] Dr Guy Sauvageau's group has pioneered the use of UM molecules; initial studies in mice and with human and nonhuman primate CB cells with pyrimidoindole-derived UM molecules were very promising.[7] Ongoing studies are currently exploring the UM171 compound in a clinical phase I study for CB expansion in patients with hematologic malignancies undergoing transplants. Dr Shpall's research group pioneered an expansion strategy co-culturing CB with bone marrow–derived mesenchymal stem cells and cytokines, reporting a 30-fold expansion of CD34+ cells.[11–13] Transplantation of an expanded unit combined with an unmanipulated unit was associated with a reduced time to neutrophil engraftment compared with historical controls. The Bernstein and Delaney group has shown that incubation of CD34+ CB cells with immobilized Delta-1 (Notch ligand) and cytokines expanded CD34+ cells.[14,15] This approach is safe and was associated with a decreased time to neutrophil recovery in the expansion group. A variety of other stem cell-active factors, including copper chelator tetraethylenepentamine, prostaglandin E2,[10] angiopoietin-like 5,[16] IGFBP2, pleiotrophin, and HoxB4 have been explored for CB expansion.[17] Dr Rafii's research group has developed a model using specialized endothelial cells, which form a vascular niche that can supply a complex repertoire of angiocrine factors supporting HSCs and progenitors throughout life.[18] Using this approach, we have recently published encouraging results in a large animal nonhuman primate model and shown engraftment of EC-expanded nonhuman primate bone marrow cells.[19]

Selection of gene-edited and chemoprotected hematopoietic stem cells in vivo

Despite promising strategies for ex vivo HSC and CB expansion, to date there are no convincing data available that this can be accomplished with adult bone marrow or mobilized peripheral blood HSCs. Hence, a second approach to increase the level of engraftment of gene-edited HSCs is to provide a means for postengraftment selection. We will focus on the MGMTP140K system, because other systems using a dimerizer-based approach did not result in reliable HSC selection in large animal studies and have not been advanced to any clinical studies.[1–3,20] The basic concept of MGMTP140K selection is shown in **Fig. 2**. Successful genetic chemoprotection of HSCs using wild-type *MGMT* as a selectable marker gene has been demonstrated in murine models, but was less effective in the clinical setting.[21] *MGMT* mutants, which are highly resistant to the inhibitory action of O^6-benzylguanine (O^6BG), have also been described.[22,23] The use of these mutants has allowed the combination of O^6BG with either TMZ or BCNU to enhance the in vivo selection or chemoprotection. We have performed extensive studies in a canine model to show safe and efficient selection in both the autologous and the allogeneic HSC setting.[24–28] We have shown safe and efficient selection long-term in secondary canine recipients, indicating that these MGMTP140K-selected cells were not exhausted and could provide for long-term hematopoiesis. We have also demonstrated that gene-modified allogeneic canine CD34$^+$ cells can engraft even after low-dose total body irradiation conditioning and cytotoxic drug treatment, producing a significant and sustained multilineage increase in gene-modified repopulating cells.[24] We have also reported efficient and stable MGMTP140K-mediated multilineage selection in two nonhuman primate models.[29] We were able to show that treatment with both O^6BG and BCNU stably increased the percentage of transgene-expressing cells from very low levels (as low as 1%) to levels greater than 75% for both myeloid and lymphoid cells. We have

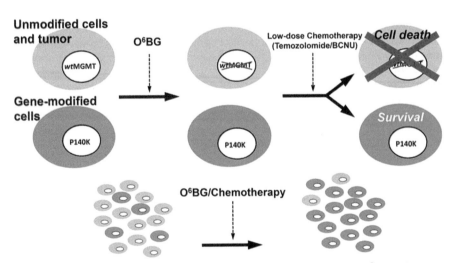

Fig. 2. MGMTP140K-mediated in vivo selection and chemoprotection. O^6-benzylguanine (O^6BG) binds to and inactivates MGMT, thereby sensitizing tumor cells and blood cells to treatment with temozolomide (TMZ) or N,N′-bis(2-chloroethyl)-N-nitroso-urea (BCNU). MGMTP140K modification prevents O^6BG binding and the inactivation of the protein, rendering MGMTP140K-expressing blood and immune cells resistant to the combination O^6BG and TMZ or BCNU. This approach can be used in the treatment of cancers (eg, glioblastoma).

several years of follow-up in many of these animals and we could demonstrate effective multilineage protection and selection in the long term. We also performed extensive retrovirus integration site analyses before and after drug treatments, which confirmed the presence of multiple clones and established the safety of this approach. Overall, these data from clinically relevant animal models demonstrated that *MGMTP140K*-transduced HSCs can engraft and provide effective marrow protection from chemotherapy. As discussed elsewhere in this article, this approach could be applied more broadly for HSC gene therapy targeting human diseases of a malignant, genetic, and infectious nature, including human immunodeficiency virus.[30–32]

Examples of Hematopoietic Stem Cell Gene Therapy for Cancer

MGMTP140K-resistant blood cells and cancer therapies: Glioblastoma

GBM, the most common and aggressive primary brain tumor in adults, is almost uniformly fatal, carrying a 47% chance of survival at 1 year from diagnosis and a median overall survival of approximately 14 months.[33,34] Several significant prognostic factors have been identified, but even in the most favorable groups survival beyond 2 years is unusual.[34–37] Over the past decade, new therapies in GBM have accomplished little to improve overall survival. Radiation prolongs survival after initial surgical resection. Chemotherapeutics such as BCNU and TMZ have been the most effective agents to treat GBM to date, with TMZ being used in the current standard chemotherapy regimen.[34,37] *MGMT* expression has been shown to be important in mediating treatment resistance in human central nervous system tumors. Expression levels are regulated by the promoter controlling *MGMT*. High expression is a result of an unmethylated *MGMT* promoter status in tumor cells and low expression occurs with a methylated *MGMT* promoter status. The majority of GBM diagnoses have an unmethylated *MGMT* promoter, and are resistant to TMZ owing to the increased levels of MGMT expression and subsequent enhanced ability to repair TMZ-induced DNA damage. These patients have poor median survival (12.6 months vs 23.4 months in methylated *MGMT* promoter patients).[34,37] It is important to point out that *MGMT* overexpression and alkylating agent resistance is also found in many other tumor types (reviewed in Refs.[38,39]). The small nucleoside inhibitor, O^6BG, has been shown to block MGMT activity effectively and, thus, concurrent administration of O^6BG with TMZ restores tumor cell sensitivity to the alkylating agent, and has been investigated previously as a strategy to improve TMZ efficacy in recurrent GBM patients.[40,41] However, early phase studies showed that severe off-target myelosuppression owing to concurrent administration of O^6BG with TMZ was a significant obstacle. The hematopoietic-specific toxicity was attributed to low-to-nonexistent levels of MGMT detected in HSCs, which was further reduced by the use of O^6BG.[23] This formed the basis for our clinical study using chemoprotected HSCs, which we hypothesized should be able to tolerate this treatment approach combining the O^6BG tumor sensitizing agent with the chemotherapy TMZ or BCNU. We studied this approach in a prospective phase I and II study (ClinicalTrials.gov; NCT00669669) using MGMTP140K gene-modified and chemoprotected hematopoietic $CD34^+$ cells to prevent hematopoietic toxicity during combination O^6BG and TMZ chemotherapy. Patients diagnosed with unmethylated *MGMT* promoter malignant gliomas (World Health Organization grade IV) received radiation therapy without concomitant TMZ, because this treatment is unlikely to significantly benefit patients with *MGMT* promoter unmethylated tumors and would compromise the HSC pool available for subsequent gene modification. Radiation therapy was followed by peripheral blood stem cell mobilization and leukapheresis. Autologous peripheral blood $CD34^+$ cells were enriched and modified genetically with a gammaretroviral vector encoding the MGMTP140K transgene and reinfused within 24 to 48 hours after administration of single-agent BCNU at a dose of 600 mg/m^2 to facilitate engraftment of gene-modified cells. After hematopoietic recovery from BCNU, patients received combination TMZ and O^{6}BG chemotherapy at or above the previously established maximum tolerated dose of TMZ at 472 mg/m^2. The results of the first 7 patients from this study have been reported elsewhere.[42,43]

Table 1 shows the demographics, treatment, and survival of the first 8 patients enrolled. Seven of these patients were able to undergo treatment; 1 patient did not mobilize the required minimum number of CD34$^+$ cells per kilogram. We found that hematopoietic suppression associated with BCNU conditioning was moderate, and no complications requiring intervention during the engraftment period were observed. Myelosuppression after O^{6}BG and TMZ chemotherapy was observed in 5 of the 7 patients and this occurred most frequently after the first, second, and third cycles. There was a single incidence of significant chemotherapy-associated myelosuppression in a patient with little to no gene-modified (ie, chemoprotected) blood cells at the time of chemotherapy. No significant myelosuppression was observed after the first 100 days of infusion of the chemoprotected cells in the patient with the longest follow-up. This patient had evidence of long-term engraftment of gene-modified cells and received a total of 9 cycles of combination O^{6}BG and TMZ chemotherapy at or above the previously established maximum tolerated dose for TMZ (472 mg/m^2 and 590 mg/m^2, respectively). Marking levels and chemotherapy protection for 7 treated patients is shown in **Fig. 3**. Transient increases in gene-modified granulocytes after chemotherapy corresponded with transient increases observed in total white blood cell populations and coincided with nadir neutropenia and thrombocytopenia after each cycle, demonstrating protection of gene-modified peripheral blood cells. In 3 patients, we observed a loss of detectable gene-modified cells in the peripheral blood between 40 and 100 days after transplantation, which was likely owing to the use of a particular commercial lot of culture medium used during ex vivo gene transfer into CD34$^+$ cells from these patients. There were otherwise no observable significant differences in cell fitness at the time of transplant based on cell dose, cell viability, efficiency of gene transfer, or colony-forming capacity. The observed decline in gene-modified cells over time and after discontinuation of selective chemotherapy treatment in the remaining 4 patients could also be owing to stem cell cytotoxicity associated with high MGMT expression driven by the strong MND viral promoter, as has been suggested by Milsom and colleagues.[44] Patients were evaluated per Revised Assessment in Neuro-Oncology[45] criteria while on study treatment. One patient received 9 cycles of chemotherapy and demonstrated complete response. Of 7 remaining patients, 6 demonstrated progressive disease with a median progression-free survival from diagnosis of 9 months. Median overall survival was 20 months for the 7 patients treated to date, and we observed 100% survival of enrolled patients at 1 year from diagnosis. Three of the 7 treated patients were alive at 2 years, resulting in a significant improvement compared with historical GBM patients with unmethylated MGMT promoter status (1 of 54; $P = .02$).[34] Moreover, all 7 patients surpassed the median survival for patients in the same recursive portioning class.[46] **Fig. 4** shows stable disease by magnetic resonance imaging in 2 patients at 1 year after diagnosis.[42] Published results of this phase I study indicate that gene modification with MGMTP140K can chemoprotect the blood and bone marrow from the myelosuppression associated with combined O^{6}BG and TMZ chemotherapy. The superior treatment response in study patients provides strong evidence of therapeutic benefit over standard of care regimens for GBM patients with unmethylated MGMT promoter status, supporting continued investigation of this approach. This study is currently being continued and we plan to expand to a phase II study.

Table 1
Patient demographics, treatment and survival

GBM Patient	EOR	Age/RPA Class/Gender	KPS at Diagnosis	Tumor MGMT Promoter Status	Initial Treatment[a]	No. Adjuvant O6BG/TMZ Cycles	Adjuvant TMZ Dose(s), mg/m^2	PFS (mo)	OS (mo)	Best Response[b]
1	GTR	57/IV/M	100	Unmethylated	RT only	9	472–590	57[c]	57[d]	PR[e]
2	STR[f]	52/IV/F	100	Unmethylated	RT only	3	472	8	18	SD
3	GTR	53/IV/M	90	Unmethylated	RT only	4	472	12	23	SD
4	GTR	64/IV/F	90	Unmethylated	RT only	2	472	6	14	SD
5	GTR	41/III/M	100	Unmethylated	RT only	5	472	9	28	SD
6	GTR	61/IV/F	100	Unmethylated	RT only	4	472	3.5	20	PD
7	GTR	61/IV/M	90	Unmethylated	RT only	4	472–590	9	17[d]	SD
8	STR[f]	50/V/M	90	Unmethylated	RT only	N/A[g]	N/A	N/A	N/A	N/A

Abbreviations: EOR, extent of surgical resection; GBM, glioblastoma multiforme; GTR, gross total resection; KPS, Karnofsky performance score; MGMT, methylguanine methyltransferase; N/A, not applicable; O6BG, O6-benzylguanine; OS, overall survival; PD, progressive disease; PFS, progression-free survival; PR, partial response; RPA, Radiation Therapy Oncology Group (RTOG) recursive partitioning analysis class; RT, radiation therapy; SD, stable disease; STR, subtotal resection; TMZ, temozolomide.

a 60 Gy.

b Best responses listed were those observed while patients were receiving treatment on study and were evaluated by the Revised Assessment in Neuro-Oncology criteria.

c Patient has not demonstrated progression to date and is currently alive 57 mo from diagnosis.

d Currently alive.

e Patient received no further treatment and most recent off-study response evaluation demonstrated complete response by Revised Assessment in Neuro-Oncology criteria.

f Greater than 50% resection of the primary tumor was achieved with confidence, residual tumor apparent on post-resection magnetic resonance imaging.

g Insufficient CD34+ cells collected; patient was removed from study and received standard care adjuvant TMZ dosing without O6BG.

From Adair JE, Johnston SK, Mrugala MM, et al. Gene therapy enhances chemotherapy tolerance and efficacy in glioblastoma patients. J Clin Invest 2014;124(9):4084; with permission.

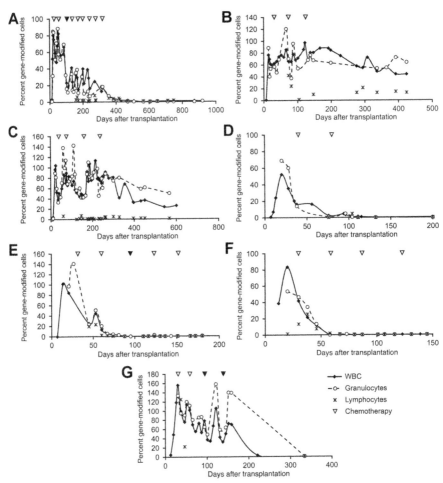

Fig. 3. Persistence of MGMTP140K gene-modified cells in vivo. Percentage of gene-modified white blood cells (WBCs), calculated as the measured gammaretroviral vector copy number × 100, assuming a single vector copy per cell within circulating peripheral blood of patients 1 to 7 are represented in *A* to *G*, respectively. Each graph represents circulating bulk white blood cell (*black diamonds*), granulocytes (*white circles*), and lymphocytes (*asterisks*), with integrated transgene-containing provirus by polymerase chain reaction assay (y axis) over time (x axis). Chemotherapy (*inverted triangles*) is shown as well, with colored triangles representing escalated doses of temozolomide. (*From* Adair JE, Johnston SK, Mrugala MM, et al. Gene therapy enhances chemotherapy tolerance and efficacy in glioblastoma patients. J Clin Invest 2014;124(9):4087; with permission.)

Drs Sloan and Gerson from Case Western have also reported on their results from a phase I clinical trial using the MGMTP140K system approach.[47] The investigators treated 10 newly diagnosed GBM patients with standard surgery and radiation, followed by transplantation with autologous MGMTP140K-engineered CD34+ cells. A significant difference from our study was the use of a self-inactivating lentiviral vector rather than a gammaretroviral vector and different promoters driving the MGMTP140K transgene cassette. The MGMTP140K cassette, however, is the same. They assessed chemoprotection by monitoring the patients' blood counts during the chemotherapy

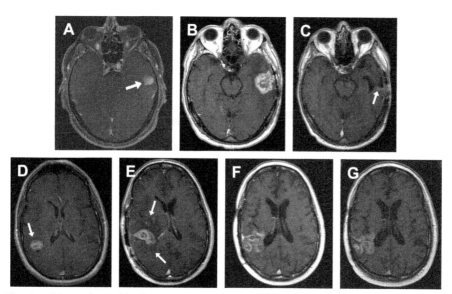

Fig. 4. Evidence for stable disease in 2 patients at 1 year after diagnosis. (*A–C*) Magnetic resonance imaging (MRI) of the brain (patient 1). (*A*) Area of enhancement seen in the left temporal lobe at initial presentation (*arrow*). Gross total resection was performed and histology confirmed glioblastoma, World Health Organization grade IV. (*B*) Area of enhancement and surrounding edema in the left temporal lobe 6 months after diagnosis (interpreted as pseudoprogression). (*C*) Stable disease with faint area of linear enhancement at the posterior margin of the resection cavity (*arrow*) 12 months after initial diagnosis (6 months after second craniotomy) after 4 additional cycles of O^6-benzylguanine (O^6BG)/temozolomide (TMZ) chemotherapy. (*D–G*) MRI of the brain (patient 3). (*D*) Enhancing lesion in the right parietal lobe (*arrow*) at initial presentation. (*E*) First postradiation scan, enlargement of the enhancing area, and associated vasogenic edema (*arrowheads*) are present (interpreted as possible pseudoprogression). (*F*) Six months after the original diagnosis, after 2 cycles of O^6BG/TMZ chemotherapy, the area of enhancement has enlarged, but the surrounding edema has diminished and the patient was stable clinically. (*G*) Eleven months from original diagnosis, after 2 additional doses of O^6BG with TMZ chemotherapy. Image shows area of contrast enhancement, which is stable when compared with the previous scan. (*From* Adair JE, Beard BC, Trobridge GD, et al. Extended survival of glioblastoma patients after chemoprotective HSC gene therapy. Sci Transl Med 2012;4(133):133ra157; with permission.)

treatment. Lentiviral vector transduction efficiencies before infusion of gene-modified cells were between 2.5% and 75%. After infusion, gene marking in the peripheral blood and bone marrow cells increased 3- to 26-fold with only mild myelosuppression, consistent with chemoselection and chemoprotection. Survival ranged from 20 to 36 months, which also exceeded their predicted survival suggesting clinical benefit.

In both studies, genetic modification requires culture of the enriched CD34$^+$ cells under HSC-supportive conditions for a period of 2 to 4 days before reinfusion in a dedicated facility operating under current Good Manufacturing Practices. Thus, for widespread distribution, significant scale-up will be required. One possibility is to centralize current Good Manufacturing Practices–compliant manufacturing facilities, but issues of timing, shipment conditions, and product viability remain. Another option is to downsize the current Good Manufacturing Practices facility requirement into a closed system, automated technology, which can be transported and operated by clinic staff at the point of patient care. We recently described one such option using commercially available technology for immunomagnetic bead-based cell separation and manipulation.[19]

Hematopoietic stem cells and immunotherapy

Another very appealing and exciting approach is the use of HSCs for the generation of genetically modified lymphocytes with genes encoding TCRs or CARs recognizing tumor-associated antigens. The use of CARs is revolutionizing the treatment of patients with certain hematologic malignancies especially CD19-positive leukemias and lymphomas.[48–51] These studies highlight the enormous potential of CAR T-cell–based therapies. One important challenge is the limited in vivo survival of T cells engineered to express a CAR or TCR in patients. Different culture conditions and novel conditioning regimens, including fludarabine and cyclophosphamide, have been explored to prolong in vivo survival.[50,51] However, the use of autologous HSCs with engineered TCRs or CARs may solve both the problem of cell persistence and also potentially the issue of TCR mispairing with endogenous TCR chains.[52–56] In most cases, CD34$^+$ cells are selected for cell engineering and manipulation similar to the study described for patients with glioblastoma. Expression of the delivered transgene can be driven by a constitutive promoter or a lineage-specific regulatory element can be used to restrict expression to specific cell types, such as erythroid, myeloid, or lymphoid.[57,58] After successful modification, HSCs may provide a long-lasting supply of effector T cells engineered against the antigen of interest. TCR- or CAR-modified HSCs would continuously produce T-lymphocyte progenitors that would undergo thymopoiesis and development, increasing the potential for development of immunologic memory. This is in contrast with current infusions of mature T cells, which have a finite lifespan. Another potential advantage of using HSCs for TCR engineering is a reduced risk of mispairing of the engineered TCRs, because HSCs have not yet rearranged their germline TCR loci and, thus, the engineered TCR can suppress rearrangement of the endogenous TCR loci.[56] However, there is the potential that TCRs for self-antigens could be eliminated by the thymus. Stärck and colleagues[59] recently compared TCR engineered T cells with HSCs and found comparable efficacy in controlling tumors in mice. Both retroviral or lentiviral introduction of prearranged cancer antigen–specific TCR or CAR to HSCs have been used to provide an ongoing source of targeted T cells and, perhaps, other effectors. Although infusions of TCR- or CAR-modified mature T cells have an antineoplastic impact within days to weeks, production of antitumor effector cells from engineered, transplanted HSCs may take longer, with de novo T lymphopoiesis occurring only after several months. Stable engraftment of TCR- or CAR-modified HSCs will likely lead to sustained production of targeted effector cells, potentially providing sustained antitumor activity.[52,60] More recently, Dr Kohn's research group has performed studies using a lentiviral vector carrying the cDNA for a human TCR recognizing the NY-ESO-1 tumor-associated antigen.[61] Investigators used CD34$^+$ cells from mobilized peripheral blood as a clinically relevant HSC source. Higher doses of CD34$^+$ cells were needed to effectively engraft the NSG mice compared with CB-derived CD34$^+$ cells; however, production of T cells expressing the anti–NY-ESO-1 TCR in transplanted mice was observed. In contrast with the TCR against MART-1 expressed on both CD4$^+$ and CD8$^+$ T cells, expression of the NY-ESO-1 TCR has been restricted to CD8$^+$ T cells, indicating that the specific TCR plays an instructive role in T-cell development.[62] These examples suggest the use of HSCs as a vehicle to continuously produce TCR-modified T cells may be a feasible approach for immunotherapy in patients with cancer.

In contrast with TCR genes introduced into HSCs, a major potential advantage of CARs is that their expression will not be limited to T cells, because the surface display of CARs does not require CD3 coexpression. Thus, CARs may be expressed on multiple hematopoietic lineages (T, natural killer [NK], and myeloid), amplifying the potential graft-versus-cancer activity.[63,64] Generation of T cells from transplanted HSCs may be slow and limited in adult recipients, but myeloid and NK cells should be produced rapidly after transplantation, providing an early source of antitumor immunity.[22,28,29] The CAR-expressing T cells are likely the most efficient cytotoxic effector cells against tumor because of their longer lifespan, greater activation and proliferation properties, and potential for immunologic memory. Several studies, however, have reported similar antigen-specific cytotoxicity of CAR-modified NK and myeloid cells compared with CAR-modified T cells.[63–65] Myeloid and NK cells also do not depend on thymopoiesis to become active cytotoxic effectors and could exponentially amplify the antitumor immune response directed by CAR. In addition, CAR-modified HSCs can be infused at the time of transplantation, when chemotherapy or radiation-based conditioning would create favorable conditions for the efficacy of this approach, that is, engraftment of gene-modified cells, as well as decreasing tumor burden and the risks of immunogenicity of the CAR molecules. Thus, CAR modification of a portion of the donor HSC may provide additional antileukemic effects. Several issues, however, will have to be evaluated with the HSC approach. There is a possibility that the presence of the CAR will have adverse effects on de novo T-cell production, by causing negative selection, or suppression of endogenous TCR gene rearrangement by allelic exclusion, as has been shown with TCRs, or the potential for diverse CAR-expressing leukocytes to cause unique toxicities.

The use of HSCs for CAR or TCR gene therapy will require pretransplant conditioning with agents that have myeloablative or at least marrow cytoreductive activity, such as total body irradiation or busulfan. This is in contrast with T-cell–based CAR therapy, where lymphodepletion is required with either cyclophosphamide and/or fludarabine. Thus, HSC-based immunotherapy would be preferably combined with an autologous or allogeneic stem cell transplantation to optimize engraftment and minimize any additional toxicities. Recent data suggest that adult HSCs are more myeloid skewed, which could affect the ability to generate T cells from engineered HSCs.[66] In addition, age likely affects thymic function with advancing age diminishing the potential for de novo thymopoiesis.[67,68] Prior treatments, such as chemotherapy or radiation therapy, may also affect thymic function. Fortunately, the use of HSCs would still allow for efficient production of myeloid or NK CAR cells. A possible concern for HSC-based immunotherapy in hematologic malignancies is the risk of gene-modifying malignant cells in the $CD34^+$ cell product. Ideally, HSC collection should be performed after treatment and documented remission to reduce this risk. The identification of additional markers to purify healthy HSC from blasts would be beneficial. Current clinical trials have focused on T-cell–based immunotherapy and, thus, it will likely take some time until we learn more about the potential benefits of HSC-based CAR or TCR therapy.

SUMMARY

HSCs remain attractive targets for cancer gene therapy approaches. The chemoprotection described herein for GBM is currently moving into a phase II study using a lentiviral vector. This approach could also benefit patients with other tumors displaying unmethylated MGMT promoters or high MGMT expression levels. The use of HSCs for immunotherapy with engineered CARs and TCRs is still in the early phases and might be ideally combined initially unnecessary comma an autologous transplant is part of the treatment of the underlying disease, such as in multiple myeloma. Here one could envision engineering a fraction of the autologous HSCs with an antitumor TCR or CAR construct, and then infusing the modified cells together with the unmodified stem cells after the appropriate conditioning. Unique benefits of HSC transplantation and immunotherapy are suggested by recent data demonstrating that HSC transplantation can facilitate the recruitment of tumor-specific T cells to malignant gliomas.[69]

REFERENCES

1. Neff T, Horn PA, Valli VE, et al. Pharmacologically regulated in vivo selection in a large animal. Blood 2002;100(6):2026–31.
2. Richard RE, De Claro RA, Yan J, et al. Differences in F36VMpl-based in vivo selection among large animal models. Mol Ther 2004;10(4):730–40.
3. Gori JL, Beard BC, Williams NP, et al. In vivo protection of activated Tyr22-dihydrofolate reductase gene-modified canine T lymphocytes from methotrexate. J Gene Med 2013;15(6–7):233–41.
4. Cowan MJ, Kiem HP. Devouring the hematopoietic stem cell: setting the table for marrow cell transplantation (Commentary). Mol Ther 2016;24(11):1892–4.
5. Chhabra A, Ring AM, Weiskopf K, et al. Hematopoietic stem cell transplantation in immunocompetent hosts without radiation or chemotherapy. Sci Transl Med 2016;8(351):351ra105.
6. Palchaudhuri R, Saez B, Hoggatt J, et al. Non-genotoxic conditioning for hematopoietic stem cell transplantation using a hematopoietic-cell-specific internalizing immunotoxin. Nat Biotechnol 2016;34(7):738–45.
7. Fares I, Chagraoui J, Gareau Y, et al. Cord blood expansion. Pyrimidoindole derivatives are agonists of human hematopoietic stem cell self-renewal. Science 2014;345(6203):1509–12.
8. Wagner JE Jr, Brunstein CG, Boitano AE, et al. Phase I/II trial of StemRegenin-1 expanded umbilical cord blood hematopoietic stem cells supports testing as a stand-alone graft. Cell Stem Cell 2016;18(1):144–55.
9. Boitano AE, Wang J, Romeo R, et al. Aryl hydrocarbon receptor antagonists promote the expansion of human hematopoietic stem cells. Science 2010;329(5997):1345–8.
10. Goessling W, Allen RS, Guan X, et al. Prostaglandin E2 enhances human cord blood stem cell xenotransplants and shows long-term safety in preclinical nonhuman primate transplant models. Cell Stem Cell 2011;8(4):445–58.
11. de Lima M, McNiece I, Robinson SN, et al. Cord-blood engraftment with ex vivo mesenchymal-cell coculture. N Engl J Med 2012;367(24):2305–15.
12. McNiece I, Harrington J, Turney J, et al. Ex vivo expansion of cord blood mononuclear cells on mesenchymal stem cells. Cytotherapy 2004;6(4):311–7.
13. Robinson SN, Simmons PJ, Yang H, et al. Mesenchymal stem cells in ex vivo cord blood expansion [review]. Best Pract Res Clin Haematol 2011;24(1):83–92.
14. Delaney C, Varnum-Finney B, Aoyama K, et al. Dose-dependent effects of the Notch ligand Delta1 on ex vivo differentiation and in vivo marrow repopulating ability of cord blood cells. Blood 2005;106(8):2693–9.
15. Delaney C, Heimfeld S, Brashem-Stein C, et al. Notch-mediated expansion of human cord blood progenitor cells capable of rapid myeloid reconstitution. Nat Med 2010;16(2):232–7.
16. Zhang CC, Kaba M, Iizuka S, et al. Angiopoietin-like 5 and IGFBP2 stimulate ex vivo expansion of human cord blood hematopoietic stem cells as assayed by NOD/SCID transplantation. Blood 2008;111(7):3415–23.

17. Amsellem S, Pflumio F, Bardinet D, et al. Ex vivo expansion of human hematopoietic stem cells by direct delivery of the HOXB4 homeoprotein. Nat Med 2003; 9(11):1423–7.

18. Seandel M, James D, Shmelkov SV, et al. Generation of functional multipotent adult stem cells from GPR125+ germline progenitors. Nature 2007;449(7160): 346–50.

19. Gori JL, Butler JM, Kunar B, et al. Endothelial cells promote expansion of long-term engrafting marrow hematopoietic stem and progenitor cells in primates. Stem Cells Transl Med 2017;6(3):864–76.

20. Okazuka K, Beard BC, Emery DW, et al. Long-term regulation of genetically modified primary hematopoietic cells in dogs. Mol Ther 2011;19(7):1287–94 [Erratum appears in Mol Ther 2011;19(11):2102 Note: Torok-Storb, Beverly [added]].

21. Cornetta K, Croop J, Dropcho E, et al. A pilot study of dose-intensified procarbazine, CCNU, vincristine for poor prognosis brain tumors utilizing fibronectin-assisted, retroviral-mediated modification of CD34+ peripheral blood cells with O6-methylguanine DNA methyltransferase. Cancer Gene Ther 2006;13(9): 886–95.

22. Dolan ME, Pegg AE, Dumenco LL, et al. Comparison of the inactivation of mammalian and bacterial O6-alkylguanine-DNA alkyltransferases by O6-benzylguanine and O6-methylguanine. Carcinogenesis 1991;12(12):2305–9.

23. Allay JA, Dumenco LL, Koc ON, et al. Retroviral transduction and expression of the human alkyltransferase cDNA provides nitrosourea resistance to hematopoietic cells. Blood 1995;85(11):3342–51.

24. Neff T, Horn PA, Peterson LJ, et al. Methylguanine methyltransferase-mediated in vivo selection and chemoprotection of allogeneic stem cells in a large-animal model. J Clin Invest 2003;112(10):1581–8.

25. Horn PA, Keyser KA, Peterson LJ, et al. Efficient lentiviral gene transfer to canine repopulating cells using an overnight transduction protocol. Blood 2004;103(10): 3710–6.

26. Neff T, Beard BC, Peterson LJ, et al. Polyclonal chemoprotection against temozolomide in a large-animal model of drug resistance gene therapy. Blood 2005; 105(3):997–1002.

27. Gerull S, Beard BC, Peterson LJ, et al. In vivo selection and chemoprotection after drug resistance gene therapy in a nonmyeloablative allogeneic transplantation setting in dogs. Hum Gene Ther 2007;18:451–6.

28. Beard BC, Sud R, Keyser KA, et al. Long-term polyclonal and multilineage engraftment of methylguanine methyltransferase P140K gene-modified dog hematopoietic cells in primary and secondary recipients. Blood 2009;113(21): 5094–103.

29. Beard BC, Trobridge GD, Ironside C, et al. Efficient and stable MGMT-mediated selection of long-term repopulating stem cells in nonhuman primates. J Clin Invest 2010;120(7):2345–54.

30. Peterson CW, Haworth KG, Burke BP, et al. Multilineage polyclonal engraftment of Cal-1 gene-modified cells and in vivo selection after SHIV infection in a nonhuman primate model of AIDS. Mol Ther Methods Clin Dev 2016;3:16007.

31. Younan PM, Polacino P, Kowalski JP, et al. Positive selection of mC46-expressing CD4+ T cells and maintenance of virus specific immunity in a primate AIDS model. Blood 2013;122(2):179–87.

32. Younan PM, Polacino P, Kowalski JP, et al. Combinatorial hematopoietic stem cell transplantation and vaccination reduces viral pathogenesis following SHIV89.6P-challenge. Gene Ther 2015;22(12):1007–12.

33. Tanaka S, Louis DN, Curry WT, et al. Diagnostic and therapeutic avenues for glioblastoma: no longer a dead end? Nat Rev Clin Oncol 2012;10(1):14–26.

34. Stupp R, Hegi ME, Mason WP, et al. Effects of radiotherapy with concomitant and adjuvant temozolomide versus radiotherapy alone on survival in glioblastoma in a randomised phase III study: 5-year analysis of the EORTC-NCIC trial. Lancet Oncol 2009;10(5):459–66.

35. Davis FG, Kupelian V, Freels S, et al. Prevalence estimates for primary brain tumors in the United States by behavior and major histology groups. Neuro Oncol 2001;3(3):152–8.

36. Davis FG, McCarthy BJ, Freels S, et al. The conditional probability of survival of patients with primary malignant brain tumors: surveillance, epidemiology, and end results (SEER) data. Cancer 1999;85(2):485–91.

37. Stupp R, Mason WP, van den Bent MJ, et al. Radiotherapy plus concomitant and adjuvant temozolomide for glioblastoma. N Engl J Med 2005;352(10):987–96.

38. Liu L, Gerson SL. Targeted modulation of MGMT: clinical implications [review]. Clin Cancer Res 2006;12(2):328–31.

39. Sharma S, Salehi F, Scheithauer BW, et al. Role of MGMT in tumor development, progression, diagnosis, treatment and prognosis. Anticancer Res 2009;29(10):3759–68.

40. Quinn JA, Jiang SX, Reardon DA, et al. Phase II trial of temozolomide plus o6-benzylguanine in adults with recurrent, temozolomide-resistant malignant glioma. J Clin Oncol 2009;27(8):1262–7.

41. Quinn JA, Jiang SX, Reardon DA, et al. Phase I trial of temozolomide plus O6-benzylguanine 5-day regimen with recurrent malignant glioma. Neuro Oncol 2009;11(5):556–61.

42. Adair JE, Beard BC, Trobridge GD, et al. Extended survival of glioblastoma patients after chemoprotective HSC gene therapy. Sci Transl Med 2012;4(133):133ra157.

43. Adair JE, Johnston SK, Mrugala MM, et al. Gene therapy enhances chemotherapy tolerance and efficacy in glioblastoma patients. J Clin Invest 2014;124(9):4082–92.

44. Milsom MD, Jerabek-Willemsen M, Harris CE, et al. Reciprocal relationship between O6-methylguanine-DNA methyltransferase P140K expression level and chemoprotection of hematopoietic stem cells. Cancer Res 2008;68(15):6171–80.

45. Wen PY, Macdonald DR, Reardon DA, et al. Updated response assessment criteria for high-grade gliomas: response assessment in neuro-oncology working group. J Clin Oncol 2010;28(11):1963–72.

46. Li J, Wang M, Won M, et al. Validation and simplification of the Radiation Therapy Oncology Group recursive partitioning analysis classification for glioblastoma. Int J Radiat Oncol Biol Phys 2011;81(3):623–30.

47. Sloan AE, Fung H, Reese J, et al. 141 phase I trial of genetically modified hematopoietic progenitor cells facilitate bone marrow chemoprotection and enabling TMZ/O6BG dose escalation resulting in improved survival. Neurosurgery 2016;63(Suppl 1):157.

48. Porter DL, Levine BL, Kalos M, et al. Chimeric antigen receptor-modified T cells in chronic lymphoid leukemia. N Engl J Med 2011;365(8):725–33.

49. Grupp SA, Kalos M, Barrett D, et al. Chimeric antigen receptor-modified T cells for acute lymphoid leukemia. N Engl J Med 2013;368(16):1509–18.

50. Turtle CJ, Hanafi LA, Berger C, et al. Immunotherapy of non-Hodgkin's lymphoma with a defined ratio of CD8+ and CD4+ CD19-specific chimeric antigen receptor-modified T cells. Sci Translational Med 2016;8(355):355ra116.

51. Turtle CJ, Hanafi LA, Berger C, et al. CD19 CAR-T cells of defined CD4+:CD8+ composition in adult B cell ALL patients. J Clin Invest 2016;126(6):2123–38.

52. Gschweng E, De Oliveira S, Kohn DB. Hematopoietic stem cells for cancer immunotherapy. Immunol Rev 2014;257(1):237–49.

53. Corrigan-Curay J, Kiem HP, Baltimore D, et al. T-cell immunotherapy: looking forward. Mol Ther 2014;22(9):1564–74.

54. Vatakis DN, Koya RC, Nixon CC, et al. Antitumor activity from antigen-specific CD8 T cells generated in vivo from genetically engineered human hematopoietic stem cells. Proc Natl Acad Sci U S A 2011;108(51):E1408–16.

55. Kitchen SG, Zack JA. Engineering HIV-specific immunity with chimeric antigen receptors. AIDS Patient Care STDS 2016;30(12):556–61.

56. Vatakis DN, Arumugam B, Kim SG, et al. Introduction of exogenous T-cell receptors into human hematopoietic progenitors results in exclusion of endogenous T-cell receptor expression. Mol Ther 2013;21(5):1055–63.

57. Papapetrou EP, Kovalovsky D, Beloeil L, et al. Harnessing endogenous miR-181a to segregate transgenic antigen receptor expression in developing versus post-thymic T cells in murine hematopoietic chimeras. J Clin Invest 2009;119(1):157–68.

58. Brown BD, Gentner B, Cantore A, et al. Endogenous microRNA can be broadly exploited to regulate transgene expression according to tissue, lineage and differentiation state. Nat Biotechnol 2007;25(12):1457–67.

59. Starck L, Popp K, Pircher H, et al. Immunotherapy with TCR-redirected T cells: comparison of TCR-transduced and TCR-engineered hematopoietic stem cell-derived T cells. J Immunol 2014;192(1):206–13.

60. Yang L, Baltimore D. Long-term in vivo provision of antigen-specific T cell immunity by programming hematopoietic stem cells. Proc Natl Acad Sci U S A 2005;102(12):4518–23.

61. Wargo JA, Robbins PF, Li Y, et al. Recognition of NY-ESO-1+ tumor cells by engineered lymphocytes is enhanced by improved vector design and epigenetic modulation of tumor antigen expression. Cancer Immunol Immunother 2009;58(3):383–94.

62. Chodon T, Comin-Anduix B, Chmielowski B, et al. Adoptive transfer of MART-1 T-cell receptor transgenic lymphocytes and dendritic cell vaccination in patients with metastatic melanoma. Clin Cancer Res 2014;20(9):2457–65.

63. Hege KM, Cooke KS, Finer MH, et al. Systemic T cell-independent tumor immunity after transplantation of universal receptor-modified bone marrow into SCID mice. J Exp Med 1996;184(6):2261–9.

64. Roberts MR, Cooke KS, Tran AC, et al. Antigen-specific cytolysis by neutrophils and NK cells expressing chimeric immune receptors bearing zeta or gamma signaling domains. J Immunol 1998;161(1):375–84.

65. Tran AC, Zhang D, Byrn R, et al. Chimeric zeta-receptors direct human natural killer (NK) effector function to permit killing of NK-resistant tumor cells and HIV-infected T lymphocytes. J Immunol 1995;155(2):1000–9.

66. Benz C, Copley MR, Kent DG, et al. Hematopoietic stem cell subtypes expand differentially during development and display distinct lymphopoietic programs. Cell Stem Cell 2012;10(3):273–83.

67. Mackall CL, Fleisher TA, Brown MR, et al. Age, thymopoiesis, and CD4+ T-lymphocyte regeneration after intensive chemotherapy. N Engl J Med 1995;332(3):143–9.

68. Weinberg K, Annett G, Kashyap A, et al. The effect of thymic function on immunocompetence following bone marrow transplantation. Biol Blood Marrow Transplant 1995;1(1):18–23.
69. Flores C, Pham C, Snyder D, et al. Novel role of hematopoietic stem cells in immunologic rejection of malignant gliomas. Oncoimmunology 2015;4(3):e994374.

Gene Modified T Cell Therapies for Hematological Malignancies

Ulrike Abramowski-Mock, PhD, Juliette M. Delhove, PhD,
Waseem Qasim, MBBS, PhD*

KEYWORDS

- Gene therapy • Gene editing • Adoptive immunotherapy • T cell receptor
- Chimeric antigen receptor • Lentiviral vectors • Leukemia • Lymphoma

KEY POINTS

- T cells engineered with chimeric antigen receptors mediate high levels of leukemic remission.
- Emerging gene editing techniques are now being incorporated.
- Challenges for dissemination to a larger number of patients are being addressed.

INTRODUCTION

Harnessing the immune system to actively seek and specifically eradicate tumor cells is attractive as an anticancer therapy and provides a valuable addition to existing strategies based on chemotherapy and radiotherapy. Genetic engineering of T cells for use against hematological malignances has delivered some of the most compelling evidence to date that such approaches can be effective. This article reviews recent developments in this area, considers the potential of emerging therapies, and discusses the challenges in delivering such products.

GENETIC REDIRECTION OF T CELLS AGAINST TUMOR ANTIGENS

T cells express heterodimeric antigen-specific $\alpha\beta$ receptors (TCRs) that recognize antigenic peptides, including certain tumor-associated antigens, expressed by

Disclosure: U. Abramowski-Mock and J.M. Delhove declare that they have no conflict of interest. W. Qasim holds contract research/ trials funding from Cellectis/Servier, Miltenyi Biotec, Bellicum, and Autolus Ltd, and has received consulting fees from Autolus and Orchard Therapeutics; W. Qasim has a patent application pending for gene-edited T cells. W. Qasim/ U. Abramowski-Mock supported by National Institute for Health Research (grant no: NIHR RP 2014-05-007), which also supports the Biomedical Research Centre at UCL Great Ormond Street Institute of Child Health. J.M. Delhove is supported by Innovate UK (grant no: 167152). Molecular and Cellular Immunology Unit, University college London, UCL Great Ormond Street Institute of Child Health, 30 Guilford Street, London WC1N 1EH, UK
* Corresponding author.
E-mail address: w.qasim@ucl.ac.uk

cell-surface MHC molecules. In general, helper T cells with CD4 expression interact with peptides expressed by MHC class II, and cytotoxic CD8 T cells interact with MHC class I:peptide complexes. Expression of recombinant TCRs with defined MHC:peptide specificity can redirect immunity and result in targeted killing of malignant cells. This approach is restricted to intracellular peptides derived from tumor antigens and requires MHC loading and surface presentation to allow immune synapse formation. Efforts to confer durable, high-level T cell modification have largely relied on genetic transfer of TCR genes by integrating γ-retroviral or lentiviral vectors. Early examples included retroviral transfer of genes encoding TCR αβ chains against melanoma antigen MART1, where melanoma regression was reported in 2 of 15 initial subjects treated,[1] and subsequent studies where NY-ESO-1 was targeted in patients with melanoma and synovial cell sarcoma.[2] Mindful of the risks of aberrant cross-pairing between recombinant TCR chains and their endogenous counterparts, additional disulphide bridges or murine constant chain domains have been used to mitigate against the risk of generating novel autoreactive TCRs. Further improvements include modification of TCR complementarity determining regions (CDRs) with enhanced-avidity TCRs and predictive strategies to determine on-target and off-target adverse effects. Alternatively, cross-pairing can be excluded by knocking out the endogenous TCR chains using designer nucleases such as zinc-finger nucleases[3,4] and transcription activator-like effector nucleases (TALENs).[5] An example of unpredicted effects caused by off-target antigen cross-recognition was encountered when an HLA-A01 restricted affinity-enhanced MAGE-A3 TCR-mediated unexpected cardiac toxicity through detection of the peptide antigen, titin.[6,7] Unanticipated neural complications have arisen because of MAGE expression in the central nervous system, where TCR-engineered cells mediated on-target recognition.[8]

In the context of hematological malignancies, suitable target antigens that discriminate between malignant and nonmalignant cells have proven elusive. Clinical trials targeting Wilms tumor antigen 1 (WT1) on acute myeloid leukemia (AML) and myelodysplastic syndromes (MDS) are underway in the United Kingdom[9,10] and the United States.[11–15] A similar approach is being developed to target certain viral infections, with programs for the application of cytomegalovirus, Epstein Barr virus and hepatitis B-related disease.[16]

A key limitation of TCR-based cellular therapy is the need to generate receptor combinations for multiple HLA/peptide populations. Chimeric antigen specific receptors (CARs) have the advantage of not being HLA restricted and independent of antigen processing and presentation. CAR epitopes include surface expressed proteins such as cluster of differentiation (CD) molecules but also lipid antigens. CARs comprise an extracellular antigen-binding domain (usually a single-chain antigen-recognition domain) with a transmembrane anchor (eg, derived from immunoglobulin G [IgG] or CD8), and intracellular signaling motifs from CD3 molecules linked to costimulatory domains from CD28, 4-1BB, OX40, and other elements.[17]

Costimulatory configurations based on 4-1BB-CD3ζ signaling have reported some remarkable results in trials where lentiviral delivery of CAR receptors specific for the B cell antigen, CD19, have produced significant leukemic remissions.[18–20] Cell infusions following lymphodepleting conditioning using chemotherapy (combinations of cyclophosphamide, bendamustine, pentostatin, and etoposide) in subjects with CLL and ALL may be critical in supporting expansion and persistence of incoming effector populations. Anti-CD19 CARs with alternative CD28-CD3ζ activation domains in T cells transduced by gamma-retroviral vectors have been investigated at National Cancer Institute (NCI)-mediated clinical responses in 6 of 8 patients with CLL and follicular lymphoma[21,22] and have also been applied in trials of allogeneic donor CAR T cells following transplant.[23] Similar studies for ALL[24] and NHL[25] were undertaken with complete response rates of 14 of 16 (88%) and 10 of 20 (50%) respectively. Modified allogeneic T cells generated by coculture with EBV-LCLs have also been used, anticipating that virus-specific T cells generated in this fashion would persist long term without significant graft versus host disease (GvHD). Antitumor responses were evident in 2 of 6 relapsed subjects with persistence of 8 to 9 weeks documented.[26] Although most studies have used viral vector delivery for stable transgene integration, 1 alternative is the plasmid-based Sleeping Beauty (SB) system. Here, stable transposition of CAR19 DNA from plasmid delivered by electroporation of T cells is being investigated in early phase studies.[27,28] The safety profile of T cells modified with integrating vectors has to date been reassuring, with no reports of genotoxicity caused by vector integration. Toxicities caused by cell-mediated effects, including cytokine release phenomena and neurotoxicity have been problematic in several studies. Strategies to minimize adverse effects include the incorporation of suicide genes or cell elimination pathways, or adopting approaches such as mRNA delivery for temporary effects. This could be particularly useful for transient effects against AML antigens such as CD33 and CD123, which are also expressed by normal progenitors.[29]

One limitation of immune-based therapies against tumors is the evolution of escape phenomena over time. Strategies targeting a single antigen are prone to circumvention and evasion if antigen expression is lost. Relapse of leukemia after CAR19 therapy following loss of CD19 epitope expression have been reported in 10% to 20% of children. Hemizygous deletions, frameshift or missense mutations, or alternatively spliced CD19 isoforms have been detected in such relapses.[30] Loss of target epitopes could be addressed by targeting multiple antigens with different CARs, as demonstrated in models simultaneously targeting CD19 and CD123,[31] but additional evasion strategies including suppressive effects and manipulation of the microenvironment may also need to be addressed for sustained leukemic eradication. A summary of key published clinical trials using CAR T cells is available in **Table 1**.

GENE-EDITING ANTILEUKEMIC T CELLS

Genome editing technologies are advancing at a remarkable pace, with the first clinical applications using T cell therapies underway. Broadly, reagents incorporating customizable sequence-specific DNA-binding elements linked to nucleases can mediate highly specific double-stranded DNA breaks (DSB) that trigger endogenous NHEJ or HDR DNA repair pathways. The former can be exploited for knock-out effects through indels causing frame-shift and nonsense mutations and the latter for more sophisticated gene repair or targeting gene insertion strategies. Earlier-stage reagents include meganucleases, homing endonucleases derived from *I-CreI,* and zinc finger nucleases (ZFNs) comprising *Fok*I cleavage domains linked to sequence-specific zinc finger proteins. More recently, TALENs and alternative nucleotide-mediated CRISPR/Cas9 and CRISPR/Cpf1 systems have become available. The latter combine bacterial Cas9 with synthetic guide RNA (gRNA) complementary to the target genome for highly specific cleavage of double-stranded DNA.

One early application of editing technology has been to address endogenous TCR expression in engineered cells, both for autologous TCR trials and allogeneic, non-HLA matched settings. The latter are important given the difficulties in manufacturing CAR T cells for heavily treated patients. CAR T cells can be generated from allogeneic HLA-matched donors, if available, as part of a transplant strategy,[23,57] but the products still have to be manufactured in a bespoke manner. The availability of

Table 1
Clinical experience using CAR-T cells redirected toward hematological malignancies

Target	Malignancy	Gene Transfer Method	Costimulatory Domain	T Cell Origin	Cell Dosage	N	Center	Reference
CD19	FL	Electroporation	CD3ζ	Autologous	$1-2 \times 10^9/m^2$	2	NCI	Jensen et al,[32] 2010
CD19	FL	Retroviral	CD28	Autologous	$5 \times 10^6/kg$	1	NCI	Kochenderfer et al,[21] 2010
CD19	FL; CLL; SMZL	Retroviral	CD28	Autologous	$5-55 \times 10^6/kg$	8	NCI	Kochenderfer et al,[22] 2012
CD19	CLL; MCL; DLBCL	Retroviral	CD28	Allogeneic	$1-100 \times 10^6/kg$	10	NCI	Kochenderfer et al,[23] 2013
CD19	CLL	Retroviral	CD28	Autologous	$1-4 \times 10^6/kg$	4	NCI	Kochenderfer et al,[33] 2015
CD19	ALL	Retroviral	CD28	Autologous	$1, 3 \times 10^6/kg$	21	NCI	Lee et al,[34] 2015
CD19	CLL; ALL	Retroviral	CD28	Autologous	$2-30 \times 10^6/kg$	9	MSKCC	Brentjens et al,[35] 2011
CD19	ALL	Retroviral	CD28	Autologous	$1.5-3 \times 10^6/kg$	5	MSKCC	Brentjens et al,[36] 2013
CD19	CLL, ALL	Retroviral	CD28	Autologous	$0.4, 1, 3 \times 10^7/kg$	10	MSKCC	Brentjens et al,[35] 2011
CD19	FL; DLBCL	Retroviral	CD28	Autologous	$2-20 \times 10^7/m^2$	6	BCM	Savoldo et al,[37] 2011
CD19	ALL, CLL	Retroviral	CD28	Allogeneic	$1.5, 4.5, 12 \times 10^7/m^2$	8	BCM	Cruz et al,[26] 2013
CD19	CLL; ALL	Retroviral	CD28	Autologous	$0.2, 1, 2 \times 108/m^2$	14	BCM	Xu et al,[38] 2014
CD19	CLL; ALL; DLBCL; FL; MCL	Retroviral	4-1BB	Autologous	$1.5-500 \times 10^7$ cells	110	Upenn	Maude et al,[39] 2014
CD19	CLL	Lentiviral	4-1BB	Autologous	$0.15-16 \times 10^6/kg$	3	Upenn	Porter et al,[18] 2011; Kalos et al,[19] 2011
CD19	ALL	Lentiviral	4-1BB	Autologous	$10-100 \times 10^6/kg$	2	Upenn	Maude et al,[39] 2014
CD19	MM	Lentiviral	4-1BB	Autologous	$1-5 \times 10^7$ cells	10	Upenn	Garfall et al,[40] 2015
CD19	CLL, SLL, MM	Lentiviral	4-1BB	Autologous	$1-5 \times 10^{7/8}$ cells	42	Upenn	Fraietta et al,[41] 2016

CD19	ALL	Lentiviral	4-1BB	Autologous	$0.76–20.6 \times 10^6/kg$	30	Upenn	Maude et al,[39] 2014
CD19	NHL	Sleeping Beauty Transposition	CD28	Autologous Allogeneic	$1 \times 10^6/m^2$ $1 \times 10^6/m^2$	Auto (7) Allo (19)	MDACC	Kebriaei et al,[28] 2016
CD20	MCL; NHL	Electroporation	CD28-4-1BB	Autologous	$0.1–3.3 \times 10^9/m^2$	3	FHCRC	Till et al,[42] 2012
CD20	DLBCL	Lentiviral	4-1BB	Autologous	$\sim0.3–2.2 \times 10^7/kg$	7	CPLAGH	Wang et al,[43] 2014
CD22	FL; DLBCL; NHL; B-ALL	Lentiviral	4-1BB	Autologous	$0.3–1 \times 10^7/kg$	9	NCI	Haso et al,[44] 2013
CD30	HHL; NHL	Retroviral	CD28	Autologous	$2 \times 10^7 - 1 \times 10^8/m^2$	28	BCM	Rothe et al,[45] 2015
CD30	HL	Lentiviral	4-1BB	Autologous	$3.2 \times 10^5/kg$	11	CPLAGH	Wang et al,[46] 2015
CD33	AML	Lentiviral	4-1BB	Autologous	1.19×10^9 cells	10	CPLAGH	Wang et al,[46] 2015
CD123	AML	Lentiviral	CD28	Autologous Allogeneic	—	30	COHNMC	Mardiros et al,[47] 2015
CD138	MM	Lentiviral	4-1BB	Autologous	$0.44–3.78 \times 10^7/kg$	5	CPLAGH	Guo et al,[48] 2016
BCMA	MM	Retroviral	CD28	Autologous	$0.3 \times 15 \times 10^6/kg$	12	NCI	Ali et al,[49] 2016
ROR1	CLL; SLL	Sleeping Beauty	4-1BB	Autologous	$1 \times 10^5/kg$	48	MDACC	Deniger et al,[50] 2015
IgK	NHL; CLL; MM	Retrovirus	CD28	Autologous	$0.2–2 \times 10^8/m^2$	16	BCM	Ramos et al,[51] 2016
LeY	AML	Retroviral	CD28	Autologous	$0.5–1.3 \times 10^9$ cells	5	PMCCC	Ritchie et al,[52–56] 2013

Abbreviations: ALL, acute lymphoblastic leukemia; BCM, Baylor College of Medicine; BCMA, B-cell maturation antigen; BL, burkitt lymphoma; CLL, chronic lymphocytic leukemia; COHNMC, City of Hope National Medical Center; CPLAGH, Chinese PLA General Hospital (China); DLBCL, diffuse large B-cell lymphoma; FHCRC, Fred Hutchinson Cancer Research Center; FL, follicular lymphoma; HL, Hodgkin's lymphoma; LeY, Lewis Y antigen; MCL, mantle cell lymphoma; MDACC, MD Anderson Cancer Center; MDS, myelodysplastic syndrome; MM, multiple myeloma; MSKCC, Memorial Sloan Kettering Cancer Center; NHL, non-Hodgkin lymphoma; NCI, National Cancer Institute; PMCCC, Peter MacCallum Cancer Center (Australia); ROR1, receptor tyrosine kinase like orphan receptor 1; SLL, small lymphocytic lymphoma; Upenn, University of Pennsylvania.

Reported enrollment numbers (N) as detailed for registered trials at clinicaltrials.gov.

premanufactured, off-the-shelf CAR T cells could overcome these limitations, but such an approach has the risk of GvHD and/or host-mediated rejection of mismatched cell infusions. In order to generate a universal product, gene-editing reagents, including ZFNs, meganucleases, TALENs, and CRISPR/Cas9, are all being employed to disrupt expression of TCR, HLA, and other relevant cell surface molecules[3,5,58] (**Fig. 1**). For example, ZFNs against both TCR α and β chains have been used to prevent endogenous expression and restricted cells from displaying an introduced WT1-specific TCR.[4] TALENs targeting the constant domain of the endogenous T cell receptor alpha chain (TRAC) and simultaneously disrupting CD52 have been combined with lentiviral delivery of CAR19. Knockout of TRAC creates T cells that can be infused despite HLA-mismatch with reduced risk of GvHD.[59–61] The destruction of CD52 leaves cells resistant toward alemtuzumab treatment, a commonly used anti-CD52 monoclonal antibody used for lymphodepletion as part of transplant conditioning. Two infants with relapsed pediatric B-ALL following conventional myeloablative allo-SCT and other experimental interventions successfully achieved molecular remission after receiving infusions of such allogeneic cells. Two studies are now underway using universal, gene-edited CAR19 T cells (UCART19) in pediatric (NCT02808442) and adult patients (NCT02746952) in the United Kingdom. Similar CRISPR/Cas9-based approaches are planned to reduce the risk of TCR cross-pairing in trials using autologous T cells.[62] Other early targets include immune checkpoint pathways. These are usually crucial for maintaining self-tolerance to prevent autoimmunity and regulation of immune responses against pathogens. In certain tumors, this physiologic safety mechanism can be used to escape detection by the immune system by dampening effector T cell responses and upregulating regulatory suppressive effects. Important examples of immune checkpoint receptors include programmed cell death protein 1 (PD-1) and cytotoxic T-lymphocyte-associated antigen 4 (CTLA-4).[63] Interference with these inhibitory pathways by monoclonal antibodies against CTLA-4, PD-1, and its ligand PD-L1 enhances antitumor response by loosening the immunologic brake on endogenous T cells[64,65] and increasing T effector to Treg ratios.[66,67] Therapies targeting immune checkpoints have been shown to be effective in a variety of tumors including melanoma, prostate cancer, renal cell carcinoma, and nonsmall-cell lung cancer, either alone or in combination.[68,69] Naturally, these pathways are also attractive targets for disruption by gene editing, several centers are at an advanced stage of planning trials using checkpoint-disrupted cells. For example, knock-out of the PD-1-gene using CRIPSR/Cas9 to generate activated tumor-infiltrating T cells with extended persistence and less prone to exhaustion is proposed for lung cancer (NCT02793856), prostate cancer (NCT02867345), invasive bladder cancer (NCT02863913), and metastatic renal carcinoma (NCT02867332). A combination of PD-1 and TCR gene disruption in T cells engineered to express receptors against melanoma antigen NY-ESO-1 could both enhance expression of the introduced TCR and prolong persistence. It is generally anticipated that genetic targeting of PD-1 will lead to more potent and sustained effects compared with antibody treatments, although this may also increase the risk of autoimmunity as tolerance is breached.[70]

MANUFACTURING, DISSEMINATION, AND COMMERCIALIZATION

Manufacturing of complex cellular therapeutic product is still challenging and only feasible in laboratories with relevant manufacturing experience, infrastructure, and staff. The production of engineered T cells requires a series of manipulation steps including cell preparation (eg, Ficoll gradient separation and washing steps), enrichment (using magnetic bead separation), activation (using soluble or bead conjugated anti-CD3/

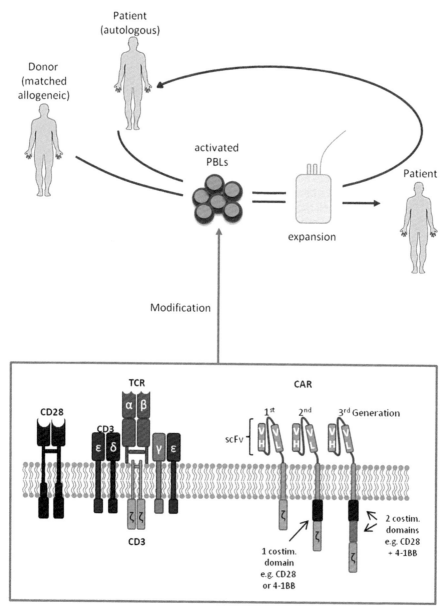

Fig. 1. Modification of lymphocytes for cancer immunotherapy. Autologous or allogeneic peripheral blood lymphocytes (PBLs) isolated by leukapharesis are activated in culture and modified to express recombinant T cell receptors (TCRs) or chimeric antigen receptor (CAR) genes. TCRs recognize their antigen in the context of major histocompatibility complex (MHC) and signal through a multimeric CD3 complex. CARs comprise an antibody-derived recognition domain fused to a CD3zeta signaling domain alone (first generation) or in combination with costimulatory elements from CD28 or 4-1BB (second generation) or both (third generation).

CD28-antibodies), transduction with the respective viral vector, and culture supporting sufficient expansion to achieve target doses. Expansion in gas-permeable bags or bioreactor devices, including the Wave bioreactor, is commonplace to achieve therapeutic doses. Where metallic activation beads are used, these are removed by magnetic separation ahead of final product formulation. Alternative activation reagents, including soluble antibody or TransAct, can be removed by simple washing steps.[71] Additional gene-editing steps have recently been incorporated into some products, and usually involve an electroporation step for the delivery of nuclease reagents. At the end of production, samples are requird for release characterization including sterility, screening for replication-competent vector, potency, and other assessments. Doses are usually cryopreserved in target doses based on weight or surface area using controlled rate freezing, and stability data accumulated over time (**Fig. 2**). Recently, aspects of CAR-T cell manufacturing have been automated (eg, the CliniMACS Prodigy has been shown to support lentiviral T cell modification with minimal hands-on time),[72,73] and phase I testing of cells manufactured in such a system is underway in the allogeneic transplant setting in London (clinicaltrials.gov, NCT02893189).

Effector function and cell persistence are critical for effective immunotherapy. Both features are influenced strongly by the phenotype of cells following manufacture, which usually involves multiple manipulations, activation, culture, and cryopreservation. Isolated peripheral blood T cells can be differentiated into the following phenotypes: naïve T cells (T_N), stem cell memory T cells (T_{SCM}), central memory T cells (T_{CM}), effector memory T cells (T_{EM}), and terminally differentiated effector T cells (T_{EFF}). Stem cell memory T cells show the highest potential for self-renewal and survival,[74] whereas effector memory T cells show the greatest effector function and cytotoxicity and have an increased ability to respond to chemokines for homing to peripheral tissue.[75] Based on a self-renewal effector model, naïve T cells differentiate into T_{SCM} upon antigen recognition, which then differentiate further into T_{CM} and T_{EM} and finally into short-lived effector T cells[74] (**Fig. 3**). More differentiated populations have shorter telomeres and consequently reduced persistence. Interim data for the T_{CM}-enriched cells in the NHL-setting showed good engraftment, although persistence of the cells was limited to no more than 28 days, comparable to similar pan-T cell trials.[76] As T_{SCM} can give rise to all memory T cell subsets they may be most promising for long-term anti-tumor responses.[77] However, because of the low proportion of these cells within peripheral blood (2%–3%),[74] specific targeting of this subset of cells for manufacturing purposes is currently challenging, and clinical approaches are broadly limited to larger enriching CD4 and CD8 subsets.[25,78]

Clinical centers and commercial partners are cooperating to foster wider dissemination of engineered cell therapies. At NCI, Kite Pharma is investigating CAR19 vectors with CD28 and CD3ζ signaling domains in refractory NHL and other B cell lymphomas. Novartis, in association with University of Pennsylvania, has advanced lentiviral CAR19 programs (with 4-1BB- CD3ζ) in relapsed refractory ALL. Celgene/Bluebird Bio is also testing lentiviral CAR vectors with 4-1BB domains in relapsed refractory multiple myeloma patients. Juno Therapeutics & Celgene are utilizing γ-retroviral CAR19 with a CD28 costimulatory in similar populations, while Ziopharm Oncology/Intrexon at MD Anderson has focused on Sleeping Beauty CAR19. In Europe, Servier/Pfizer has initiated trials of UCART19 in pediatric ALL at Great Ormond Street Hospital and adult ALL at Kings College Hospital. Catapult TCR has adopted a γ-retroviral TCR study against WT1 for relapsed AML and MDS. Academic trials at University College London and Autolus are also investigating CAR19 and other vectors in B cell malignancies.

The clinical success of T cell therapies, particularly against CD19-expressing hematological cancers, has spurred the development of T cell therapies targeting an array of

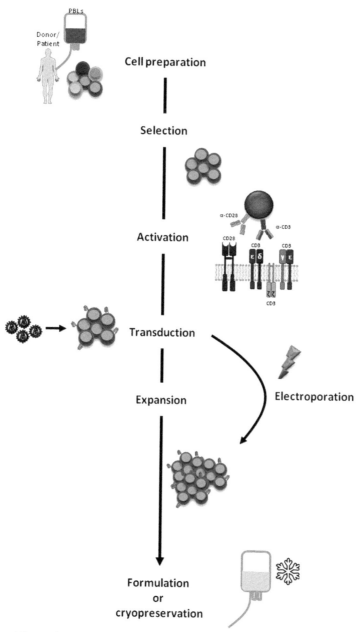

Fig. 2. Workflow of manufacturing genetically modified T cells. Cell preparation may include selection of specific T cell subsets (eg, CD8, CD62L) by magnetic bead enrichment. Activation follows in specialist media with anti- CD3-specific antibody, usually in combination with anti-CD28 antibody, using iron-coated beads or other nanoscale structures. Lentiviral or gamma-retroviral vectors are a common choice for stable transduction of TCR or CAR genes, or mRNA may be electroporated for transient expression. Transduced cells are then expanded, processed to remove activation beads, and washed and cryopreserved in specified dose formulations.

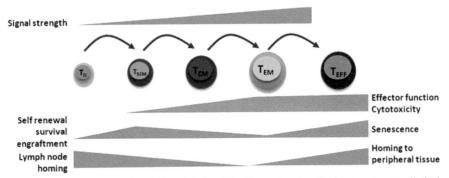

Fig. 3. T cell subsets. Peripheral blood derived T cells can be classified into naïve T cells (T_N), stem cell memory T cells (T_{SCM}), central memory T cells (T_{CM}), effector memory T cells (T_{EM}), and terminally differentiated effector T cells (T_{EFF}). Upon antigen recognition, naive T cells proliferate and gradually differentiate into more memory-type T cells. During this process, T cells lose their capacity for self-renewal, survival, engraftment, and homing to lymph nodes but gain effector function and improve their cytotoxicity as well as homing to peripheral tissue. (*Adapted from* Restifo NP, Dudley ME, Rosenberg SA. Adoptive immunotherapy for cancer: harnessing the T cell response. Nat Rev Immunol 2012;12(4):276; with permission.)

antigens. Genome editing has further diversified the applicability of immunotherapies with universal therapies for allogeneic transplantation being made a reality. Further improvements to the manufacturing process and better expansion of the most efficacious subset of T cells should permit increased scalability and commercialization of T cell products in the future.

REFERENCES

1. Morgan RA, Dudley ME, Wunderlich JR, et al. Cancer regression in patients after transfer of genetically engineered lymphocytes. Science 2006; 314(5796):126–9.
2. Robbins PF, Morgan RA, Feldman SA, et al. Tumor regression in patients with metastatic synovial cell sarcoma and melanoma using genetically engineered lymphocytes reactive with NY-ESO-1. J Clin Oncol 2011;29(7):917–24.
3. Torikai H, Reik A, Liu PQ, et al. A foundation for universal T-cell based immunotherapy: T cells engineered to express a CD19-specific chimeric-antigen-receptor and eliminate expression of endogenous TCR. Blood 2012;119(24): 5697–705.
4. Provasi E, Genovese P, Lombardo A, et al. Editing T cell specificity towards leukemia by zinc finger nucleases and lentiviral gene transfer. Nat Med 2012;18(5): 807–15.
5. Berdien B, Mock U, Atanackovic D, et al. TALEN-mediated editing of endogenous T-cell receptors facilitates efficient reprogramming of T lymphocytes by lentiviral gene transfer. Gene Ther 2014;21(6):539–48.
6. Linette GP, Stadtmauer EA, Maus MV, et al. Cardiovascular toxicity and titin cross-reactivity of affinity-enhanced T cells in myeloma and melanoma. Blood 2013; 122(6):863–71.
7. Cameron BJ, Gerry AB, Dukes J, et al. Identification of a Titin-derived HLA-A1-presented peptide as a cross-reactive target for engineered MAGE A3-directed T cells. Sci Transl Med 2013;5(197):197ra103.

8. Morgan RA, Chinnasamy N, Abate-Daga D, et al. Cancer regression and neurological toxicity following anti-MAGE-A3 TCR gene therapy. J Immunother 2013; 36(2):133–51.

9. Xue S, Gillmore R, Downs A, et al. Exploiting T cell receptor genes for cancer immunotherapy. Clin Exp Immunol 2005;139(2):167–72.

10. Ochi T, Fujiwara H, Okamoto S, et al. Novel adoptive T-cell immunotherapy using a WT1-specific TCR vector encoding silencers for endogenous TCRs shows marked antileukemia reactivity and safety. Blood 2011;118(6):1495–503.

11. Schmitt TM, Aggen DH, Stromnes IM, et al. Enhanced-affinity murine T-cell receptors for tumor/self-antigens can be safe in gene therapy despite surpassing the threshold for thymic selection. Blood 2013;122(3):348–56.

12. Long AH, Haso WM, Shern JF, et al. 4-1BB costimulation ameliorates T cell exhaustion induced by tonic signaling of chimeric antigen receptors. Nat Med 2015;21(6):581–90.

13. Hassan R, Ho M. Mesothelin targeted cancer immunotherapy. Eur J Cancer 2008; 44(1):46–53.

14. Morgan RA, Yang JC, Kitano M, et al. Case report of a serious adverse event following the administration of T cells transduced with a chimeric antigen receptor recognizing ERBB2. Mol Ther 2010;18(4):843–51.

15. Beatty GL, Haas AR, Maus MV, et al. Mesothelin-specific chimeric antigen receptor mRNA-engineered T cells induce anti-tumor activity in solid malignancies. Cancer Immunol Res 2014;2(2):112–20.

16. Qasim W, Brunetto M, Gehring AJ, et al. Immunotherapy of HCC metastases with autologous T cell receptor redirected T cells, targeting HBsAg in a liver transplant patient. J Hepatol 2015;62(2):486–91.

17. Sadelain M, Brentjens R, Riviere I. The basic principles of chimeric antigen receptor design. Cancer Discov 2013;3(4):388–98.

18. Porter DL, Levine BL, Kalos M, et al. Chimeric antigen receptor-modified T cells in chronic lymphoid leukemia. N Engl J Med 2011;365(8):725–33.

19. Kalos M, Levine BL, Porter DL, et al. T cells with chimeric antigen receptors have potent antitumor effects and can establish memory in patients with advanced leukemia. Sci Transl Med 2011;3(95):95ra73.

20. Grupp SA, Kalos M, Barrett D, et al. Chimeric antigen receptor-modified T cells for acute lymphoid leukemia. N Engl J Med 2013;368(16):1509–18.

21. Kochenderfer JN, Wilson WH, Janik JE, et al. Eradication of B-lineage cells and regression of lymphoma in a patient treated with autologous T cells genetically engineered to recognize CD19. Blood 2010;116(20):4099–102.

22. Kochenderfer JN, Dudley ME, Feldman SA, et al. B-cell depletion and remissions of malignancy along with cytokine-associated toxicity in a clinical trial of anti-CD19 chimeric-antigen-receptor-transduced T cells. Blood 2012;119(12): 2709–20.

23. Kochenderfer JN, Rosenberg SA. Treating B-cell cancer with T cells expressing anti-CD19 chimeric antigen receptors. Nat Rev Clin Oncol 2013;10(5):267–76.

24. Davila ML, Riviere I, Wang X, et al. Efficacy and toxicity management of 19-28z CAR T cell therapy in B cell acute lymphoblastic leukemia. Sci Transl Med 2014;6(224):224ra225.

25. Turtle CJ, Hanafi LA, Berger C, et al. Immunotherapy of non-Hodgkin's lymphoma with a defined ratio of CD8+ and CD4+ CD19-specific chimeric antigen receptor-modified T cells. Sci Transl Med 2016;8(355):355ra116.

26. Cruz CR, Micklethwaite KP, Savoldo B, et al. Infusion of donor-derived CD19-redirected virus-specific T cells for B-cell malignancies relapsed after allogeneic stem cell transplant: a phase 1 study. Blood 2013;122(17):2965–73.

27. Singh N, Liu X, Hulitt J, et al. Nature of tumor control by permanently and transiently modified GD2 chimeric antigen receptor T cells in xenograft models of neuroblastoma. Cancer Immunol Res 2014;2(11):1059–70.

28. Kebriaei P, Singh H, Huls MH, et al. Phase I trials using sleeping beauty to generate CD19-specific CAR T cells. J Clin Invest 2016;126(9):3363–76.

29. Kenderian SS, Ruella M, Shestova O, et al. CD33-specific chimeric antigen receptor T cells exhibit potent preclinical activity against human acute myeloid leukemia. Leukemia 2015;29(8):1637–47.

30. Sotillo E, Barrett DM, Black KL, et al. Convergence of acquired mutations and alternative splicing of CD19 enables resistance to CART-19 immunotherapy. Cancer Discov 2015;5(12):1282–95.

31. Ruella M, Barrett DM, Kenderian SS, et al. Dual CD19 and CD123 targeting prevents antigen-loss relapses after CD19-directed immunotherapies. J Clin Invest 2016;126(10):3814–26.

32. Jensen MC, Popplewell L, Cooper LJ, et al. Antitransgene rejection responses contribute to attenuated persistence of adoptively transferred CD20/CD19-specific chimeric antigen receptor redirected T cells in humans. Biol Blood Marrow Transplant 2010;16(9):1245–56.

33. Kochenderfer JN, Dudley ME, Kassim SH, et al. Chemotherapy-refractory diffuse large B-cell lymphoma and indolent B-cell malignancies can be effectively treated with autologous T cells expressing an anti-CD19 chimeric antigen receptor. J Clin Oncol 2015;33(6):540–9.

34. Lee DW, Kochenderfer JN, Stetler-Stevenson M, et al. T cells expressing CD19 chimeric antigen receptors for acute lymphoblastic leukaemia in children and young adults: a phase 1 dose-escalation trial. Lancet 2015;385(9967):517–28.

35. Brentjens RJ, Riviere I, Park JH, et al. Safety and persistence of adoptively transferred autologous CD19-targeted T cells in patients with relapsed or chemotherapy refractory B-cell leukemias. Blood 2011;118(18):4817–28.

36. Brentjens RJ, Davila ML, Riviere I, et al. CD19-targeted T cells rapidly induce molecular remissions in adults with chemotherapy-refractory acute lymphoblastic leukemia. Sci Transl Med 2013;5(177):177ra138.

37. Savoldo B, Ramos CA, Liu E, et al. CD28 costimulation improves expansion and persistence of chimeric antigen receptor–modified T cells in lymphoma patients. J Clin Invest 2011;121(5):1822–6.

38. Xu Y, Zhang M, Ramos CA, et al. Closely related T-memory stem cells correlate with in vivo expansion of CAR. CD19-T cells and are preserved by IL-7 and IL-15. Blood 2014;123(24):3750–9.

39. Maude SL, Frey N, Shaw PA, et al. Chimeric antigen receptor T cells for sustained remissions in leukemia. N Engl J Med 2014;371(16):1507–17.

40. Garfall AL, Maus MV, Hwang WT, et al. Chimeric antigen receptor T cells against CD19 for multiple myeloma. N Engl J Med 2015;373(11):1040–7.

41. Fraietta JA, Beckwith KA, Patel PR, et al. Ibrutinib enhances chimeric antigen receptor T-cell engraftment and efficacy in leukemia. Blood 2016;127(9):1117–27.

42. Till BG, Jensen MC, Wang J, et al. CD20-specific adoptive immunotherapy for lymphoma using a chimeric antigen receptor with both CD28 and 4-1BB domains: pilot clinical trial results. Blood 2012;119(17):3940–50.

43. Wang Y, Zhang WY, Han QW, et al. Effective response and delayed toxicities of refractory advanced diffuse large B-cell lymphoma treated by CD20-directed chimeric antigen receptor-modified T cells. Clin Immunol 2014;155(2):160–75.
44. Haso W, Lee DW, Shah NN, et al. Anti-CD22–chimeric antigen receptors targeting B-cell precursor acute lymphoblastic leukemia. Blood 2013;121(7):1165–74.
45. Rothe A, Sasse S, Topp MS, et al. A phase 1 study of the bispecific anti-CD30/ CD16A antibody construct AFM13 in patients with relapsed or refractory Hodgkin lymphoma. Blood 2015;125(26):4024–31.
46. Wang QS, Wang Y, Lv HY, et al. Treatment of CD33-directed Chimeric Antigen Receptor-modified T Cells in One Patient With Relapsed and Refractory Acute Myeloid Leukemia. Mol Ther 2015;23(1):184–91.
47. Mardiros A, Forman SJ, Budde LE. T cells expressing CD123 chimeric antigen receptors for treatment of acute myeloid leukemia. Curr Opin Hematol 2015; 22(6):484–8.
48. Guo B, Chen M, Han Q, et al. CD138-directed adoptive immunotherapy of chimeric antigen receptor (CAR)-modified T cells for multiple myeloma. J Cell ImJ Clin Oncolmunother 2016;2(1):28–35.
49. Ali SA, Shi V, Maric I, et al. T cells expressing an anti-B-cell maturation antigen chimeric antigen receptor cause remissions of multiple myeloma. Blood 2016; 128(13):1688–700.
50. Deniger DC, Yu J, Huls MH, et al. Sleeping beauty transposition of chimeric antigen receptors targeting receptor tyrosine kinase-like orphan receptor-1 (ROR1) into diverse memory T-cell populations. PLoS One 2015;10(6):e0128151.
51. Ramos CA, Savoldo B, Torrano V, et al. Clinical responses with T lymphocytes targeting malignancy-associated kappa light chains. J Clin Invest 2016;126(7): 2588–96.
52. Ritchie DS, Neeson PJ, Khot A, et al. Persistence and efficacy of second generation CAR T cell against the LeY antigen in acute myeloid leukemia. Mol Ther 2013;21(11):2122–9.
53. Urnov FD, Rebar EJ, Holmes MC, et al. Genome editing with engineered zinc finger nucleases. Nat Rev Genet 2010;11(9):636–46.
54. Joung JK, Sander JD. TALENs: a widely applicable technology for targeted genome editing. Nat Rev Mol Cell Biol 2012;14(1):49–55.
55. Sander JD, Joung JK. CRISPR-Cas systems for editing, regulating and targeting genomes. Nat Biotechnol 2014;32(4):347–55.
56. Komor AC, Kim YB, Packer MS, et al. Programmable editing of a target base in genomic DNA without double-stranded DNA cleavage. Nature 2016;533(7603): 420–4.
57. Brudno JN, Somerville RP, Shi V, et al. Allogeneic T cells that express an anti-CD19 chimeric antigen receptor induce remissions of B-cell malignancies that progress after allogeneic hematopoietic stem-cell transplantation without causing graft-versus-host disease. J Clin Oncol 2016;34(10):1112–21.
58. Osborn MJ, Webber BR, Knipping F, et al. Evaluation of TCR gene editing achieved by TALENs, CRISPR/Cas9, and megaTAL nucleases. Mol Ther 2015; 24(3):570–81.
59. Poirot L, Philip B, Schiffer-Mannioui C, et al. Multiplex genome-edited T-cell manufacturing platform for "Off-the-Shelf" adoptive T-cell immunotherapies. Cancer Res 2015;75(18):3853–64.
60. Qasim W, Zhan H, Samarasinghe S, et al. Molecular remission of infant B-ALL after infusion of universal TALEN gene-edited CAR T cells. Sci Transl Med 2017; 9(374) [pii:eaaj2013].

61. Qasim W, Amrolia PJ, Samarasinghe S, et al. First clinical application of talen engineered universal CAR19 T cells in B-ALL. Blood 2015;126(23):2046.

62. Reardon S. First CRISPR clinical trial gets green light from US panel. Nature News 2016.

63. Pardoll DM. The blockade of immune checkpoints in cancer immunotherapy. Nat Rev Cancer 2012;12(4):252–64.

64. Leach DR, Krummel MF, Allison JP. Enhancement of antitumor immunity by CTLA-4 blockade. Science 1996;271(5256):1734–6.

65. Iwai Y, Ishida M, Tanaka Y, et al. Involvement of PD-L1 on tumor cells in the escape from host immune system and tumor immunotherapy by PD-L1 blockade. Proc Natl Acad Sci U S A 2002;99(19):12293–7.

66. Quezada SA, Peggs KS, Curran MA, et al. CTLA4 blockade and GM-CSF combination immunotherapy alters the intratumor balance of effector and regulatory T cells. J Clin Invest 2006;116(7):1935–45.

67. Wang W, Lau R, Yu D, et al. PD1 blockade reverses the suppression of melanoma antigen-specific CTL by CD4+ CD25(Hi) regulatory T cells. Int Immunol 2009; 21(9):1065–77.

68. Sharma P, Allison JP. Immune checkpoint targeting in cancer therapy: toward combination strategies with curative potential. Cell 2015;161(2):205–14.

69. Sledzinska A, Menger L, Bergerhoff K, et al. Negative immune checkpoints on T lymphocytes and their relevance to cancer immunotherapy. Mol Oncol 2015; 9(10):1936–65.

70. Cyranoski D. Chinese scientists to pioneer first human CRISPR trial. Nature 2016; 535:476–7.

71. Casati A, Varghaei-Nahvi A, Feldman SA, et al. Clinical-scale selection and viral transduction of human naive and central memory CD8+ T cells for adoptive cell therapy of cancer patients. Cancer Immunol Immunother 2013;62(10):1563–73.

72. Priesner C, Aleksandrova K, Esser R, et al. Automated enrichment, transduction and expansion of clinical-scale CD62L+ T cells for manufacturing of GTMPs. Hum Gene Ther 2016;27(10):860–9.

73. Mock U, Nickolay L, Philip B, et al. Automated manufacturing of chimeric antigen receptor T cells for adoptive immunotherapy using CliniMACS prodigy. Cytotherapy 2016;18(8):1002–11.

74. Gattinoni L, Lugli E, Ji Y, et al. A human memory T cell subset with stem cell-like properties. Nat Med 2011;17(10):1290–7.

75. Sallusto F, Lenig D, Forster R, et al. Pillars article: two subsets of memory T lymphocytes with distinct homing potentials and effector functions. Nature. 1999. 401: 708–712. J Immunol 2014;192(3):840–4.

76. Wang X, Popplewell LL, Wagner JR, et al. Phase 1 studies of central memory-derived CD19 CAR T-cell therapy following autologous HSCT in patients with B-cell NHL. Blood 2016;127(24):2980–90.

77. Gattinoni L, Klebanoff CA, Restifo NP. Paths to stemness: building the ultimate antitumour T cell. Nat Rev Cancer 2012;12(10):671–84.

78. Turtle CJ, Hanafi LA, Berger C, et al. CD19 CAR-T cells of defined CD4+:CD8+ composition in adult B cell ALL patients. J Clin Invest 2016;126(6):2123–38.

UNITED STATES POSTAL SERVICE ® Statement of Ownership, Management, and Circulation
(All Periodicals Publications Except Requester Publications)

1. Publication Title	2. Publication Number	3. Filing Date
HEMATOLOGY/ONCOLOGY CLINICS OF NORTH AMERICA	002 – 473	9/18/2017

4. Issue Frequency	5. Number of Issues Published Annually	6. Annual Subscription Price
FEB, APR, JUN, AUG, OCT, DEC	6	$397.00

7. Complete Mailing Address of Known Office of Publication (Not printer) (Street, city, county, state, and ZIP+4®)

ELSEVIER INC.
230 Park Avenue, Suite 800
New York, NY 10169

Contact Person
STEPHEN R BUSHING
Telephone (Include area code)
215-239-3688

8. Complete Mailing Address of Headquarters or General Business Office of Publisher (Not printer)

ELSEVIER INC.
230 Park Avenue, Suite 800
New York, NY 10169

9. Full Names and Complete Mailing Addresses of Publisher, Editor, and Managing Editor (Do not leave blank)

Publisher (Name and complete mailing address)

ADRIANNE BRIGIDO, ELSEVIER INC.
1600 JOHN F KENNEDY BLVD. SUITE 1800
PHILADELPHIA, PA 19103-2899

Editor (Name and complete mailing address)

STACY EASTMAN, ELSEVIER INC.
1600 JOHN F KENNEDY BLVD. SUITE 1800
PHILADELPHIA, PA 19103-2899

Managing Editor (Name and complete mailing address)

PATRICK MANLEY, ELSEVIER INC.
1600 JOHN F KENNEDY BLVD. SUITE 1800
PHILADELPHIA, PA 19103-2899

10. Owner (Do not leave blank. If the publication is owned by a corporation, give the name and address of the corporation immediately followed by the names and addresses of all stockholders owning or holding 1 percent or more of the total amount of stock. If not owned by a corporation, give the names and addresses of the individual owners. If owned by a partnership or other unincorporated firm, give its name and address as well as those of each individual owner. If the publication is published by a nonprofit organization, give its name and address.)

Full Name	Complete Mailing Address
WHOLLY OWNED SUBSIDIARY OF REED/ELSEVIER, US HOLDINGS	1600 JOHN F KENNEDY BLVD. SUITE 1800 PHILADELPHIA, PA 19103-2899

11. Known Bondholders, Mortgagees, and Other Security Holders Owning or Holding 1 Percent or More of Total Amount of Bonds, Mortgages, or Other Securities. If none, check box ▶ ☐ None

Full Name	Complete Mailing Address
N/A	

12. Tax Status (For completion by nonprofit organizations authorized to mail at nonprofit rates) (Check one)
The purpose, function, and nonprofit status of this organization and the exempt status for federal income tax purposes:
☒ Has Not Changed During Preceding 12 Months
☐ Has Changed During Preceding 12 Months (Publisher must submit explanation of change with this statement)

13. Publication Title	14. Issue Date for Circulation Data Below
HEMATOLOGY/ONCOLOGY CLINICS OF NORTH AMERICA	AUGUST 2017

PS Form 3526, July 2014 [Page 1 of 4 (see instructions page 4)] PSN: 7530-01-000-9931 PRIVACY NOTICE: See our privacy policy on www.usps.com

15. Extent and Nature of Circulation		Average No. Copies Each Issue During Preceding 12 Months	No. Copies of Single Issue Published Nearest to Filing Date
a. Total Number of Copies (Net press run)		327	285
b. Paid Circulation (By Mail and Outside the Mail)	(1) Mailed Outside-County Paid Subscriptions Stated on PS Form 3541 (Include paid distribution above nominal rate, advertiser's proof copies, and exchange copies)	95	102
	(2) Mailed In-County Paid Subscriptions Stated on PS Form 3541 (Include paid distribution above nominal rate, advertiser's proof copies, and exchange copies)	0	0
	(3) Paid Distribution Outside the Mails Including Sales Through Dealers and Carriers, Street Vendors, Counter Sales, and Other Paid Distribution Outside USPS®	59	69
	(4) Paid Distribution by Other Classes of Mail Through the USPS (e.g. First-Class Mail®)	0	0
c. Total Paid Distribution (Sum of 15b (1), (2), (3), and (4))	▶	154	171
d. Free or Nominal Rate Distribution (By Mail and Outside the Mail)	(1) Free or Nominal Rate Outside-County Copies included on PS Form 3541	90	114
	(2) Free or Nominal Rate In-County Copies Included on PS Form 3541	0	0
	(3) Free or Nominal Rate Copies Mailed at Other Classes Through the USPS (e.g. First-Class Mail)	0	0
	(4) Free or Nominal Rate Distribution Outside the Mail (Carriers or other means)	0	0
e. Total Free or Nominal Rate Distribution (Sum of 15d (1), (2), (3) and (4))	▶	90	114
f. Total Distribution (Sum of 15c and 15e)	▶	244	285
g. Copies not Distributed (See Instructions to Publishers #4 (page 83))	▶	83	0
h. Total (Sum of 15f and g)	▶	327	285
i. Percent Paid (15c divided by 15f times 100)	▶	63.11%	60%

* If you are claiming electronic copies, go to line 16 on page 3. If you are not claiming electronic copies, skip to line 17 on page 3.

16. Electronic Copy Circulation		Average No. Copies Each Issue During Preceding 12 Months	No. Copies of Single Issue Published Nearest to Filing Date
a. Paid Electronic Copies	▶	0	0
b. Total Paid Print Copies (Line 15c) + Paid Electronic Copies (Line 16a)	▶	154	171
c. Total Print Distribution (Line 15f) + Paid Electronic Copies (Line 16a)	▶	244	285
d. Percent Paid (Both Print & Electronic Copies) (16b divided by 16c × 100)	▶	63.11%	60%

☒ I certify that 50% of all my distributed copies (electronic and print) are paid above a nominal price.

17. Publication of Statement of Ownership
☒ If the publication is a general publication, publication of this statement is required. Will be printed
in the OCTOBER 2017 issue of this publication.
☐ Publication not required.

18. Signature and Title of Editor, Publisher, Business Manager, or Owner

STEPHEN R. BUSHING - INVENTORY DISTRIBUTION CONTROL MANAGER

Stephen R. Bushing   Date 9/18/2017

I certify that all information furnished on this form is true and complete. I understand that anyone who furnishes false or misleading information on this form or who omits material or information requested on the form may be subject to criminal sanctions (including fines and imprisonment) and/or civil sanctions (including civil penalties).

PS Form 3526, July 2014 (Page 2 of 4) PRIVACY NOTICE: See our privacy policy on www.usps.com

Moving?

Make sure your subscription moves with you!

To notify us of your new address, find your **Clinics Account Number** (located on your mailing label above your name), and contact customer service at:

Email: journalscustomerservice-usa@elsevier.com

800-654-2452 (subscribers in the U.S. & Canada)
314-447-8871 (subscribers outside of the U.S. & Canada)

Fax number: 314-447-8029

Elsevier Health Sciences Division
Subscription Customer Service
3251 Riverport Lane
Maryland Heights, MO 63043

*To ensure uninterrupted delivery of your subscription, please notify us at least 4 weeks in advance of move.

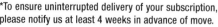

ELSEVIER

Printed and bound by CPI Group (UK) Ltd, Croydon, CR0 4YY

03/10/2024

01040392-0004